DERMATOLOGY: CLINICAL & BASIC SCIENCE SERIES

ETHNIC SKIN
AND HAIR

DERMATOLOGY
CLINICAL & BASIC SCIENCE SERIES

Series Editor
Howard I. Maibach, M.D.
University of California at San Francisco School of Medicine
San Francisco, California, U.S.A.

1. Health Risk Assessment: Dermal and Inhalation Exposure and Absorption of Toxicants, *edited by Rhoda G. M. Wang, James B. Knaack, and Howard I. Maibach*
2. Pigmentation and Pigmentary Disorders, *edited by Norman Levine and Howard I. Maibach*
3. Hand Eczema, *edited by Torkil Menné and Howard I. Maibach*
4. Protective Gloves for Occupational Use, *edited by Gunh A. Mellstrom, Jan E. Wahlberg, and Howard I. Maibach*
5. Bioengineering of the Skin (Five Volume Set), *edited by Howard I. Maibach*
6. Bioengineering of the Skin: Water and the Stratum Corneum, Volume I, *edited by Peter Elsner, Enzo Berardesca, and Howard I. Maibach*
7. Bioengineering of the Skin: Cutaneous Blood Flow and Erythema, Volume II, *edited by Enzo Berardesca, Peter Elsner, and Howard I. Maibach*
8. Skin Cancer: Mechanisms and Human Relevance, *edited by Hasan Mukhtar*
9. Bioengineering of the Skin: Methods and Instrumentation, Volume III, *edited by Enzo Berardesca, Peter Elsner, Klaus-P. Wilhelm, and Howard I. Maibach*
10. Dermatologic Research Techniques, *edited by Howard I. Maibach*
11. The Irritant Contact Dermatitis Syndrome, *edited by Pieter van der Valk, Pieter Coenrads, and Howard I Maibach*
12. Human Papillomavirus Infections in Dermatovenereology, *edited by Gerd Gross and Geo von Krogh*
13. Bioengineering of the Skin: Skin Surface, Imaging, and Analysis, Volume IV, *edited by Klaus-P. Wilhelm, Peter Elsner, Enzo Berardesca, and Howard I. Maibach*
14. Contact Urticaria Syndrome, *edited by Smita Amin, Howard I. Maibach, and Arto Lahti*
15. Skin Reactions to Drugs, *edited by Kirsti Kauppinen, Kristiina Alanko, Matti Hannuksela, and Howard I. Maibach*
16. Dry Skin and Moisturizers: Chemistry and Function, *edited by Marie Lodén and Howard I. Maibach*
17. Dermatologic Botany, *edited by Javier Avalos and Howard I. Maibach*
18. Hand Eczema, Second Edition, *edited by Torkil Menné and Howard I. Maibach*

19. Pesticide Dermatoses, *edited by Homero Penagos, Michael O'Malley, and Howard I. Maibach*

20. Bioengineering of the Skin: Skin Biomechanics, Volume V, *edited by Peter Elsner, Enzo Berardesca, Klaus-P. Wilhelm, and Howard I. Maibach*

21. Nickel and the Skin: Absorption, Immunology, Epidemiology, and Metallurgy, *edited by Jurij J. Hostýnek and Howard I. Maibach*

22. The Epidermis in Wound Healing, *edited by David T. Rovee and Howard I. Maibach*

23. Bioengineering of the Skin: Water and the Stratum Corneum, Second Edition, *edited by Joachim W. Fluhr, Peter Elsner, Enzo Berardesca, and Howard I. Maibach*

24. Protective Gloves for Occupational Use, Second Edition, *edited by Anders Boman, Tuula Estlander, Jan E. Wahlberg, and Howard I. Maibach*

25. Latex Intolerance: Basic Science, Epidemiology, and Clinical Management, *edited by Mahbub M. U. Chowdhry and Howard I. Maibach*

26. Cutaneous T-Cell Lymphoma: Mycosis Fungoides and Sezary Syndrome, *edited by Herschel S. Zackheim*

27. Dry Skin and Moisturizers: Chemistry and Function, Second Edition, *edited by Marie Lodén and Howard I. Maibach*

28. Ethnic Skin and Hair, *edited by Enzo Berardesca, Jean-Luc Lévêque, and Howard Maibach*

29. Sensitive Skin Syndrome, *edited by Enzo Berardesca, Joachim W. Fluhr, and Howard I. Maibach*

30. Copper and the Skin, *edited by Jurij J. Hostýnek, and Howard I. Maibach*

31. Bioengineering of the Skin: Skin Imaging and Analysis, Second Edition, *edited by Klaus-P. Wilhelm, Peter Elsner, Enzo Berardesca, and Howard I. Maibach*

DERMATOLOGY: CLINICAL & BASIC SCIENCE SERIES

ETHNIC SKIN AND HAIR

Edited by

Enzo Berardesca
San Gallicano Dermatological Institute
Rome, Italy

Jean-Luc Lévêque
L'Oréal Recherche
Clichy, France

Howard I. Maibach
University of California at San Francisco School of Medicine
San Francisco, California, U.S.A.

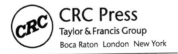

CRC Press
Taylor & Francis Group
Boca Raton London New York

CRC Press is an imprint of the
Taylor & Francis Group, an **informa** business

CRC Press
Taylor & Francis Group
6000 Broken Sound Parkway NW, Suite 300
Boca Raton, FL 33487-2742

First issued in paperback 2019

© 2011 by Taylor & Francis Group, LLC
CRC Press is an imprint of Taylor & Francis Group, an Informa business

No claim to original U.S. Government works

ISBN-13: 978-0-8493-3088-9 (hbk)
ISBN-13: 978-0-367-38999-4 (pbk)

A CIP record for this book is available from the British Library.

Library of Congress Cataloging-in-Publication Data available on application

**Visit the Taylor & Francis Web site at
http://www.taylorandfrancis.com**

**and the CRC Press Web site at
http://www.crcpress.com**

Preface

Dermatological knowledge has been based, since its early beginning, on investigating and understanding physiology and pathology of skin conditions related to Caucasian (or white) skin. It was assumed that skin of different color(s) behave in the same manner of white skin; this is true, indeed, for the majority of skin diseases and the major basic pathophysiological pathways. However, the more we know in depth skin reactions, the more we understand that skin color can play an important role in diversifying skin responses, not only as a consequence of cultural, social and economic factors, but also in terms of real biological differences due, first of all, to genetic influences including melanin content and structural differences in skin barrier.

The purpose of this book, written by leading authors in ethnic-related skin research is the first attempt to gather all the scientific data available today for better understanding, classifying, and treating ethnic skin conditions. This is important not only in general terms for skin science, but practically for thousands of dermatologists working worldwide in a multiethnic and multicultural society with no more boundaries.

The book should be helpful for all scientists needing to better understand skin mechanisms related to ethnic differences as well as involved in designing tailored cosmetics or therapeutic strategies for treating ethnic skin disorders. The book, in particular, will focus on differences in hair structure and development, aging mechanisms, barrier function, skin reactivity, differences due to topically applied substances, and skin disease expression in different ethnic groups. Therefore, dermatologists, cosmetologists, pharmacologists, and toxicologists should enjoy reading it; hopefully, to achieve a better understanding of all known mechanisms involved in generating different ethnic responses.

Enzo Berardesca
Jean-Luc Lévêque
Howard I. Maibach

Contents

Preface iii
Contributors ix

1. **Anthropology of Skin Colors** *1*
   Aldo Morrone

2. **Biophysical Properties of Ethnic Skin** *13*
   Grazia Primavera and Enzo Berardesca

3. **Light Penetration and Melanin Content in Ethnic Skin** . . . *19*
   Nikiforos Kollias and Paulo R. Bargo

4. **Photoreactivity of Ethnic Skin** *47*
   Giovanni Leone and Alessia Pacifico

5. **Hair Anthropology** *55*
   Leszek J. Wolfram, E. Dika, and Howard I. Maibach

6. **The Transverse Dimensions of Human Head Hair** *79*
   J. Alan Swift

7. **Influence of Ethnic Origin of Hair on**
   Water-Keratin Interaction *93*
   Alain Franbourg, Frédéric Leroy, Marielle Escoubés, and
   Jean-Luc Lévêque

8. **The Age-Dependent Changes in Skin Condition in Ethnic Populations from Around the World** *105*
   Greg G. Hillebrand, Mark J. Levine[†], and Kukizo Miyamoto

9. **Update on Racial Differences in Susceptibility to Skin Irritation and Allergy** *123*
   Michael K. Robinson

10. **Ethnic Itch** *135*
    Daniela A. Guzman-Sanchez, Christopher Yelverton, and Gil Yosipovitch

11. **Age-Related Changes in Skin Microtopography: A Comparison Between Caucasian and Japanese Women** *141*
    Sophie Gardinier, Hassan Zahouani, Christiane Guinot, and Erwin Tschachler

12. **Inter- and Intraethnic Differences in Skin Micro Relief as a Function of Age and Site** *153*
    Stephane Diridollou, Jean de Rigal, Bernard Querleux, Therese Baldeweck, Dominique Batisse, Isabelle Des Mazis, Grace Yang, Frédéric Leroy, and Victoria Holloway Barbosa

13. **Stratum Corneum Lipids and Water Holding Capacity: Comparison Between Caucasians, Blacks, Hispanics and Asians** *169*
    Alessandra Pelosi, Enzo Berardesca, Joachim W. Fluhr, Philip Wertz, Jocélia Lago Jansen, Angela Anigbogu, Tsen-Fang Tsai, and Howard I. Maibach

14. **The Impact of Skin Disease in "Ethnic" Skin** *179*
    Gary J. Brauner

15. **Acne and Scarring** *197*
    Andrew F. Alexis and Susan C. Taylor

[†] Deceased.

16. **Black Skin Cosmetics: Specific Skin and Hair Problems of African Americans and Cosmetic Approaches for Their Treatment** *205*
  Christian Oresajo and Sreekumar Pillai

17. **Ethnical Aspects of Skin Pigmentation** *223*
  Olivier de Lacharrière and Rainer Schmidt

18. **Sensitive Skin—An Ethnic Overview** *235*
  Olivier de Lacharrière

19. **Diversity of Hair Growth Parameters** *245*
  Geneviève Loussouarn

Index *263*

Contributors

Andrew F. Alexis   Skin of Color Center, St. Luke's-Roosevelt Hospital and Columbia University College of Physicians and Surgeons, New York, New York, U.S.A.

Angela Anigbogu   Department of Dermatology, University of California at San Francisco School of Medicine, San Francisco, California, U.S.A.

Therese Baldeweck   L'Oréal Recherche, Aulnay, France

Victoria Holloway Barbosa   L'Oréal Recherche, Institute for Ethnic Hair and Skin Research, Chicago, Illinois, U.S.A.

Paulo R. Bargo   J & J Consumer and Personal Products Worldwide, Skillman, New Jersey, U.S.A.

Dominique Batisse   L'Oréal Recherche, Chevilly, France

Enzo Berardesca   Department of Dermatology, San Gallicano Dermatological Institute (IRCCS), Rome, Italy

Gary J. Brauner   Mount Sinai School of Medicine, New York, New York, U.S.A.

Olivier de Lacharrière   Life Sciences, L'Oréal Recherche, Clichy, France

Jean de Rigal   L'Oréal Recherche, Chevilly, France

Isabelle Des Mazis   L'Oréal Recherche, Chevilly, France

E. Dika   Department of Dermatology, University of California at San Francisco School of Medicine, San Francisco, California, U.S.A.

Stephane Diridollou   L'Oréal Recherche, Institute for Ethnic Hair and Skin Research, Chicago, Illinois, U.S.A.

Marielle Escoubés   Laboratores des Biomatériaux et Polymères, CNRS-Lyon, Lyon, France

Joachim W. Fluhr   Department of Dermatology, San Gallicano Dermatological Institute (IRCCS), Rome, Italy, and Friedrich Schiller University, Jena, Germany

Alain Franbourg   L'Oréal Recherche, Centre Charles Zviak, Clichy, France

Sophie Gardinier   CE.R.I.E.S., Neuilly Sur Seine Cedex, France

Christiane Guinot   CE.R.I.E.S., Neuilly Sur Seine Cedex, and Computer Science Department, Ecole Polytechnique, Université de Tours, Tours, France

Daniela A. Guzman-Sanchez   Department of Dermatology, Wake Forest University School of Medicine, Salem, North Carolina, U.S.A.

Greg G. Hillebrand   The Procter & Gamble Company, Cincinnati, Ohio, U.S.A., and Kobe, Japan

Jocélia Lago Jansen   Department of Dermatology, University of California at San Francisco School of Medicine, San Francisco, California, U.S.A.

Nikiforos Kollias   J & J Consumer and Personal Products Worldwide, Skillman, New Jersey, U.S.A.

Giovanni Leone   Phototherapy Unit, San Gallicano Dermatological Institute (IRCCS), Rome, Italy

Frédéric Leroy   L'Oréal Recherche, Aulnay, France

Jean-Luc Lévêque   L'Oréal Recherche, Centre Charles Zviak, Clichy, France

Mark J. Levine[†] The Procter & Gamble Company, Cincinnati, Ohio, U.S.A., and Kobe, Japan

Geneviève Loussouarn L'Oréal Recherche, Clichy, France

Howard I. Maibach Department of Dermatology, University of California at San Francisco School of Medicine, San Francisco, California, U.S.A.

Kukizo Miyamoto The Procter & Gamble Company, Cincinnati, Ohio, U.S.A., and Kobe, Japan

Aldo Morrone Department of Preventive Medicine of Migration, Tourism, and Tropical Dermatology, San Gallicano Dermatological Institute (IRCCS), Rome, Italy

Christian Oresajo Engelhard Corporation, Stony Brook, New York, U.S.A.

Alessia Pacifico Phototherapy Unit, San Gallicano Dermatological Institute (IRCCS), Rome, Italy

Alessandra Pelosi Department of Dermatology, San Gallicano Dermatological Institute (IRCCS), Rome, Italy

Sreekumar Pillai Engelhard Corporation, Stony Brook, New York, U.S.A.

Grazia Primavera San Gallicano Dermatological Institute (IRCCS), Rome, Italy

Bernard Querleux L'Oréal Recherche, Aulnay, France

Michael K. Robinson The Procter & Gamble Company, Cincinnati, Ohio, U.S.A.

Rainer Schmidt Life Sciences, L'Oréal Recherche, Clichy, France

J. Alan Swift Department of Textiles and Paper, University of Manchester, Manchester, U.K.

Susan C. Taylor Skin of Color Center, St. Luke's-Roosevelt Hospital and Columbia University College of Physicians and Surgeons, New York, New York, U.S.A.

[†] Deceased.

Tsen-Fang Tsai   Department of Dermatology, University of California at San Francisco School of Medicine, San Francisco, California, U.S.A.

Erwin Tschachler   CE.R.I.E.S., Neuilly Sur Seine Cedex, France and Department of Dermatology, University of Vienna Medical School, Vienna, Austria

Philip Wertz   Dows Institute, University of Iowa, Iowa City, Iowa, U.S.A.

Leszek J. Wolfram   Department of Dermatology, University of California at San Francisco School of Medicine, San Francisco, California, U.S.A.

Grace Yang   L'Oréal Recherche, Institute for Ethnic Hair and Skin Research, Chicago, Illinois, U.S.A.

Christopher Yelverton   Department of Dermatology, Wake Forest University School of Medicine, Salem, North Carolina, U.S.A.

Gil Yosipovitch   Department of Dermatology, Wake Forest University School of Medicine, Salem, North Carolina, U.S.A.

Hassan Zahouani   Laboratoire de Tribology et Dynamique des Systèmes, UMR CNRS 5513, Ecole Centrale de Lyon–ENI Saint–Etienne, Institut Européen de Tribologie, Ecully Cedex, France

1

Anthropology of Skin Colors

Aldo Morrone

Department of Preventive Medicine of Migration, Tourism, and Tropical Dermatology, San Gallicano Dermatological Institute (IRCCS), Rome, Italy

INTRODUCTION

"Southern frontier. This border was defined in year VIII of the Reign of Sesostris III, King of Upper and Lower Egypt, who lives forever and for eternity. Crossing this border by land or water, by boat or with herds, is forbidden to all black people, with the exception of those who cross for the purposes of selling or buying at warehouses."

These words were written on a stone slab found in southern Egypt that dates back to the 19th century B.C. It is perhaps one of the first documents to legitimize discrimination based on skin color (1).

For a long time skin color has been an indicator of one's "race." Although the origin of the word "race" is considered to date back to the 15th century—it is not clear whether it comes from the Latin word "generatio" or "ratio," in the sense of nature, quality—the study of human races started much earlier.

The Egyptians were probably the first to try a classification of the human populations based on skin color. The words engraved on the 19th century B.C. stone found in the south of Egypt validate one of the first discriminations between peoples based on skin color (1,2).

Later, Lynnaeus and Blumenbach classifications divided the human populations into four and five varieties, respectively, and since then the concept of "Caucasian" to indicate the Western population started to break through.

Indeed, the gene maps of the living beings reveal striking realities. People apparently very far from each other show, however, only few differences, while people who seem quite close are in fact much more dissimilar. The somatic characteristics, such as the skin color for example, do not characterize a race but are a consequence of a complex biological and cultural adaptation (3).

The world's mobile human population—people who temporarily or permanently cross borders for reasons of employment, politics, or tourism—comprised 1.4 billion persons in 2005. In particular, 200 million people traveled in search of employment. This demonstrates increasing desperation in the world: in the 80s the number was 70 million. Mobility has always been a necessity for humanity and has constantly been mixing human geography and state of health. Traveling always includes danger and the risk of illness; the word itself possesses a relationship to illness. In fact, the Greek noun and the verb originally meant journeying to arrive and settle in a foreign land. The profoundly rooted idea that traveling is an experience that builds character and tests the health of the traveler is seen clearly in the German adjective *bewandert* that today means "shrewd" or "expert," but in the 15th century simply meant "well-traveled." The English verbs *to fare* and *to fear* have the same etymological root and have the experiential terrain in common, within the idea of traveling (4,5).

THE CONCEPT OF RACE

From a scientific point of view, does it make sense to speak about *race*? Is there scientific value in continuing to use racial subdivisions in medicine? Who is Caucasian? Have Caucasians ever existed? The results of studies in genetics, anthropology, and molecular biology confirm that beneath our skin we are biologically indistinguishable (6).

According to the anthropologist Alan Goodman, the concept of race is completely obsolete and should have been discarded at the beginning of the last century. Race is an unstable and indefinable concept on which scientific theories cannot be built.

In the April 1997 edition of *Science* magazine, Goodman wrote:

> "*Even acknowledging that the idea of race is a legend we will not eradicate racism. Until researchers, even in good faith, go on using the concept of race without clearly defining it, they will sustain the idea of race on a biological basis, thus misleading public opinion and encouraging racist attitudes.*"

Thirty years ago the American paleontologist George Gaylord Simpson declared that all definitions of human beings predating Darwinian theory were groundless. In his opinion they should be completely ignored (7). The scientific concept of race, derived from the Greek concept of the great chain of being and from the Platonic idea of ideal forms, was definitely antievolutionist and had to be thrown away (8).

This should have happened at the beginning of the century, when anthropologist Franz Boas demonstrated that race, language, and culture do not follow the same path, as other authors had previously maintained. However, the concept survived. It should then have died down in the 30s, when the "new evolutionary synthesis" helped explain subtle variations in human biology (9). Nevertheless, between 1899, when *Races of Europe* by William Z. Ripley was published, and 1939, when a book of the same title was published by the anthropologist Carleton S. Coon, the concept of race has remained more or less intact (6).

"Race" should have disappeared in the 1950s and 1960s, when scientists passed from studying pure genetic lines to studying genetic variations as a response to the forces of evolution. But the concept of race, along with racism, did not die. For Coon, "races" were merely transformed into populations with particular problems of adaptation. Most doctors, biologists, and anthropologists now admit that from the medical, biological, and genetic point of view "race" is an imaginary concept. Unfortunately, the idea still survives in many different forms (7,10).

RACISM AND MEDICINE

In the Greek cities where they practiced, Hippocratic doctors treated men and women, citizens and outsiders, freemen and slaves, Greeks or foreigners, whoever was in need. In the Hippocratic doctor's eyes, they were all human beings. Tangible proof of this humanity is offered by the vocabulary used—the Greek word, meaning human being, appears frequently in the writings of Hippocratic doctors, who used the word to refer to the patient (11). Everything referring to differences of sex, social status, or racial origin was secondary; the sick person was paramount and had to be restored to health (12). In contradistinction to this tradition, there is a deep and long-lasting connection between medicine and racism. This relationship has manifested itself in two distinct ways, which, though they may seem unrelated, were, nevertheless, to coincide in particular circumstances and with horrendous consequences. Firstly, as a scientific discipline, medicine sought to establish a *scientific basis* for comprehending perceived racial differences. Secondly, doctors have used prisoners and concentration camp inmates for so-called "scientific" experiments, notably, but not only, under Nazi regimes. In these circumstances, humans have been reduced to the level of laboratory animals and have been subjected to experiments that often ended in death—and which were often intended to do so (10,13).

Also significant is the tendency to associate the appearance or spread of a disease or epidemic with the presence of a particular group. Thus following the return of the plague to Toulon in 1348, Jews were accused of spreading the disease and were persecuted on this account. More generally, syphilis has typically been named after the people held responsible for its spread, so that in France it was known as "the Neapolitan disease" and in Naples as "the French disease." Much more recently, when AIDS appeared in the early 1980s, it was immediately branded a "gay" syndrome, because people were convinced that it was spread (only) by homosexuals. Despite the Hippocratic oath, doctors have taken and continue to take part in crimes against humanity—sometimes on the pretext that this is in pursuit of "scientific discovery" and thus somehow defensible. Notable in this context are the experiments carried out by the Nazis on those defined as "subhuman"—principally, concentration camp inmates and prisoners of war of certain nationalities, though also those defined by the Nazis as "feeble-minded." Such experiments were not merely widespread, but routine. These experiments encompassed skilled amputations and transplants which, given their purpose, were carried out in absurdly hygienic conditions; injections of pus into the legs and breasts to "study" the effects of sulfanilamide; being forced to drink sea water to "test" the effects of thirst; being left for hours in baths of ice to "observe" the effects of cold on the body. The Shutz Staffel (SS) doctors involved (not more than 100, as against the 150,000 German "civilian" doctors) believed in the importance this work would have for future medicine, but above all they believed in the need to create a new "SS medical science." It has been argued that if there had been at least some positive results, perhaps such experiments might be understood, if not justified though few would accept such an argument and many would see it as a dangerous position to take. However, in the event, a careful evaluation of all the experiments conducted by doctors such as Fischer, Romberg, Gebhardt, Mengele, and Schumann (all condemned to death at the Nuremberg Trials), not a single experiment has added in the slightest to the progress of postwar medical science (14). Even today doctors and psychologists in many countries are used in the interrogation and torture of detainees. Their special responsibility is not to prevent torture, but to halt it before there is any "visible" damage, which might be seen in the event of a visit by an international commission (11).

AN IMPRECISE ALPHABET

Why can't race function as a kind of shorthand alphabet for biological difference? The answer lies in the structure of human variation and in the chameleonic nature of the concept of race (15).

Many genetic traits show very small variations in different geographical areas. Imagine a merchant from the 15th century traveling on foot from Stockholm, Sweden, to Cape Town, South Africa. That merchant would have noticed that skin color becomes darker approaching the Equator, and lighter when moving away. Taking a different route, from Siberia towards Singapore, he would have seen the same phenomenon, even though none of the people he met would today be classified as white or black as for us they are all "Asian." Race, in other words, does not determine skin color and vice versa.

There are more variations in genetic traits within a race than between races. About 30 years ago, the population geneticist Richard C. Lewontin, from Harvard University, made a statistical study on blood samples from the two most common blood groups. He discovered that, on average, 94% of genetic variation in the group was found within a single so-called race, less than 6% could be explained as a variation between races. Consequently, applying generalizations derived from our judgments of a race to individuals is imprecise.

According to the American biologist Donald E. Muir, those who continue to see race in biology, without bad intentions, are nothing more than "good racists," although, by scientifically legitimizing race, they automatically help "bad racists." Unfortunately, there are still many scientists who belong to both these groups (16).

According to Michael Rustin, "race" is an empty category and one of the most destructive and powerful social categorizations (17).

Humans do not all have the same appearance, yet paradoxically those who are biologically the closest, are the most hostile to each other. For instance, Irish and English, Hutu and Tutsi, Arabs and Israelis, Huron and Iroquois, Bosnians, Croatians, and Serbs. Their animosities, rivalries and wars originate from economic, political, social, and cultural differences, not from biological variations. However, biology is often used to justify the differences, thus making "Evil" appear as a consequence of nature, although nature in itself has nothing to do with it (16,18).

LINNAEUS'S CLASSIFICATION

The desire to organize knowledge has pushed many researchers to classify human beings, similarly to classifications of flora and fauna. One of the first to attempt this task was Carl von Linné, or Linnaeus (1707–1778).

Linnaeus scientifically formalized, in 1758, differences between populations on the various continents (19). Primate orders (which Linnaeus invented) were divided into various types, including our genus, *Homo*. According to Linnaeus, *Homo* included two species, *Homo sapiens* (us) and *Homo nocturnus* (chimpanzees), so how many subspecies did *H. sapiens* include?

The naturalist decided that there were five: *H. sapiens monstruosus*, which included all individuals affected by congenital malformations, and four "geographic" types:

- *H. sapiens americanus*
- *H. sapiens europaeus*

- *H. sapiens asiaticus*
- *H. sapiens afer*

As an "objective" scientist, Linnaeus claimed to be applying the same rules to the human race that had been applied to other species. However, we must recognize that the characteristics of each geographic subspecies defined by Linnaeus were ridiculous generalizations, slanderous, and generally without biological justification. So, *Homo sapiens americanus* is tenacious, satisfied, free, red-skinned, impassive, and of bad character. *Homo europaeus* is athletic, lively, and inventive. *Homo asiaticus* is simple, proud, and greedy, while *Homo afer* is astute, slow, and negligent. Linnaeus was, of course, a product of his age, which considered Europeans to be superior to all other peoples. But in that era particularly, the idea of humans grouped into four types became scientific knowledge. Today we know that the subspecies of the 18th century are neither fundamental nor biological groupings of our species. This is the main illusion introduced by Linnaeus: a scientific legitimization of a division of human beings into a small number of distinct and homogeneous groups (17).

In any case, although his correlation between physical and mental attributes was arbitrary, and despite its aura of racism, Linnaeus never used the term "race," but rather "variety."

The term "race" was introduced by Georges Louis Leclerc de Buffon (1707–1788), who described human groups using both biological characteristics and "moral" characteristics (a term which at that time evoked more than today the derivation from the Latin "mores") (20).

BLUMENBACH AND CAUCASIANS

The first person to propose a classification of humans based on skin color and other visible exterior characteristics was Johan Friedrich Blumenbach (1752–1840). Blumenbach is also the first to use the term Caucasian in clinical–anthropological language. His first publication in Latin was his doctorate thesis, delivered in 1775, in which he grouped humans according to skin color (21). Later, in 1776 and 1781, he highlighted in two separate books this classification by which five "varieties" are distinguished (22,23):

1. Caucasian (pale skin, brown hair, with nonprominent malar bones, straight, narrow and quite long nose, and full, rounded chin), living in Europe (except in Lapland and other Finnish regions), in Western Asia up to the Ganges river and in Northern Africa.
2. Mongolian (yellow-brown skin, black hair, flat nose, narrow eyelid opening with a medial fold), living in Asian territory not occupied by Europeans and including the Finns, Laplanders, and Inuit.

3. Ethiopian (black skin, woolly hair, narrow face, pointy chin, etc.), including all of the African populations except those from the North of the continent.
4. American (copper-colored skin and black hair), including the inhabitants of both Americas except the Inuit.
5. Malaysian (dark-brown skin, black hair, wide nose, and large mouth), including all inhabitants of the Pacific islands.

In the third edition (1795) of his text *"De generis humani varietate nativa liber"* (24) and successively in 1798 in the first edition in German of his treatise, (25) Blumenbach used the term "Caucasian" taking it from an interesting book by a French traveler, Jean Chardin (1643–1713) who had crossed the Caucasus towards the end of the 18th century. In the preface to his travel diary, he wrote about his enthusiasm for traveling and especially the two trips he had made to India (*the extreme passion that I have always had for traveling took me twice to Western India*). He declared that *"the blood of Georgia is the most beautiful in the West and, I think, the world. I never saw an ugly face in that land, neither male nor female; rather I saw the faces of Angels…"* (26). No mention of skin color is made. However, over the centuries, the beauty of female Circassian slaves (almost a synonym for Caucasian, when referring to the nearby residents of this region of Caucasus) was renowned in the Orient ("who are the prizes of Muslim seraglios").

Chardin uses the term "Caucasian" to refer to the beauty of this population, whose name derives from the Caucasus mountain that lies north of the region of Georgia where these people are found. He does not refer to the color of their skin, but to their beauty by highlighting this variety.

The expression "Caucasian" was later used to describe populations with white skin. It entered into medical language as a generic designation of white people. However, we must be aware of the fact that there are Caucasian populations who are not, in fact, white (6). There is quite a distinction between Ireland and the Punjab or the borders of Ethiopia and the land of Falasha Jews. In fact, there are light- and dark-skinned populations on all continents. Dermatologists, so concerned with skin phototype, must remember that there are populations living in extreme conditions of ultraviolet radiation, such as the high altitudes of Tibet or those of South America, who do not have the darkest skin colors (6). An inhabitant of Punjab or Baluchistan may be much darker, despite being Caucasian. Blumenbach understood this and for this reason preferred the term "variety," revealing the impossibility of tracing a clear dividing line between skin colors (6). There is no human "variety" characterized by skin color or other physical features so well defined that it cannot be linked to some other "variety." Today we must rather speak of groups of populations or ethnic groups, eliminating the term "race," not only because it does not exist on a biological plane but because it lacks all scientific foundation and is, therefore, useless on a clinical level.

When we say or write "Caucasian," we must remember the historical origin of this term, of its erroneous use, of the age in which it entered scientific literature and the meaning that we intend to give it today.

NOAH'S CHILDREN

The human race cannot be subdivided or compartmentalized like zoological species. There is no fixed number of human "types." If we look at people from distant regions, for example, Norway, Nigeria and Vietnam it is clear that they do not resemble each other. But what do these differences mean? A couple of centuries ago, different people were thought to be the descendants of Noah's children, who had moved to the four corners of the earth and multiplied. Today, however, there is no reason to think that in a certain era there were people living only near Oslo, Lagos, or Saigon; nor any reason to believe that the most extreme variations of humanity represent a primordial purity. As far as we know, there have always been many people distributed in all parts of the Old World (7,27).

It is easy, therefore, to dispute the classification system created by Linnaeus. The inhabitants of southern Asia, India, and Pakistan are generally dark-skinned like Africans, but present European features and live in Asia. Where do they fall in such classification? And if we put them in a separate group, what should we do with those who are different from the majority: Polynesians, the inhabitants of New Guinea, aboriginal Australians, North Africans? (7,27).

THE AFRICAN EXAMPLE

In Africa there are populations with extremely varied somatic traits, morphology, and skin color. The continent houses tall, thin individuals in Kenya (Nilotics), small people in Congo (pygmies), and others in South Africa. Thus, African physical stereotypes are extremely diverse as their ancestors from South-East Asia. Despite the diversity of the African population, there is a tendency to classify them into one category of human race (African/black/negroid) for the purpose of isolating them from the European or mid-Eastern populations (European/white/Caucasoid). In fact, the "Africans" of Somalia look much more similar to the inhabitants of Saudi Arabia or Iran—countries near Somalia—than, for example, to the Ghanaians on the West African coast. Likewise, the Iranians and the Saudis are more similar to the Somalis than to the Norwegians. Thus, associating the Ghanaians and the Somalis on the one hand and the Saudis and Norwegians on the other creates an artificial model which is contradicted by all empirical studies of human biology (7,27).

ANTHROPOLOGY OF SKIN COLORS

We know today that race does not determine the color of the skin, and that the color of the skin does not define a race. We can clearly assert that a "caucasic race" does not exist, just as a "black race" does not exist, and that the color of the skin of an individual depends on the interaction of various biological, genetic, environmental, and cultural factors. Moreover, we must emphasize the fact that a "black skin" is not black, just as a "white skin" is not really white, and that certainly a "yellow skin" does not exist. In fact, the different colors of the skin rather represent variations in the red spectrum (28,29).

Among all the primates, only human beings have a skin almost completely hairless, a skin that can take on various shades of color. All scientists today agree in affirming that the various colors of the skin present among the inhabitants of the world are not in the least casual; rather, they are produced by evolutionary processes of adaptation. In fact the populations with a darker skin tend to concentrate near the equator, while those with a fairer skin are nearer the poles. For a long time we thought that the dark skin had evolved in order to offer protection from cutaneous carcinomas, but a series of recent discoveries leads us today toward a new interpretation of human pigmentation. Bio-anthropological and epidemiological data indicate that the distribution on a world scale of the color of human skin is due to natural selection, which operates to regulate the effects of ultraviolet radiation on some nutritional substances (folates and vitamin D), which are essential for the reproductive process of human beings (30).

All over the world the human pigmentation has evolved in such a way that the skin could become dark enough not to allow the sunlight to destroy the folates, but sufficiently fair to favor the production of vitamin D.

The evolution of cutaneous pigmentation is correlated with the progressive disappearance of hairs. Human being have been evolving independently of superior monkeys at least for seven million years, i.e., since the time when our nearest ancestors separated from their closest relatives, the chimpanzees.

Chimpanzees have changed very little over such a long time, compared to human being.

The chimpanzee's skin is fair and covered with thick hairs. The younger individuals' face, hands, and feet are rosy, and become darker only over the years due to prolonged exposure to sunlight. Primitive human beings had almost certainly a fair skin covered with hairs, the loss of which has been presumably the initial event, and only at a later stage the color of the skin has also changed (30).

SKIN COLOR(S)

Supporting the multigenic hypothesis is the fact that the color "black" is not dominant in nature. A descendant of a mixed family often demonstrates significant difference in skin color from other family members. In addition, skin pigmentation can vary over the course of an individual's life, due to the reduction in the number of active 3,4-dihydroxy-L-phenylalanine (DOPA), positive melanocytes that accompanies aging.

But then, what are the differences that we observe among individuals due to?

We can reduce these to three main elements: genetic factors, adaptation to ecological conditions, and adaptation to climatic conditions, while not forgetting that, as Cavalli-Sforza affirms, it is not easy to distinguish between biological inheritance and cultural inheritance (3,31–33).

It is always possible that the causes of a difference are of biological, or better genetic origin, or that they are due to adaptation, meaning cultural, or that both contribute. It is to this adaptation that the somatic characteristics of Earth's inhabitants may be correlated, diversifying in skin color, eye color, hair color, nose shape, and body size (3,31–33).

Black skin protects those who live near the equator from the ultraviolet radiation that may produce skin cancer. According to Cavalli-Sforza, in hot, humid climates, like tropical rain forests, it is advantageous to be small, in order to increase one's surface area in relation to body volume and thereby reducing energy requirements and producing less heat. Curly hair holds sweat longer and prolongs the cooling effect of perspiration. In this way, the possibility of overheating, the cause of heat-stroke, is reduced.

In more temperate climates, a diet based almost exclusively on cereals would cause vitamin D deficiency in Europeans, given the lack of this vitamin in cereal products. However, light-skinned people can produce enough vitamin D, using components contained in cereals, because their skin allows the penetration of ultraviolet light, which transforms these elements into vitamin D (34,35).

In colder climates, the face and body are constructed in such a way as to protect against the cold. The body and especially the head tend to be rounded and body volume is greater. This reduces surface area in relation to volume, thereby reducing loss of heat. The nose is small, with a lower danger of freezing, as are the nostrils, in order to allow more time to warm and humidify the air before it reaches the lungs (34,35).

Eyes are protected from the cold, thanks to the eyelids, which are like small pockets of fat, providing excellent thermal isolation and leaving a narrow opening through which one can see, while remaining protected from cold Siberian winds (34,35).

If we look beyond visible characteristics, it is absurd to believe that relatively "pure" races exist. In the past, people did not know that, in order to obtain racial "purity" or genetic homogeneity (which in any case, can never be complete in superior animals), crossbreeding should take place between close relatives such as brother and sister, or parents and children, for at least 20 generations. This would have devastating consequences on the ability to reproduce and on the health of children and has never occurred in human history, with the exception of brief periods and under particular conditions, such as during some Egyptian or Persian dynasties.

Race and its purity are inexistent, impossible, and completely undesirable (36).

During the 20th and 21st centuries some diseases have manifested themselves in populations which only marginally had suffered from them in the past, and in particular:

1. Early cutaneous aging, cutaneous carcinomas in fair-skinned subjects.
2. Rickets in dark-skinned subjects.

The progressive ability of the skin to adapt to the various types of environment, to which human beings have moved, reflects the importance that the color of the skin has for the survival itself (30). On the other hand, its unstable nature also makes it one of the least useful characteristics for the determination of the evolutive relationships among the various human groups.

REFERENCES

1. Morrone A. L'altra faccia di Gaia. Roma: Armando Editore, 1999.
2. Rackham H. (ed.) Pliny: Natural History, Harvard University Press, libri I and II, Cambridge, Massachusetts: 1979.
3. Cavalli Sforza LL, Menozzi P, Piazza A. History and Geography of Human Genes. Princeton, New Jersey: Princeton University Press, 1994.
4. Morrone A, Veraldi S. "Salgari's syndrome": a new syndrome for dermatologists. J Eur Acad Dermatol Venereol 2002; 16(Suppl 1):221.
5. Morrone A, Hercogova J, Lotti T. Dermatology of Human Mobile Population. MNL, Bologna, 2004.
6. Holubar K. What is a Caucasian. J Invest Derm 1996; 106:800.
7. Goodman AH. Bred in the Bone. The Sciences 1997; 2:20.
8. Levinas E. Totality and Infinity. Pittsburgh: Duquesne University Press, 1969.
9. Boas F. Race, Language, and Culture. New York, New York: Collier Macmillan, 1940.
10. Mosse GL. Nationalization of the Masses: Political Symbolism and Mass Movements in Germany from the Napoleonic Wars Through the Third Reich. Ithaca: Cornell University Press, 1991.
11. Morrone A. Racism and Medecine. In: Bolaffi G, Bracalenti R, Braham P, Gindro P, Gindro S, eds. Dictionary of Race, Ethnicity and Culture. London, SAGE, 2003:182.
12. Mann MJ, Gruskin S, Grodin MA, Annas GJ. Health and Human Rights: A Reader. New York, New York: Routledge, 1999.
13. Annas GJ, Grodin MA. The Nazi Doctors and the Nuremberg Code: Human Rights in Human Experimentation. New York, New York: Oxford University Press, 1992.

14. Katz, J. Experimentation with human beings. New York: Russell Sage Foundation, 1967.
15. Darwin C. On the Origin of Species by Means of Natural Selection or the Preservation of Favored Races in the Struggle of Life. London: Murray, 1959.
16. Rush B. Observations intended to favor a supposition that the black Color (as it is called) of Negroes is derived from Leprosy. American Philosophical Society Transactions 1799; 4:289–297.
17. Wieviorka M. The arena of racism. London: Sage Pub., 1995.
18. Takaki R. Reflections on Racial Patterns in America: Ethnicity and Public Policy, University of Wisconsin, 1982:1–23.
19. Tentori T. Il rischio della certezza. Pregiudizio, Potere, Cultura. Studium, Roma, 1987:314.
20. Gobineau de JA. Essai sur l'inégalité des races humaines. Paris: L'Harmattan, 1967.
21. Blumenbach IF. De generis umani variegate nativa. Thesis, Rosenbusch, Goettingae, 1775b.
22. Blumenbach IF. De generis umani variegate nativa liber. Vandenhoek, Goettingae, 1776.
23. Blumenbach IF. Editio altera longe auctior et emendatior. Vandenhoek, Goettingae, 1781.
24. Blumenbach IF. De generis umani variegate nativa liber, editio termia Vandenhoek e Ruprecht, Goettingae, 1795a.
25. Blumenbach IF. Über die natürlichen Verschiedenheiten im Menschengeschlechte. Breitkopf und Härtel, Leipzig, 1798.
26. Chardin John. Travels in Persia 1673–1677. London: Argonaut Press, 1927.
27. Marks J. La race, théorie populaire de l'hérédité. La Recherches 1997; 10:17–23.
28. Mahé A. Dermatologie sur peau noire. Paris: Doin Éditeurs, 2000.
29. Mahé A. Dry skin and black skin: what are the facts? Ann Dermatol Venereol 2002; 129(1 Pt 2):152–157.
30. Jablonski NG, Chaplin G. The evolution of human skin coloration. J Human Evol 2000; 39:1–27.
31. Cavalli Sforza LL, Feldman MW. The application of molecular genetic approaches to the study of human evolution. Nat Gen Suppl 2003; 33:266–275.
32. Cavalli Sforza LL, Piazza A. Demic expansions and human evolution. Science 1993; 256:639–646.
33. Cavalli Sforza LL. Genes, people, and languages. Proc Natl Acad Sci USA 1997; 94:7719–7724.
34. Cavalli Sforza LL. Genetic and cultural diversity in Europe. J Anthr Res 1997; 53:383–404.
35. Cavalli Sforza LL, Cavalli Sforza F. The Great Human Diaspora: the history of diversity and evolution. New York, New York: Perseus Press, 1996.
36. Szasz T. The Manufacture of Madness. New York: Harper & Row, 1970: 154–155.

2

Biophysical Properties of Ethnic Skin

Grazia Primavera

San Gallicano Dermatological Institute (IRCCS), Rome, Italy

Enzo Berardesca

Department of Dermatology, San Gallicano Dermatological Institute (IRCCS), Rome, Italy

INTRODUCTION

Even though it is well established that all humans belong to the same species, many physical differences exist among human populations. The use of bioengineering techniques is useful to investigate these differences that could be due to genetic, socioeconomic, and environmental factors (1).

BARRIER FUNCTION

Stratum corneum is equally thick in different races (2–5). However, Weigand et al. demonstrated that the stratum corneum in blacks contains more cell layers and requires more cellophane tape strips to be removed than the stratum corneum of Caucasians (6), while Kampaore and Tsuruta showed that Asian skin was significantly more sensitive to stripping than black skin (7). Weigand also found great variance in values obtained from black subjects, whereas data from white subjects were more homogeneous. No correlation was found between the degree of pigmentation and the number of cell layers. These data could be explained due to the greater intercellular cohesion in blacks, resulting in an increased number of cell layers and an increased resistance to stripping. This mechanism may involve lipids (8), because the lipid content of the stratum corneum ranges from 8.5% to 14%, with higher values in blacks (5,9). This result was confirmed by Weigand et al. who showed that delipidized specimens of stratum corneum were equal in weight in the two races (6). Johnson and Corah found that the mean electrical resistance of an adult black skin is doubled in adult white skin, suggesting an increased cohesion of the stratum corneum (10). Infact, La Ruche and Cesarini found that, in comparison with white skin, the black skin stratum corneum is equal in thickness but more compact: about 20 cell layers are observed in blacks versus 16 layers in whites (5).

Corcuff et al. (11) investigated the corneocyte surface area and the spontaneous desquamation and found no differences between black, white, and oriental skin. However, an increased desquamation (up to 2.5 times) was found in blacks. They concluded that the differences might be related to a different composition of the intercellular lipids of the stratum corneum. Sugino et al. (12) found significant differences in the amount of ceramides in the stratum corneum, with the lowest levels in blacks followed by Caucasian, Hispanics, and Asians. In this experiment, ceramide levels were inversely correlated with transepidermal water loss (TEWL) and directly correlated with water content (WC). Meguro et al. confirmed these correlations (13). These data may partially explain the controversial findings in the literature on the mechanisms of skin sensitivity.

Changes in skin permeability and barrier function have been reported. Kompaore et al. (7,14) evaluated TEWL and lag time after application of a vasoactive compound (methyl nicotinate) before and after removal of the stratum corneum by tape stripping. Before tape stripping, TEWL was 1.3 times greater in blacks and Asians compared to Caucasians. No difference was found between blacks and Asians, whereas after stripping they found a significantly higher TEWL in blacks and Asians than in Whites. In particular, after stripping Asians showed the highest TEWL (Asians 1.7 times greater than Caucasians). They conclude that, similar to previous studies (15,16), skin permeability measured by TEWL, is higher in blacks than in Caucasians. They also conclude that Asian skin has the highest permeability among the groups studied. However, these findings have not yet been confirmed by other groups. Infact, Sugino et al. (12) also included Asians in their study but found that baseline TEWL was, in decreasing order, blacks greater than Caucasians greater than or equal to Hispanics greater than or equal to Asians. Another study (17) about Asian skin, has compared TEWL in Asians and Caucasians and found no statistically significant differences at baseline or after stripping; however, no vasoactive substance was applied.

Reed et al. (18) found differences in the recovery of the barrier between subjects with skin type II/III compared to skin type V/VI, but no differences between Caucasians in general and Asians. Darker skin recovered faster after barrier damage induced by tape stripping.

BIOPHYSICAL PARAMETERS

TEWL, skin conductance, and skin mechanical properties have been measured under basal conditions in Whites, Hispanics, and blacks to assess whether skin color (melanin content) could induce changes in skin biophysical properties (19). Differences appear in skin conductance are more evident in biomechanical features such as skin extensibility, skin elastic modulus, and skin recovery. They differ in dorsal and ventral sites according to races and highlight the influence of solar irradiation on skin and the role of melanin in maintaining it unaltered.

Wilson et al. (15) demonstrated higher in vitro TEWL values in black compared to White skin taken from cadavers. They also found differences in black and White skin physiology; infact the TEWL increased with skin temperature. In their own study, they concluded that black skin would have a greater rise to achieve the same temperature and, therefore, a higher TEWL. Because TEWL depends on passive water vapor loss that is theoretically directly related to the ambient relative humidity and temperature (20), then, the increased TEWL in black skin could be asssociated with an increase in temperature because it is well established that a difference in black and Caucasian temperature exists.

Most studies using the forearm, back, and inner thigh (12–16,21,22) show a greater TEWL in blacks compared to Whites; however, Warrier et al. (23) have demonstrated, studying a larger sample size, that TEWL is lower in blacks than Whites when measuring on the cheeks and legs. No racial differences in TEWL exist either on the volar or dorsal forearms. However, WC is increased in Hispanics on the volar forearm and decreased in Whites (compared only to blacks) on the dorsal forearm. These findings partially confirm previous observations (16,24). Skin lipids may play a role in modulating the relation between stratum corneum WC and TEWL resulting in higher conductance values in blacks and Hispanics.

Racial differences in skin conductance are difficult to interpret in terms of stratum corneum WC, because other physical factors, such as the skin surface or the presence of hair, can modify the quality of the skin-electrode contact. In all races, significant differences exist between the volar and dorsal forearms (19). These results are in apparent contrast with TEWL recordings. Indeed, increased stratum corneum WC, correlates with a higher TEWL (25). These data may be explained on the basis of the different intercellular cohesion or lipid composition. A greater cell cohesion with a normal TEWL could result in increased skin WC.

Racial variability should be considered in terms of different skin responses to topical and environmental agents. Race provides a useful tool to investigate and compare the effects of lifetime sun exposure and ambient relative humidity. Evolution provided over 100,000 years of genetical advantage to survive for those races living in a specific area with specific climatic conditions. Survivering in harmful environment requires an optimal adaptation of outermost layers of our body, the skin on structural, biochemical, and molecular level. It is evident that melanin protection decreases sun damage; differences between sun-exposed and sun-protected areas are not detectable in races with dark skin.

However, TEWL studies are characterized by a large interindividual variability and biased by environmental effects and eccrine sweating. To bypass these influences, an in vitro technique for measuring TEWL was used to compare TEWL in two racial groups (blacks and whites) (15). Black skin had a significantly higher mean TEWL than white skin. In both groups, a significant correlation between skin temperature and increased TEWL was found. The data confirm differences between races found in in vivo studies (16,24). The TEWL measurements with regard to Asian skin may be deemed inconclusive as baseline measurements have found Asian skin to have TEWL values that are equal to black skin and greater than Caucasian skin (14), less than other ethnic groups (12), and no different than other ethnic groups (17).

IRRITATION

Irritation, as measured by TEWL (16,24), revealed a different pattern of reaction in whites after chemical exposure to sodium lauryl sulfate. Blacks and Hispanics developed stronger irritant reactions after exposure. We applied 0.5% and 2.0% sodium lauryl sulphate (SLS), to untreated, preoccluded, and predelipidized black and Caucasian skin and quantified the resulting level of irritation using WC, TEWL, and laser doppler velocimetry (LDV) of the stratum corneum (16). There were only a statistical difference in irritation measuring TEWL after 0.5% SLS application to the preoccluded area between the two groups. Infact, blacks had 2.7 times higher TEWL levels than Caucasians, suggesting that blacks in the preoccluded state are more susceptible to irritation than Caucasians. In another study, we compared differences in irritation between Hispanic and Caucasian skin (16). We found higher values of TEWL for Hispanics compared to Whites after SLS-induced irritation. However, these values were not statistically significant. The reaction of Hispanic skin to SLS resembles black skin when irritated with the same substance. Therefore, these data oppose the traditional clinical view, based on observing erythema, that blacks are less reactive to irritants than Whites.

CONCLUSION

Ethnic (racial) differences in skin physiology have been minimally investigated. The current experimental human model for skin is largely based upon physical and biochemical properties known about Caucasian skin.

Thus, anatomical or physiological properties in skin of different races that may alter a disease process or a treatment of that disease are not being accounted for. Therefore, we still cannot answer the question "how resistant is black skin compared to white?" There exists reasonable evidence to support that black skin has a higher TEWL compared to white skin by means of objective measurements. Although some deductions have been made about Asian and Hispanic skin, the results are contradictory and further evaluation of Asian and Hispanic skin needs to be done. Perhaps more specificity about the origin of their heritage should also be included because "Asian" and "Hispanic" encompasses a broad spectrum of people. Although we remain optimistic that further knowledge will lead to refined claim support and more appropriated formulation for race based skin care.

REFERENCES

1. Shriver MD. Ethnic variation as a key to the biology of human disease. Ann Intern Med 1997; 127:401–403.
2. Freeman RG, Cockerell EG, Armstrong J, et al. Sunlight as a factor influencing the thickness of epidermis. J Invest Dermatol 1962; 39:295–297.
3. Thomson ML. Relative efficiency of pigment and horny layer thickness in protecting the skin of European and Africans against solar ultraviolet radiation. J Physiol (Lond) 1955; 127:236.
4. Lock-Andersen J, Therkildsen P, de Fine Olivarius F, et al. Epidermal thickness, skin pigmentation and constitutive photosensitivity. Photodermatol Photoimmunol Photomed 1997; 13(4):153–158.
5. La Ruche G, Cesarini JP. Histology and Physiology of black skin. Ann Dermatol Venereol 1992; 119(8):567–574.
6. Weigand DA, Haygood C, Gaylor JR. Cell layers and density of Negro and Caucasians stratum corneum. J invest Dermatol 1974; 62:563–565.
7. Kompaore F, Tsuruta H. In vivo differences between Asian, black and white in the stratum corneum barrier function. Int Arch Occup Environ Health 1993; 65(suppl 1):S223–S225.
8. Coderch L, Lopez O, De La Maza A, Parra JLV Ceramides and skin function. Am J Clin Dermatol 2003; 4(2):107–129.
9. Rienertson RP, Wheatley VR. Studies on the chemical composition of human epidermal lipids. J Invest Dermatol 1959; 32:49–51.
10. Johnson LC, Corah NL. Racial differences in skin resistance. Science 1963; 139:766–769.
11. Corcuff P, Lotte C, Rougier A, Maibach H. Racial differences in corneocytes. Acta Derm Venereol (Stockh) 1991; 71:146–148.
12. Sugino K, Imokawa G, Maibach H. Ethnic difference of stratum corneum lipid in relation to stratum corneum function. J Invest Dermatol 1993; 100: 597.
13. Meguro S, Arai Y, Masukawa Y, Uie K, Tokimitsu I. Relationship between covalently bound ceramides and transepidermal water loss (TEWL). Arch Dermatol Res 2000; 292(9):463–468.

14. Kompaore F, Marty JP, Dupont CH. In vivo evaluation of the stratum corneum barrier function in Blacks, Caucasians and Asians with two noninvasive methods. Skin Pharmacol 1993; 6:200–207.
15. Wilson D, Berardesca E, Maibach HI. In vitro transepidermal water loss: differences between black and white human skin. Brit J Dermatol 1988; 199:647–652.
16. Berardesca E, Maibach HI. Racial differences in sodium lauryl sulphate induced cutaneous irritation: black and white. Contact Dermatitis 1988; 18:136–140.
17. Yosipovitch G, Theng CTS. Asian skin: Its Architecture, Function, and Differences from Caucasian Skin. Cosmet Toiletr 2002; 117(9):57–62.
18. Reed JT, Ghadially R, Elias PM. Effect of race, gender and skin type on epidermal permeability barrier function. J Invest Dermatol 1994; 102:537.
19. Berardesca E, de Rigal J, Leveque JL, Maibach HI. In vivo biophysical characterization of skin physiological differences in races. Dermatologica 1991; 182:89–93.
20. Baker H. The skin as a barrier. In: Rook A, ed. Textbook of dermatology. Oxford:Blackwell Scientific, 1986:355.
21. Reed JT, Ghadially R, Elias PM. Skin type, but neither race nor gender, influence epidermal permeability function. Arch Dermatol 1995; 131(10):1134–1138.
22. Berardesca E, Pirot F, Singh M, Maibach HI. Differences in stratum corneum pH gradient when comparino white Caucasian and black African-American skin. Brit J Dermatol 1998; 139:855–857.
23. Warrier AG, Kligman AM, Harper RA, Bowman J, Wickett RR. A comparison of black and white skin using noninvasive methods. J Soc Cosmet Chem 1996; 47:229–240.
24. Berardesca E, Maibach HI. Racial differences in sodium lauryl sulphate induced cutaneous irritation: black and white. Contact Dermatitis 1988; 18:65–70.
25. Rietschel RL. A method to evaluate skin moisturizers in vivo. J Invest Dermatol 1978; 70:152–155.

3

Light Penetration and Melanin Content in Ethnic Skin

Nikiforos Kollias and Paulo R. Bargo

J & J Consumer and Personal Products Worldwide, Skillman, New Jersey, U.S.A.

INTRODUCTION

Melanin and Skin Types

Ethnic skin is characterized by its high melanin content and its ability to produce large amounts of pigment on demand—following insults. Light-complexioned skin on the other hand is characterized by its lack of melanin and inability to produce melanin following insults. The reactivity of the skin to sunlight is often correlated with the amount of pigment in the skin and it is assumed that the darker a person appears the less sensitive the person is to sunlight. However, there are few African Americans who have not experienced a sunburn reaction (some of severe form) with the first long exposure to the sun after the winter months. Such individuals have been misclassified as skin type V or VI based on the pigment level in their skin rather than the reactivity of their skin to sunlight—specifically solar ultraviolet (UV). The skin typing scheme proposed by Fitzpatrick was meant to assess the sensitivity of skin to UV radiation, and while heavily pigmented individuals do not burn as readily as light-complexioned individuals, it is wrong to infer a person's sensitivity to sunlight based only on skin color intensity (Fig. 1) (1–4). Skin color has been used to classify people into racial groups and has been an obvious differentiator among populations, because as humans we have the sense of sight most highly developed in comparison to all the other senses.

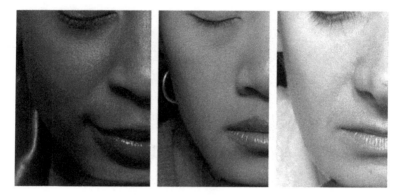

Figure 1 The shades of human skin. The faces in this figure cover the range of human color from dark-complexioned skin where melanin is abundant to light-complexioned skin where melanin is all but absent.

In general, ethnicities considered here include Africans, African Americans, East Asians, Middle East populations, South Americans, and others. In each one of these groups there exist persons of light complexion whose skin may not appear different from Caucasian skin, but its responses may be more like those of more heavily pigmented skin. Within each one of these groupings we find a full range of skin types, people who burn easily to people who never burn at their first exposure after the winter months. What is common among all these individuals is the fact that they all pigment strongly following a prolonged exposure to the sun, and even more so following multiple exposures. In this discussion, we shall not focus on oriental skin, i.e., Chinese, Japanese, Koreans, Mongolians, and others, but the comments relating to melanocompetent skin will certainly apply to these populations without explicit mention.

Hypotheses Which Are Often Considered as Rules

(i) Because of its absorption characteristics in the visible part of the spectrum, estimates of the concentration of epidermal melanin pigmentation (EMP) in the skin are considered easy to make. This approach is based strictly on the absorption properties of melanin in the visible part of the spectrum without consideration of the fact that solid melanin is also a strong scattering element in the skin because of its high index of refraction. (ii) Photoprotection in the UV is frequently predicted based on the intensity of melanin absorption in the visible part of the spectrum. (iii) An implicit assumption made in estimating the concentration of melanin in the epidermis is that we are able to differentiate melanin from the other absorbers in the skin. (iv) For practical purposes melanin is considered to be uniformly distributed in the epidermis; however, at a microscopic level melanin resides in vesicles (melanosomes) and is always in higher concentration in the keratinocytes that line the dermal papillae. (v) Finally, EMP is considered an optical barrier to observation of skin reactions in skin of color—so how are changes with disease or with treatment to be documented? These are some concepts that we revisit in this chapter. We start with a short review of melanin in the skin, then consider light distribution in skin of color, and we end with a discussion on methods of assessing melanin and skin reactions in the skin of persons of color.

MELANIN IN THE SKIN

Constitutive Pigmentation

Melanin resides in the epidermis in keratinocytes. It may also be found in the dermis (in melanophages), but only in disease states. Chemically, EMP is a heteropolymer consisting of various concentrations of monomer units that include 5,6-dihydroxyindole, 5,6-dihydroxyindole-2 carboxylic acid, dihydroxyphenylalanine (DOPA), dopachrome, and others (see discussion in Montagna, Prota, and Kenney). EMP is made from DOPA through the action of several enzymes (tyrosinase, dopachrome tautomerase, etc.) resulting in a high polymer of a very dark to black color. The reaction may be simulated in a test tube by adding tyrosinase to an aqueous solution of DOPA—this reaction does not require light. Melanin is recognized in two molecular states that are characterized grossly by the presence or absence of sulfur. Eumelanin (eu is a Greek prefix that means "good") is the melanin without sulfur and the one with sulfur is called pheomelanin (pheo is a Greek prefix that means "red"). These pigments have been identified in hair as the responsible elements for color. It has been shown that eumelanin can account for all hair colors (including blond) except red, and pheomelanin is necessary for the red color (5). Pheomelanin (red-melanin) is formed easily from DOPA in the presence of the 5-*S*-cystinyl group—the reaction has faster kinetics than the equivalent reaction for eumelanin (6). The eumelanin/pheomelanin ratio is heavily tipped towards eumelanin in darkly complexioned individuals while the opposite is true for light-complexioned individuals, with red hair; however, it is now believed that both forms of melanin exist in all skins. It should be kept in mind that pheomelanin is more photolabile than eumelanin, i.e., it reacts faster with light to produce free radicals. This reactivity of pheomelanin is considered the reason for some of the adverse effects of light on people of light complexion, and especially those with red hair. We do not know the role of pheomelanin in people with high concentrations of melanin in their skin.

The production of melanin starts in the Golgi apparatus of melanocytes where vesicles are formed (melanosomes) that become increasingly dark as they migrate away towards the dendritic processes of the melanocytes. Melanosomes are delivered to the surrounding keratinocytes where they remain through terminal differentiation and eventual desquamation. The production of melanin is regulated at the cellular level through interactions between keratinocytes and melanocytes.

Melanosomes contain tyrosinase and DOPA—the substrate—and the reaction results in EMP which may be a collection of melanin in different states of polymerization and therefore of somewhat different colors (Fig. 2). It has been suggested that the absorption spectra of melanin in different states are different (7), for example, melanin that is not fully polymerized with molecular weight of less than 1000 to 3000 D has an absorption spectrum that is like an exponential curve (becoming steeper at shorter wavelengths), while the melanin that is fully polymerized into a solid has an absorption spectrum that only gently increases at shorter wavelengths—of course this curve becomes steeper at high concentrations (Fig. 3). The absorption of the soluble fraction of melanin plays a more important role in defining the color of

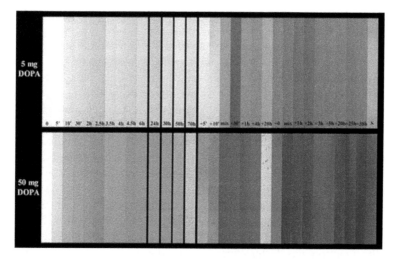

Figure 2 The colors of synthetic eumelanin (shown here in gray scale). The stripes in the figure represent images taken from a test tube into which we placed water and either 5 or 50 mg of dihydroxyphenylalanine. Tyrosinase was then added and the changes in color of the solution were observed for several days (0, 5, 10, 30 minutes, 2, 2.5, 3.5, 4, 4.5, 6, 24, 30, 50, 70 hours, 5 and 10 days; +tyr, 30 minutes, 1, 4, 20 hours, +tyr 1, 2, 3, 5, 20, 25, 38 hours). The color becomes strong early in the reaction and then it becomes gray and starts to clear because higher molecular weight melanin is formed which precipitates from the solution, making the image lighter in color and leaving a low molecular weight supernatant behind. The further addition of tyrosinase reinitiates the reaction, indicating the presence of substrate but not availability of the enzyme originally added to the solution; this operation was repeated twice. The solution becomes gray at 24 hours because it was slightly shaken, causing some precipitate to become resuspended in the solution.

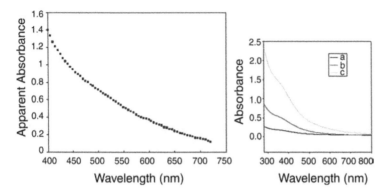

Figure 3 The absorption spectrum of epidermal melanin pigmentation. The spectrum on the left was obtained in vivo by comparing the apparent absorbance of vitiligo-involved skin with normally pigmented skin for an individual of moderately pigmented skin. The inset on the right is the absorption spectrum of three solutions of the supernatant of enzymatic eumelanin; it should be noted that the absorbance in the visible (500–700 nm) is small compared with the absorbance of native melanin.

light-complexioned people, while in dark individuals the absorption by the particulate melanin dominates, in the visible part of the spectrum. This does not mean to imply that there is less soluble melanin in persons of dark complexion.

The production of pigment during exposure to light is assumed to be due to either photo-oxidation of pre-existing pigment and/or production of new pigment from pre-existing substrates—UVA1 radiation is responsible for the induction of an immediate pigmentary response. It has been shown that exposure to UVA radiation can cause a profound pigmentary response in melanocompetent persons that occurs while the skin is being irradiated (8). This production of pigment probably depends on extensive polymerization of partially polymerized melanin. It is reasonable to assume that the melanosomes have both detectable melanin polymer and some amount of low molecular weight partially polymerized fractions. The melanosomes are organized into classes I to IV using as a criterion the amount of melanin deposition within each melanosome, where class I corresponds to no melanin deposition within the melanosomes and class IV to a vesicle that is completely full of melanin (9). Although the melanosomes are made in the melanocytes, they are transferred to the basal keratinocytes where the melanin pigment has been documented in stained histological sections—melanocytes appear usually without a large concentration of melanosomes in their cytoplasm. Melanosomes of very darkly pigmented individuals tend to appear singly dispersed, while in lighter complexioned skin they aggregate (10). There have been no studies to document the melanosome states of aggregation and melanization in individuals of dark skin tone with various levels of pigmentation—skin of color includes many shades of dark!

The melanin distribution in dark skin is highest at the basal keratino-cytes and progressively becomes lower as we approach the stratum corneum. When granular keratinocytes differentiate into flat and anucleated corneo-cytes, it is believed that the melanosome membranes break down, releasing melanin "dust" within the corneocytes (11). The amount of melanin "dust" in superficial corneocytes is essentially nil for light-complexioned individuals and increases as we go to darker complexioned individuals. We do not know if melanin dust also exists in the inter-corneocyte spaces and is discarded together with the stratum corneum lipids. We have shown that abdominal stratum corneum obtained from African American skin ex vivo was only slightly yellow when transilluminated with white light. On the other hand, the stratum corneum that is shed in a "peeling" reaction following a sun-burn is much darker (appears yellow when transilluminated with white light) even from individuals of skin types III and IV.

It has been documented in dark-complexioned individuals during the summer months that their shirt collars get soiled dark when they spend time out-of-doors, leading one to think that the dark stains are probably due to melanized corneocytes and lipids that are shed faster because of sun exposure. This phenomenon is insignificant during the winter months.

The distribution of melanosomes within the viable keratinocytes has been studied to determine the extent to which they may provide protection to the nucleus from solar UV radiation (12). Melanosomes often are con-centrated in nuclear caps that look like umbrellas, that have been shown to protect the nucleus from UV radiation. While this is frequently the case, it is not found to be so 100% of the time (Fig. 4).

The epidermis is under continuous renewal, in contrast to the dermis which to a great extent is acellular and renews very slowly. Keratinocytes are generated at the dermal–epidermal junction and then move upwards to the stratum corneum by terminally differentiating into cells that eventu-ally go through apoptosis and are shed. The trip of the keratinocytes laden with melanin from the basement membrane at the epidermal–dermal junc-tion to desquamation takes approximately 28 days, yet we find a long-term memory in the pigmentary system resulting in pigmented macules that per-sist for weeks to years. The memory of pigmented lesions in skin of color appears to be equally as long as that of light-complexioned (melanocompro-mised) individuals. The rate at which melanin is produced by melanocytes appears to be under local control and the rate persists for long periods of time. The epidermis appears to have a memory for pigment distribution most easily perceived in contrast in pigmented lesions. Some pigmented lesions, for example, may reappear with exactly the same shape following complete removal with laser therapy (e.g., café au lait spots) or with photo-dynamic therapy (PDT) (13).

We can thus visualize melanin distribution in the epidermis primarily in the basal keratinocytes and then at a smaller concentration in the

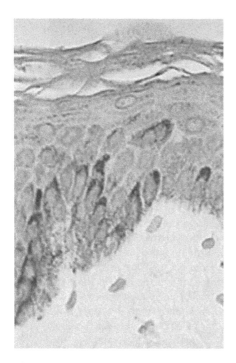

Figure 4 Distribution of melanin in basal keratinocytes. The above histological section from African American skin (stained with H&E) shows the top of the epidermis (stratum corneum, like basket weave) and the viable epidermis with keratinocytes (below) loaded with melanin distributed in caps over the nuclei, appearing to protect the nuclei from ultraviolet exposure; note that all the keratinocytes are not equally loaded with melanin. *Source*: Courtesy of C. Lin, Skin Biology Research Center, J&J.

suprabasal keratinocytes and eventually in melanin dust in the corneocytes that make up the stratum corneum. In skin of color, we find higher melanin concentration in the keratinocytes that line the dermal–epidermal junction and a lower concentration in the suprabasal keratinocytes and melanin "dust" in the stratum corneum. However, we also have to consider the organization of the epidermis; the bottom of the epidermis undulates, forming caps and troughs where dermal papillae appear to be pushing upward, always including a capillary vessel and troughs between caps (Fig. 5).

The epidermis supports a system of glyphic patterns that line its surface from birth throughout life. Melanin concentration appears to be the highest in the keratinocytes that line the papillae and its concentration becomes significantly lower in between papillae. The melanin-bearing keratinocytes also appear to avoid the bottoms of the microglyphics of the skin where there are also few papillae. The glyphic patterns become apparent as

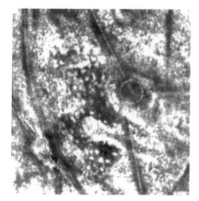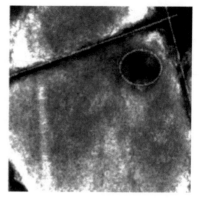

Figure 5 Melanin-laden keratinocytes. Reflectance confocal microscopy sections were obtained from normal skin in vivo at approximately equal depths. The bright objects within the image on the left are melanin-laden keratinocytes above the basement membrane separating epidermis from dermis. The image on the left was obtained from the cheek of an African American and the one on the right from a Caucasian subject. The dotted features on the left correspond to keratinocytes that are melanized; on the right there are no melanin-related structures whatsoever. The straight lines correspond to the location of glyphic lines and the circles mark the position of hair follicles.

lightly pigmented lines on a dark background when viewed at the appropriate magnification after eliminating the reflectance of the stratum corneum surface. This phenomenon of minimal pigment distribution at the bottom of glyphic troughs is most common at the deeper glyphics, (Fig. 6).

A discussion of pigmentation requires consideration of the hair follicle, as dark and thick hair contributes to the appearance of darkly complexioned people. Dark-complexioned individuals typically have black hairs of high density and of large diameters. These attributes contribute to giving the skin a darker appearance than that due to epidermal melanin alone. The darker the skin complexion the less the follicular pigmentation contributes to the skin appearance in terms of pigment. The hair follicle and its apparatus (cells, vessels, and nerves) constitute the regenerative unit of the epidermis, i.e., if the entire epidermis is damaged as in burn injury or removed as in laser resurfacing, all melanocytes are lost and the new epidermis including melanocytes regenerates from the hair follicles. Repigmentation in such lesions starts with perifollicular pigmentation then spreads out to cover the entire epidermis. The hair follicle has two types of melanocytes: one set resides below the bulb of the hair and produces and transfers the melanin that colors the cuticle, and a second group of cells that are not melanized (do not include melanosomes in their cytoplasm) reside in the vicinity of the bulge and are thought to be stand-by melanocytes which only

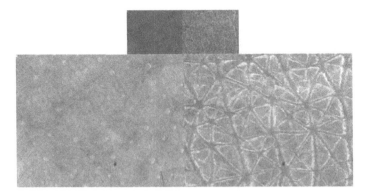

Figure 6 The influence of epidermal glyphics on the distribution of melanin. The original images are shown on the top of the frame as dark objects, the magnified views below are the same images after color adjustment (Fig. 16). In the image on the right we enhance the surface of the skin and the glyphic patterns may be visualized. In the image on the left the surface features have been eliminated by the use of an optical coupling medium allowing a clear view into the skin and the distribution of melanin at ×100. It may be noticed by comparison of the two images that the glyphic structures may be found in the image without surface details, indicating that the melanin distribution carries information about the glyphic structure of the stratum corneum.

produce pigment when they migrate to locations where they are needed to produce pigment.

In darkly pigmented African Americans and on sites exposed to the environment we frequently find perifollicular hyperpigmentation, which frequently appears as a mixture of erythema and pigmentation. This pigment forms frequently as a result of chronic perifollicular inflammation—a common phenomenon with long-term use of surfactants or with aging. Perifollicular hyperpigmentation is noticeable in African American skin when viewed in closeup or under magnification (Fig. 7). Thus, when we consider epidermal pigmentation we need to consider the basal keratinocytes loaded with melanin and the suprabasal with smaller amounts. Of the basal keratinocytes, it is the peripapillae keratinocytes that contribute greatly to the pigmented appearance of the skin. Finally, in arriving at a correct picture, we need to include the perifollicular pigmentation and the reduction in the number of pigmented keratinocytes in the glyphics that extent over the surface of the skin.

Facultative Pigmentation

So far we have considered the distribution of EMP as it is produced and controlled by genetic/hormonal stimuli—*constitutive pigmentation*. We next

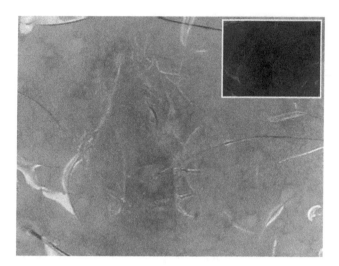

Figure 7 Hyperpigmented structures in the vicinity of hair follicles. African American facial skin of an individual with age in the range 25 to 40 years old. In the upper right corner of the image is the original image before color adjustment. The hyperpigmented structures may be easily perceived in the magnified view (×100). Around each hair follicle a hyperpigmented structure is perceivable particularly in the image obtained with an optical coupler. (Optical coupler used = KY jelly.)

consider the process that produces pigmentation with external stimuli— *facultative pigmentation* (Fig. 8). In skin of color both constitutive and facultative pigmentation may include great quantities of pigment. The melanocyte may be stimulated to produce melanin by exposure to UV radiation or chemical irritants, or through drug reactions and in light-induced dermatoses (e.g., melasma, and macular amyloidosis). It has been proposed that the melanocytes are stimulated to produce pigment by the DNA oligomeres, breakdown products of DNA degradation following exposure to UV (14). This would indicate that the melanocytes of melanocompetent individuals have an increased sensitivity to these DNA oligomers or they respond strongly to a weaker stimulus than do melanocytes in Caucasian skin.

The principal environmental cause for hyperpigmentation is exposure to sunlight, with the additional risk of photosensitization from foodstuffs or cosmetic ingredients. The reason that solar exposure has a strong effect on the pigmentation of exposed skin sites is that many people of color assume that they are not sensitive to the sun and therefore do not protect themselves adequately. Exposure of these melanocompetent individuals to the sun induces large amounts of pigment to be produced and to be accumulated. For example, chronic exposure of the face results in a face that is much more pigmented than protected sites such as the chest, which is usually covered with clothes.

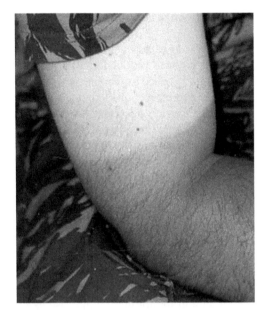

Figure 8 Facultative pigmentation induced by multiple exposures to sunlight of a melanocompetent subject with light complexion.

Exposure to UV radiation induces pigment formation both of an immediate and of a delayed nature. Delayed pigmentation appears following an exposure of the skin to a dose of short-wavelength UV radiation that is capable of inducing an inflammatory reaction—erythema. UVB (290–320 nm) and UVC (200–290 nm) both induce pigment production at three to five days after exposure *following an inflammatory response* that is maximal at 6 to 24 hours after exposure. UVA (320–400 nm) radiation induces pigment production both immediately with exposure and delayed which *may occasionally be accompanied or followed by an inflammatory response* (erythema—redness). This inflammatory response may be difficult to perceive visually because of the excessive pigment. We do not generally associate constitutive pigmentation with inflammation but rather with an innate system of signaling to the melanocytes to produce the requisite amount of pigment for each type of skin, be it African American or Caucasian. Short-wavelength (UVB and UVC) UV radiation, on the other hand, causes pigment production following an inflammatory process appearing only within the exposed skin site—these processes (erythema and pigmentation) may be overlapping in some instances, although for UVB and UVC they tend to follow each other and persist to different extents. Exposures at doses substantially higher than twice the minimum erythema dose (2 MED) may show both erythema and pigmentation reactions for extended times, sometimes for periods greater than two weeks. It is believed that in people of color, the UVB or solar erythema reaction lasts for a shorter period of time than for light-pigmented Caucasians (15).

The induction of pigment production is assessed by a threshold dose of radiation to produce minimally perceptible pigment production, and the variation of this threshold dose with wavelength is called an action spectrum for pigmentation. The action spectrum for the production of a minimal pigment reaction at seven days after exposure is similar in appearance to the action spectrum for the production of a minimal erythema reaction at 24 hours after exposure (16). The action spectrum for erythema and for pigmentation has been extensively studied for light-complexioned individuals and to a lesser extent for dark-complexioned and melanocompetent individuals (17). The action spectrum for erythema in dark-complexioned individuals would be expected to be similar to that of light-complexioned individuals except it would show a decreased sensitivity for all the wavelengths because of the presence of melanin. This would be expected to be the case if melanin acted as a neutral density filter, i.e., a filter that has the same effective absorbance at all wavelengths. If, on the other hand, melanin is considered as an absorbing molecule, then the attenuation of the sensitivity by melanin should correspond to the absorption spectrum of melanin, i.e., it should monotonically increase as we go to shorter wavelengths. What we find is that melanin is not a neutral density filter and the suppression of sensitivity that it offers does not follow the absorption spectrum of melanin (Tables 1 and 2). This would seem to indicate that melanin may not be as important a photoprotective factor as we think, because the location of some absorbers responsible for the induction of facultative pigmentation does not lie under the melanin layer in order to benefit from the absorption of melanin.

UV radiation at wavelengths longer than 340 nm and shorter than 400 nm (what is called the UVA1 range) is effective in inducing pigment reactions with little or no erythema except at high doses. Exposure of skin to UVA wavelengths shorter than 340 nm invariably induces erythema as well as pigmentation. One of the most intriguing observations about facultative pigmentation to UVA1 radiation (340–400 nm) is that the threshold dose to produce a pigment reaction immediately after exposure is the same for all skin types, irrespective of the amount of pigment in their skin! The threshold is 1.0 to 2.0 J/cm^2 while the threshold to produce a pigment reaction that lasts for at least two hours and may persist for days to weeks is about 10 times larger (11 J/cm^2). While the threshold dose is the same— independent of the pigment level of the skin—the amount of pigment that may be formed under continuous irradiation of the skin with UVA1 radiation above threshold may reach very significant levels. The amount of pigment is such that it becomes impossible to realize an erythematous reaction because of the color of the skin (Fig. 9).

The amount of pigment formed with continuous UVA1 radiation beyond the threshold is large, especially for darkly pigmented individuals,

Table 1 Comparison of Skin Sensitivity to Ultraviolet (UV) Radiation of Persons of Skin Types V and VI with Skin Types III and IV and Fair-Skinned Caucasians Given in Terms of the Dose of UV Radiation of a Specific Wavelength to Produce a Threshold Erythema Reaction 24 Hours After Exposure

	MED (mJ/cm^2) fair-skinned Caucasians	MED (mJ/cm^2) Skin types III and IV	MED (mJ/cm^2) Skin types V and VI
Wavelength (nm)	$N=17$	$N=12$	
295 ± 5	31.2 ± 25%	28.0 ± 5%	40.2 ± 65% ($N=77$)
305 ± 5	58.6 ± 25%	72.0 ± 5%[a]	134 ± 75%[a] ($N=91$)
315 ± 5	1138 ± 25%	1370 ± 5%	1383 ± 45% ($N=77$)
365 ± 10	78,000 ± 25%	168,000 ± 5%[a]	264,000 ± 25%[a] ($N=14$)

Note: By comparing the values of the MED for the various skin types we find that at 295 nm all skin types have similar sensitivity, at 305 nm the reaction of the skin is very different among skin types, at 315 nm the sensitivity is remarkably the same for all skin types, and at 365 nm the sensitivity is progressively lower for the higher pigmented skin types. It is important to note that the skin sensitivity does not decrease by more than a factor of 3 in going from skin types V to VI to fair-skinned Caucasians at any wavelength!
[a]$p < 0.0005$ when compared to the immediately previous column.
Abbreviation: MED, minimum erythema dose.
Source: The data in this table are from Ref. 17 and references therein.

Table 2 Comparison of Skin Sensitivity to Ultraviolet (UV) Radiation of Persons of Skin Types V and VI with Fair-Skinned Caucasians Given in Terms of the Dose of UV Radiation of a Specific Wavelength to Produce a Threshold Pigmentation Reaction Seven Days After Exposure

	MMD (mJ/cm^2) fair skinned Caucasians	MMD (mJ/cm^2) skin types V and VI
Wavelength (nm)	$N=17$	
295 ± 5	45.9 ± 30%	40.3 ± 65% ($N=77$)
305 ± 5	66.5 ± 25%	208 ± 60%[a] ($N=91$)
315 ± 5	1162 ± 15%	1378 ± 45%[b] ($N=77$)
365 ± 10	63,500 ± 15%	90,000 ± 35%[c] ($N=14$)

Note: The wavelength most strongly dependent on skin type is 305 nm, and 365 nm is only weakly dependent on skin type. The threshold dose to produce an immediate pigment darkening reaction (pigment that appears immediately after exposure) is completely independent of skin type.
[a]$p < 0.0005$ when compared to the previous column.
[b]$p < 0.001$.
[c]$p < 0.05$.
Abbreviation: MMD, minimum melanogenic dose.
Source: The data in this table are from Ref. 17 and 22.

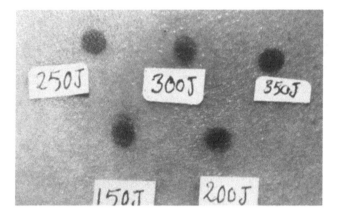

Figure 9 Ultraviolet (UV)A1-induced pigment with single prolonged exposures. A series of doses of UVA1 was delivered serially to each of the skin sites of a subject of skin type V. The amount of pigment produced was apparent when the irradiation was stopped, was of significant proportions, and lasted for more than two months.

and may occur in a single exposure to the sun. A dose of 11 J/cm² of UVA1 radiation may be delivered in 50 minutes of exposure to sunlight and corresponds to the threshold for persistent pigmentation. A frequently ignored source of facultative pigmentation is visible light. The threshold dose for visible light-induced pigmentation is much higher but the solar irradiance is also much higher. The solar irradiance in visible light is approximately 155 mW/cm² resulting in persistent pigment formation within 35 minutes of exposure to sunlight (18). Visible light-induced pigmentation is shown in Figure 10.

We have shown that the spectral absorbances of facultative pigmentation produced with different light sources (UVC, UVB, UVA1, and Visible) have different signatures and may be thus identified (Fig. 11). On dark-pigmented individuals UVC produces a pigmentary response that lasts like the UVB-induced pigment but is of lower intensity for doses of equal multiples of the MED. Exposure to UVB radiation results in a reasonably strong response at doses that generate a strong erythema response (2–3 MED); higher doses will produce a stronger response, but in some strongly pigmented individuals will also cause peeling with a loss of the additional pigmentation. UVA1 radiation produces a pigmentary response that may be very strong depending on the total dose, and has initially (at the end of the exposure) a gray appearance; the gray color becomes more like constitutive pigmentation with time, and this transformation may take from hours to one week. Visible radiation of sufficient dose to produce pigment (>300 J/cm²) results in a pigment that, unlike UV-induced pigmentation which shows sharp borders and little diffusion beyond the irradiation edge,

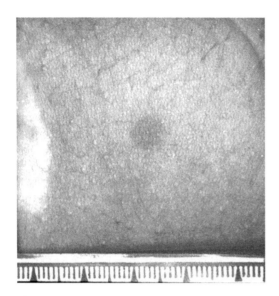

Figure 10 Visible light-induced pigmentation on a melanocompetent subject. The site that was irradiated is in the middle of the image frame and is approximately 6 mm in diameter. The dose was 400 J/cm², delivered at 0.25 W/cm².

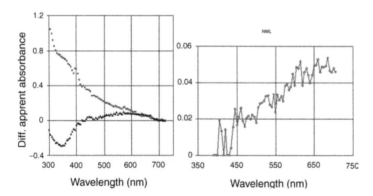

Figure 11 The spectral signatures of facultative pigmentation produced by different light sources are shown. It should be noted that UVB-induced pigmentation (left top) has a signature very close to that of native pigment, UVA1-induced pigmentation (left bottom) has a signature that resembles melanin at long wavelengths but at wavelengths below 450 nm it decreases. Unlike native pigment, visible-induced pigmentation (right) has an absorption signature that increases with increasing wavelength, i.e., exactly the opposite of native pigment.

has extended diffuse edges (~1.0 mm) and has a spectral absorption signature that is unlike constitutive melanin pigmentation, i.e., its absorbance increases weakly with wavelength (Fig. 11).

From the above discussion, it should be clear that all UV radiation as well as the visible radiation may produce an enhanced pigmentary response in skin of color, resulting in hyperpigmentation that lasts from weeks to months and beyond, depending on the dose of the original exposure and on the skin phenotype. This summarizes the information we have on acute exposures (i.e., a single exposure). However, humans tend to receive solar exposures that may occur over days or weeks, i.e., the result of multiple exposures. We know that multiple exposures given in such a fashion that they never induce erythema produce hardening in the skin so the skin may tolerate higher doses of UV radiation that usually result in increased pigment production. However, in an experiment on 90 psoriatic subjects of skin types V and VI we showed that UVB delivered at suberythemogenic doses—which were increased as the MED increased—delivered three to four times a week for 6 to 10 weeks resulted in no significant hyperpigmentation of the uninvolved skin (19). Treatment with Psoralen plus UVA irradiation (PUVA), on the other hand, on a similar group of psoriatic patients resulted in a marked increase in pigmentation of the uninvolved skin. In melano-competent subjects with psoriasis, we have observed a depigmenting action of an acute exposure to UVB radiation at 24 to 48 hours after exposure—this occurred only on a few subjects and the skin recovered within a week (personal observations).

It has been assumed because of our familiarity with this pigment (melanin) that we may easily distinguish it from the other color-bearing materials in the skin. The other molecules in the skin that absorb visible light include oxyhemoglobin and deoxyhemoglobin which exist in a roughly 60/40 ratio in the visually perceptible layers of the skin. It has been shown that visually we cannot distinguish between melanin and deoxyhemoglobin, and since deoxyhemoglobin contributes quite a bit to the color appearance of the skin, it needs to be carefully accounted for (20). The contribution of deoxy-hemoglobin to normal skin color may be experienced by applying pressure with a finger on the forearm: when the pressure is released, the color of the arm returns to "normal" as the venules are once more filled. The only way to distinguish between the two color factors is by applying pressure on the skin—e.g., with a glass slide—then if the pigment is of vascular origin it will blanch, while if it is melanin it will remain the same. This maneuver is of value on lighter pigmented subjects. In individuals with skin of color, because there is always a high concentration of melanin present, a hyperpigmented or a hypopigmented skin site may be easily taken to be due to higher or lower melanin concentration. For example, in lesions of postinflammatory hyperpigmentation, deoxyhemoglobin is frequently a contributing absorber and at times the only absorber. The only way to distinguish the pigments melanin and deoxyhemoglobin from each other is by using diffuse reflectance spectroscopy and spectral deconvolution of the skin spectrum—a process that sounds more complicated than it really is (21). Whenever a reaction of the skin involves both a vascular and a pigmentary component, it is best to attempt to assess them separately, giving a score to each.

The determination of the minimum phototoxic dose to PUVA (Psoralen plus UVA) is such a case. The skin is first sensitized with a Psoralen (either 8-methoxypsoralen (MOP) or 5-MOP) and then it is exposed to a series of doses of UVA and the MPD is determined 48 to 72 hours after exposure. At that time, for subjects of skin types V and VI, the skin reaction includes both erythema and melanin hyperpigmentation, i.e., the sites above threshold (the sites that show a response) appear both pigmented and red. It has been shown that the uncertainty in the visual determination of the threshold dose for erythema alone is 140%, invariably leading to a lower value for the MPD and a less effective treatment (22). In the case where the skin response is only erythema, as with exposure to UVB radiation at 24 hours after exposure, the determination of the threshold is easily established with equal sensitivity as in light-complexioned skin, because no matter what the enhanced pigment in the skin we know it is only due to oxyhemoglobin and deoxyhemoglobin, usually in a 3 to 1 ratio. Another interesting case where deoxyhemoglobin–melanin misdetermination plays an important role is in hypopigmented lesions where a vascular involvement may be ignored because of the apparent color of the lesion.

Finally, we may consider the question "why is there melanin in the skin?" There have been several attempts to understand the reason for the presence of melanin in the skin, especially since it exists in skin in such abundant quantities. In dark-complexioned individuals melanin absorption is of similar magnitude and often more significant than the absorption of hemoglobin and we have a good understanding of the role of the latter. We could try a thought experiment: suppose that suddenly all melanin disappeared from the skin: how would this affect its structure and function? In terms of structure, it would definitely have an effect on the appearance of the skin, but it is not clear if the function of the skin would be affected other than in photoprotection from solar UV—but if one were to remain indoors for this experiment, then the absence of melanin would have no deleterious effect. It is hard to believe that nature has endowed the biological system with such an elegant and structure—altering component that does not play any role in homeostasis. So melanin remains a factor that plays an important role in the appearance of the skin—and in photoprotection—and otherwise is an orphan in physiological function. There is a diagnostic role for this chromophore—it provides us with visual cues for areas of the skin where there may be malfunctions or deviation from physiological behavior; the only other molecule that plays a similar and important role is hemoglobin.

LIGHT DISTRIBUTION IN SKIN

The reasons to determine the light distribution in the skin are both to better understand the visual information we obtain from the skin and to devise and understand therapies based on light or drug+ light as PDT. There have been several papers in the past outlining our thinking about how light is distributed in the skin, however, those discussions have been about light-complexioned skin (23). We will try to introduce various quantities of melanin in our discussion and consider how this may change not only the distribution of light in the skin but also our perception depending on its density and distribution. We shall consider normal skin except when disease state examples help elucidate a particular distribution (geometry), e.g., dermal pigmentation.

The interaction of light with the skin may be considered in steps: first the interaction at the stratum corneum–air interface, then the interaction of light within the stratum corneum layers, followed by the interaction of light with the remaining viable epidermis and finally with the dermis. Light interactions can be thought of in terms of two processes, *absorption* and *scattering*; reflection and refraction can be thought of as special cases of scattering. In absorption, photons are taken up by the molecular species present in the light path and are converted to heat, resulting in selective attenuation of the light intensity at the absorption maxima of each encountered species, which results in a change of color of the incident beam. These changes in spectral quality may be used to identify the molecular species present and will result in a colored appearance for the object. Scattering on the other hand is responsible for changing the direction of propagation of a photon through an interaction that occurs in the interface between two media. On a macroscopic scale, we are used to describing such processes as reflection and refraction, describing how the direction and the intensity of light are altered when it goes through an interface from one medium into another (Fig. 12).

An interface defines the transition from one medium to another where the two media have different indices of refraction. The larger the change in index of refraction the larger the intensity of reflected light and the larger the angle of deviation in the direction of travel. For example, when light falls on a glass surface going from air with an index of refraction of 1.0 to glass with an index of refraction of 1.5 (like a window pane) some light is reflected and some is transmitted into the glass—this example parallels what happens when light interacts with the stratum corneum: some is reflected back and some enters into the stratum corneum. The stratum corneum surface is different from a glass surface in that it is "rough" because it is made up of flat corneocytes that are on an average 1 μm in thickness and are intercalated at the edges with each other. These cells have surfaces that may be flat (see photomicrograph, Figure 4). In pigmented individuals and particularly on exposed sites we find melanin in the stratum corneum as small particles,

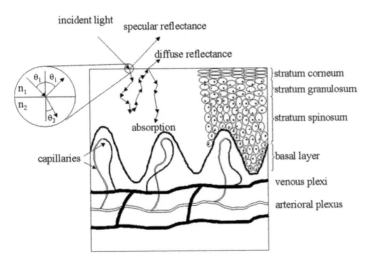

Figure 12 Schematic diagram of light interactions with skin. The insert shows the changes in light travel at the interface between two media of different indices of refraction. The small arrows indicate the tortuous path that light might follow in tissue because of scattering events with keratinocytes or cellular organelles.

of diameter less than 0.1 μm. These particles are responsible for producing forward scattering (resulting in a change in direction by approximately 10° at each scattering event), which is weakly dependent on wavelength. This forward scattering in the stratum corneum does not produce significant blurring of the subsurface structures. The presence of melanin in the stratum corneum is perceived visually by the pale yellow appearance it gives to it. If the concentration of melanin in the stratum corneum became large, so that it would become of a strong yellow-brown-gray color, then it would also limit our ability to look into the skin because it would make subsurface structures appear diffuse or foggy. This may occur only in the darkest skins and on chronically exposed sites (Fig. 12).

Light that goes through the stratum corneum enters the viable epidermis without experiencing any changes in its direction of travel, i.e., there are no changes in the index of refraction between these layers because there are no structures that separate the two layers. Since most of the melanin in skin resides in the viable epidermis it is here that we would expect the major changes in light attenuation and direction of travel to occur. Melanin granules have an index of refraction of approximately 1.7 that is the largest of any other organelle within the skin, and therefore light will scatter strongly when it interacts with them (24,25). Light that falls on one of these granules will scatter and it will also be absorbed by melanin which is a strong absorber as well. In this context, melanin might be thought of as similar to graphite: photons scatter from the surface of graphite because of its high index of refraction but photons that get beyond the surface get completely absorbed, resulting in a gray appearance rather than black. This may be observed for the darkest pigmented subjects; these individuals appear essentially silver/ black rather than brown/black. Melanin that resides in the epidermis, scatters light strongly; scattered light is of the same color as the light source, giving the skin a silvery appearance. The light that penetrates into the skin can be perceived only if it is scattered by the dermal collagen matrix. For the darkest of skins, light is strongly absorbed by the melanin present in the epidermis resulting in a small amount that makes it to the dermis. This light is then further absorbed by the epidermal melanin on its way out and results in a tiny signal. For persons with extremely high melanin concentrations in their skin, the predominant signal from the skin is from scattered light by the melanin granules and the stratum corneum, giving the skin a silverish— black appearance. Individuals whose skin appears brown do not show as strong a scattering contribution from melanin—the color brown comes from the absorption of melanin combined with some hemoglobin absorption. The richer the brown color the higher the contribution of hemoglobin and also of not fully polymerized melanin. In considering the absorption of light by melanin in the epidermis we also have to take into consideration the patterns of melanin distribution and concentration in the epidermis. Melanin is not distributed uniformly in the epidermis—this may be observed in pigmented epidermis with a videomicroscope with a magnification of ×100 (Fig. 13). Except for scattering by melanin there is some minor scattering in the epidermis

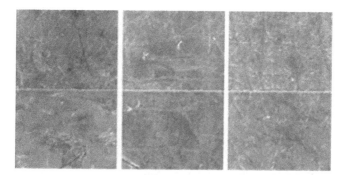

Figure 13 The three sets of images were obtained from three skin sites on an African American subject, the cheek (left), the dorsal forearm (center), and the upper inner arm (right); the upper image enhances the surface features and the lower image enhances the subsurface features of the skin. All images have been color adjusted to gray scale in order to make the details visible, the colors are not true after color correction; however, the color adjustment allows discrimination of changes in melanin distribution to become evident. Perifollicular pigmentation is visible in the image on the left, the glyphic patterns are visible in the image in the middle, and in the image in the right the pigment distribution appears to be affected by the distribution of collagen.

from cell walls and nuclei. An increase in scattering from nuclear material has been observed in epithelial tissues in tumors rich in nuclear content compared to adjacent normal tissue; this has not been documented in skin yet.

There appear to be areas where there is an abundance of pigment and other areas where there is a substantially smaller concentration of melanin pigment. It has been noted that melanin accumulates in the keratinocytes that line the dermal papillae and has been assumed that the apparent distribution of pigment in a fine network-like fashion is due to the columnar accumulation of melanin in the keratinocytes that line the dermal papillae. However, this is not the case in the above images from different body sites— the distribution of melanin is found to be also affected by the arrangement of glyphics in the stratum corneum and of dermal collagen bundles. From in vivo reflectance confocal microscopy we also find that the pigment indeed is distributed in the superficial viable epidermal layers as well as in basal keratinocytes that line dermal papillae.

When observing skin of color with a video microscope (Fig. 13) the dominant feature that can be seen is the patterns of pigment distributed in a lacework fashion with small bright spots surrounded by darker areas in a yellow-brown background. However, this is not the only pattern that may be seen: there also appear bright areas around each hair shaft with an enhancement of color just outside the bright area. This nonuniformity of pigment distribution may be perceived as a hyperpigmented circular structure surrounding each hair follicle.

Light that makes it past the epidermis enters the dermis where it is strongly scattered by the collagen and elastin matrix. The optical properties of the dermis of black skin are in no way different from those of the dermis of light-complexioned skin. Light that enters the dermis may be absorbed by the resident chromophore, hemoglobin, found in the confines of vessels and further in erythrocytes. Blood is visualized as a uniformly distributed absorber in the dermis; it should be kept in mind that this is not the case. In the vessels, hemoglobin is always in high concentrations, making vessels totally absorbing at wavelengths where the absorption spectrum of hemoglobin has strong absorption maxima, as at the Soret bands (412 and 430 nm for oxy- and deoxyhemoglobin, respectively) and the alpha, beta bands (542 and 577 nm for oxy- and 555 nm for deoxyhemoglobin). Erythrocytes are also good scatterers and may be seen in the upper dermis with a video microscope at high magnification ($> \times 400$) both as red particles and as moving scatterers by causing light intensity "flickering." Vessels are not perceivable in dark skin although they may be perceived as dark lines identifiable because of their appearance, and by association with the clearly visible vessels in light-complexioned skin. The papillary dermis may be imaged allowing the visualization of vessels and of collagen bundles; under appropriate conditions, the reticular dermis appears a diffuse pink medium that back-illuminates the papillary dermis and the epidermis.

It has been assumed that because of the dark color of black skin it is essentially impossible to study its features, or more properly to document accurately its state. Since both the absorption of melanin and of hemoglobin become greater at shorter wavelengths, the depth to which we obtain information from black skin truly depends on the wavelength to a greater degree than light skin. In light skin we know that light penetrates to a depth of approximately 70 μm at 400 nm (deep blue) and progressively increases reaching 700 μm at 700 nm (far red) (the "depth of penetration" refers to the depth in tissue at which the intensity of light has been reduced to 37% of the incident intensity) (26). The reflected light from the stratum corneum surface is approximately 4% of the incident intensity irrespective of the amount of melanin in the skin: this is due to the Fresnel reflection by the interface. For dark skin the intensity of light remitted by the skin at 400 to 450 nm is less than the intensity of the light that is reflected by the stratum corneum, i.e., less than 4%. It is only by going to the longer wavelengths in the visible part of the spectrum that the intensity of light from within the skin may rise above the stratum corneum reflectance (Fig. 14).

DOCUMENTATION OF SKIN OF COLOR

The physical attributes of the skin that are most affected by the presence of melanin are the optical parameters that relate to the appearance of the skin,

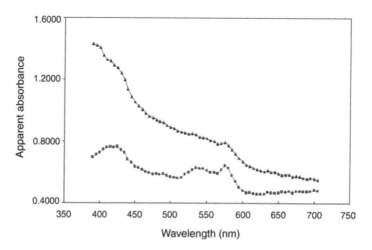

Figure 14 The apparent absorption spectra of heavily pigmented skin (top line) and light-complexioned skin (bottom line). The role of melanin becomes more important as we progress to shorter wavelengths, i.e., the spectra deviate more from each other. The absorption of hemoglobin is evident in the lightly pigmented skin both at the Soret band 415 to 430 nm and the Q-bands 540 to 580 nm; the amount of hemoglobin in the pigmented skin is of similar magnitude but is obscured by the absorption of melanin.

both in terms of surface texture and in terms of subsurface features. Standard photography (film or digital) has been used to document darkly pigmented skin, however, in studying the skin we need to document as many details about surface features and subsurface features in ethnic skin as we do about lightly-complexioned skin. A number of techniques have been developed to provide a better estimate of the distribution and concentration of absorbers and scatterers in skin; these methods have addressed primarily light-complexioned skin. These methods include both reflectance and fluorescence imaging. In reflectance, polarization of the incident light as well as of the reflected light has been used to selectively enhance surface or subsurface features. In fluorescence, excitation sources have been used in both the near UV (UVA1, 360–380 nm) and in the blue (400–460 nm) to excite fluorescence from endogenous fluorophores and to view absorbers that attenuate the fluorescence such as melanin and hemoglobin. It is clear that all the optical signals from within the skin will be severely attenuated by melanin in darkly complexioned skin; however, this does not mean that we are unable to document changes in the pigmented skin. It simply means that we might have to work a bit harder to get good signals.

There are two important facts to consider: the first is that melanin absorption is not flat across the wavelengths but increases monotonically from the red to the blue; the second is that imaging equipment is calibrated by the use of a gray card whose absorbance falls somewhere in the middle of the range most commonly used in photography (and corresponding to an average Caucasian subject, someone of a light complexion of Mediterranean extraction), as well as a white and a black standard that define the extremes in intensity. These facts may be used to modify the way imaging data may be obtained and analyzed when dealing with dark skin. Since melanin loses absorption strength as we go from the blue to the red, we might consider shifting the spectrum of the source to reduce the effective absorbance by melanin, thus making the epidermis more transparent. This is demonstrated in Figure 15 where the components of a color image are shown separately for a subject of African origin.

Thus, by shifting the wavelength of the incident light we can in effect obtain better contrast of subsurface skin features. It should be kept in mind that by going to the red in order to minimize the contribution of epidermal melanin absorbance, we also lose a great deal of the hemoglobin signals because oxyhemoglobin absorbs very weakly beyond 630 nm and deoxyhemoglobin absorbs with a strength that is very similar to that of melanin and therefore can be confused with it. In order to document erythema in dark skin we may use a process called histogram equalization, which amounts to taking the lightest and the darkest pixels in the image and then define the range of white to black to be that of the pixels of maximum and minimum intensity in the image. It should be kept in mind that in defining the darkest and the lightest pixels in the image, only pixels that belong to

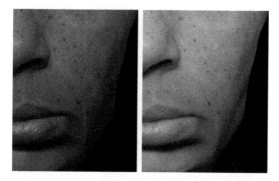

Figure 15 The image (red green blue channels) of an African American subject as obtained with a CCD camera (shown here in gray scale). On the right, the gray scale image of the red channel of the image on the left. Note that the diffuse pigment becomes less visible allowing evaluation of hyperpigmented lesions.

the image of the skin are considered and not pixels that correspond to clothing or to the image background. This is a common practice in two-dimensional graphs where we define the range of the axes to just include the range of our data. In the case of imaging we do the same thing, only we do it in a dimension that we are not used to working in, namely that of the intensity of light; here the range is from 0 to 255 or 1 to 256 for an 8-bit charged coupled device (CCD) (the detector in a camera) (8 bit refers to the number of bits of information, the dynamic range contained in each pixel that corresponds to light intensity, in this case it means 2^8, i.e., 8 binary bits). This process is outlined in Figure 16.

Histogram equalization renders the darkest of skin considerably more transparent, however, the subsurface features might be altered in this stretch of the axes and therefore attention and extra care needs to be taken when interpreting the significance of the observed features. On the other hand, surface features such as dry or "ashy" skin become easier to detect and document in dark skin because the dark epidermis provides a dark background. "Ashy" skin consists of dry corneocytes that are not well attached to the rest of the stratum corneum presenting themselves in various angles other than parallel to the stratum corneum, and therefore they desiccate further. This increases their index of refraction and the scattering of light from their surface, thus they appear white because they redirect the incident light towards the observer's eyes before it gets color modified by the absorbers in the skin. The apparent transparency of black skin when viewed with a video microscope, may be accounted for by both (1) the adjustment of the intensity of light so that a sufficient signal is obtained and (2) adjustment of the range of values of the intensity. Again we need to be careful in interpreting the observed features because they are modified by these operations—on

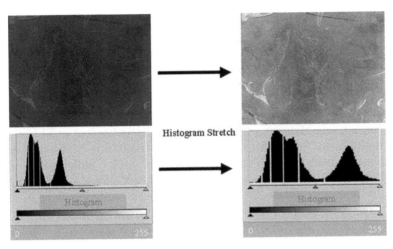

Figure 16 Demonstration of histogram equalization or histogram stretch. The brightness values of the pixels in the image of a dark African American fall in a narrow range with few if any bright values because the image is dark. We can produce a correction that allows better viewing of the image by taking the brightest pixel element and moving it to the maximum of the brightness scale, in this way stretching the axis. This operation provides a brighter image with higher discrimination between the bright and dark elements in the image. One has to be careful in performing such an operation which could lead to erroneous conclusions, because following a stretch of the image and analysis one has to return to the original with the knowledge of the information gathered following the stretch.

the other hand, these operations allow observation into the epidermis and upper dermis even of the darkest of skins.

SUMMARY

In this chapter, we propose that "ethnic" skin may be more broadly defined as melanocompetent skin, i.e., through its dynamic responses to injuries rather than through its static appearance. (i) In ethnic skin melanin is found in singly dispersed melanosomes in epidermal keratinocytes both as a higher molecular weight polymer (>15 kD) and a low molecular weight solute (<5 kD), and the lower molecular weight form is photoreactive. (ii) The melanin distribution in the epidermis forms both a diffuse background in the lowest lying keratinocytes and islands of hyperpigmentation mostly perifollicular but varying with body site. The distribution of epidermal melanin is influenced both by the glyphic structures visible on the surface of the stratum corneum and by the distribution of the superficial collagen bundles. (iii) Ethnic skin is capable of producing a very large amount of pigment following injuries both immediately after injury (e.g., UVA1 or visible light) or with a delay as in postinflammatory hyperpigmentation. (iv) The pigment responses of skin to UV injuries do not substantiate the photoprotective properties of epidermal melanin, i.e., dark skin does not appear to have a markedly lower sensitivity to shorter wavelengths, as the melanin spectrum would imply. (v) In ethnic skin, in particular, what is perceived as a pigmentary response might be due to vascular stasis or excess pigment because deoxyhemoglobin cannot be visually distinguished from melanin when the two are mixed. (vi) Melanin granules in the epidermis are responsible for both absorption of light and scattering of light. Scattering by melanin is responsible for the silver-black appearance of very dark individuals and for the discrimination of keratinocytes in images of dark skin with reflectance confocal microscopy, because melanin is the strongest scattering material in the epidermis. (vii) At a microscopic level ($\times 100$) the distribution of melanin in dark skin shows large deviations from uniform. (viii) Documentation of dark skin may be accomplished by shifting the wavelength of investigation to wavelengths where melanin is less absorbing, or by using a histogram stretch to minimize the absorption by the diffuse pigment, thus increasing the transparency of the skin. Warning procedures that alter the transparency of dark skin may also alter the perception of other features.

REFERENCES

1. Fitzpatrick TB. Soleil et peau. J Med Esthet 1975; 2:33–34.
2. Fitzpatrick TB. The validity and practicality of sun-reactive skin types I through VI. Arch Dermatol 1988; 124:869–871.
3. Thomas P, Cesarini JP. Les Phototypes. Nouv Dermatol 1984; 3:199–203.
4. Cesarini JP. Photo-induced events in the human melanocytes system: photoaggregation and photoprotection. Pigm Cell Res 1988; 1:223–233.
5. Kurtz SK, Kozikowski S, Wolfram LJ. Optical constants of solid melanins determined by reflection measurements in the visible spectrum. J Invest Dermatol 1986; 87:401.
6. Chedekel MR, Zeise L. Sunlight, melanogenesis and radicals in skin. Lipids 1988; 23:587–591.
7. Kollias N, Baqer A. Absorption mechanisms of human melanin in the visible 400–720 nm. J Invest Dermatol 1987; 89:384–388.
8. Al-Ajmi HS. The photocontact reaction. Thesis, Medical Sciences, Universisty of Dundee, 1989.
9. Montagna W, Prota G, Kenney JA Jr., Black Skin, Structure and Function. New York: Academic Press Inc., 1993.
10. Quevedo WC Jr., Fitzpatrick TB, Szabo G, Jimbow K. Biology of the melanin pigmentary system. In: Fitzpatrick TB, Eisen AZ, Wolff K, Freedberg IM, Austen FK, eds. Dermatology in General Medicine. New York: McGraw Hill, 1979.
11. Lu H, Edwards C, Gaskell S, Pearse A, Marks R. Melanin content and distribution in the surface corneocyte with skin phototypes. Brit J Dermatol 1996; 135:263–267.

12. Kobayashi N, Nakagawa A, Muramatsu T, et al. Supranuclear melanin caps reduce ultraviolet induced DNA photoproducts in human epidermis. J Invest Dermatol 1998; 110:806–810.
13. Shimbashi T, Kamide R, Hashimoto T. Long-term follow-up in treatment of solar lentigo and café-au-lait macules with Q-switched ruby laser. Aesthetic Plast Surg 1997; 21:445–448.
14. Gilchrest BA, Eller MS. DNA photodamage stimulates melanogenesis and other photoprotective responses. J Invest Dermatol Symp Proc 1999; 4:35–40.
15. Pathak MA, Fanselow DL. Photobiology of melanin pigmentation: dose/ response of skin to sunlight and its contents. J Am Acad Dermatol 1983; 9:724–733.
16. Gange RW, Park YK, Auletta M, Kagetsu N, Blackett AD, Parrish JA. Action spectra for cutaneous responses to ultraviolet radiation. In: Urbach F, Gange RW, eds. The Biological Effects of UVA Radiation. New York: Praeger Publishers, 1986:57–65.
17. Kollias N, Malallah Y, Al Ajmi H, Baqer A, Gonzalez S. Erythema and melanogenesis action spectra in heavily pigmented individuals as compared to fair-skinned Caucasians. Photodermatol Photoimmunol Photomed 1996; 12: 183–188.
18. Kollias N, Baqer A. An experimental study of the changes in pigmentation in human skin in vivo with visible and near infrared light. Photochem Photobiol 1984; 39:651–659.
19. Selim MM, Hegyi V, Al-Fouzan A. UVB phototherapy for psoriasis of skin type V. Clin Exp Dermatol 1988; 13:168–172.
20. Stamatas GN, Kollias N. Blood stasis contributes to perception of skin pigmentation. J Biomed Optics 2004; 9:315–322.
21. Stamatas GN, Zmudzka BZ, Kollias N, Beer JZ. Non-Invasive measurements of skin pigmentation in situ. Pigm Cell Res 2004; 17:618–626.
22. Kollias N, Baqer A, Sadiq I. Minimum erythema dose determination in individuals of skin type V and VI with diffuse reflectance spectroscopy. Photoderm Photoimm Photomed 1994; 10:249–254.
23. Anderson RR, Parrish JA. The optics of human skin. J Invest Dermatol 1981; 77:13–19.
24. Rajadhyaksha M, Grossman M, Esterowitz D, Webb RH, Anderson RR. In vivo confocal scanning laser microscopy of human skin: melanin provides strong contrast. J Invest Dermatol 1995; 104:946–952.
25. Langley RG, Rajadhyaksha M, Dwyer PJ, Sober AJ, Flotte TJ, Anderson RR. Confocal scanning laser microscopy of benign and malignant melanocytic skin lesions in vivo. J Am Acad Dermatol 2001; 45:365–376.
26. Kollias N. The physical basis of skin color and its evaluation in "Bioengineering methods in Dermatology." Clin Dermatol 1995; 13:361–367.

4

Photoreactivity of Ethnic Skin

Giovanni Leone and Alessia Pacifico

Phototherapy Unit, San Gallicano Dermatological Institute (IRCCS), Rome, Italy

INTRODUCTION

Our species has been divided into varying numbers of subspecies or races. These include Caucasoid (Europeans), Mongoloid (Asians), Congoid or Negroid (African Tribes), Capoid, and Australoid (Australian arborigines). This classification does not provide an exhaustive categorization of all people in the world (1).

The skin phototype system (SPS) has been used classically by dermatologists to categorize all people including those with pigmented skin. This system developed by Fitzpatrick, is based on the reaction or vulnerability of various skin types to sunlight and ultraviolet (UV) radiation and it correlates skin color with its ability to respond to UV light with burning or tanning (2,3). This classification was at the beginning used to categorize white skin. Therefore, all individuals with pigmented skin were initially classified as skin type V (4). Obviously pigmented skin includes greater color gradations and subsequently pigmented skin was divided into three subgroups: types IV to VI. These skin types rarely or never burn after sun exposure and tan readily and include subjects of many racial or ethnic backgrounds (African Americans, Caribbean Americans, and Hispanic Americans).

SPS has numerous lacks. For instance, skin photo type (SPT) has been used to predict the minimal erythema dose (MED) and may be irrelevant to people with pigmented skin. On this purpose, it has been demonstrated that in some individuals with pigmented skin there is often no relationship between constitutive skin color, skin phototype, and MED. Young et al. proved this for Korean subjects where a weak relationship between skin type and MED has been shown. In this study, skin types varied between II and V rather than only V. Furthermore, MED values ranged from 50 to 90 mJ/cm^2, whereas the skin phototypes would suggest values ranging from 25 to 90 mJ/cm^2 (5,6).

Leenuthapong showed that individuals from Thailand include photo-types II to V and that constitutive skin color does not correspond well to the Fitzpatrick classification system in the older age group. Furthermore, there is also a great variation in MED values as well as an overlap in values between different skin types (7).

Normal human skin color can be classified either as constitutive pigmentation or facultative pigmentation. Constitutive skin color is defined as the basal or genetically determined color in the absence of any external factor such as sunlight.

Constitutive pigmentation has been regarded classically as the color of the buttock skin. Facultative skin color is associated with exposure to sunlight and denotes the pigmentation of exposed skin (8).

Skin pigmentation is known to show considerable age- and sex-related changes throughout life. A recent study showed that pigmentation of sun-exposed sites increases with age and that the difference in pigmentation levels between sun-exposed sites and protected sites may indicate the degree of lifetime sun exposure in white Caucasians (9,10).

ETHNIC DIFFERENCES IN BIOLOGY OF MELANIN

The intrinsic color differences between individuals are primarily determined by the presence of biological pigments in the skin. It is generally accepted that variations in the packaging and distribution of epidermal melanin accounts for most of the ethnic variation in human skin color (11). It has been established that there are no racial differences in the number of melanocytes. It has been shown that melanocyte numbers in the skin vary considerably between different body sites; for instance, the head and forearm have the highest number (12). In this regard, an assessment of melanocyte numbers in related sites in Negroid and Caucasian subjects revealed no significant differences between these two ethnic groups (13).

Racial and ethnic differences in skin color are due to variation in the number, size, and aggregation of melanosomes within melanocytes and keratinocytes (14). Racial or ethnic differences in the size and aggregation of melanosomes within keratinocytes have been demonstrated (15). In 1969, Szabo et al. analyzed melanosome distribution in Caucasoids, Mongoloids, and Negroids. Melanosomes of Caucasian subjects were grouped or aggregated together within a surrounding membrane. The melanosomes of the Mongoloid subjects were grouped in aggregates but there was a more compact configuration compared with those of the Caucasoid subjects. In contrast, melanosomes of Negroid subjects were not aggregated but individually dispersed (16).

More recently, Olson et al. demonstrated that different groupings of melanosomes correlated with the lightness or darkness of the individual subject's skin color. In fact, dark-skinned black subjects had nonaggregated large melanosomes, whereas light-skinned black subjects had both large nonaggregated and smaller aggregated melanosomes. Melanosome groupings were affected by sun exposure. Asian skin exposed to sunlight had a predominance of nonaggregated melanosomes, whereas the unexposed skin had predominantly aggregated melanosomes. Dark-skinned white subjects with sunlight-exposed skin had nonaggregated melanosomes, whereas light-skinned white subjects with no sun exposure had aggregated melanosomes (17).

In the last 10 years, it has been confirmed by many authors that the observed ethnic differences in epidermal melanin content are due to differences in melanin production which appear to arise from a constitutively higher level of tyrosinase activity in melanocytes from darker skin types. Thus, tyrosinase protein levels do not appear to vary with ethnicity nor is there any real evidence to suggest that polymorphisms in the tyrosinase gene are responsible for this variation in activity (18).

One recent suggestion is that high tyrosinase activity is due in Negroid melanocytes to a high melanosomal pH in contrast to light Caucasian melanocytes where melanosomes have an acidic pH which effectively suppresses tyrosinase activity (19).

Another possibility is that the activity of tyrosinase is regulated by other melanosomal membrane proteins which act in various ways to maintain its function (20). One candidate is the P protein, a 110 kDa 12 membrane spanning melanosomal membrane proteins which has a high-sequence homology with various membrane anion transporters (19). At present, however, the exact function of the P protein in human melanocytes is still unclear. It has been suggested that it probably acts to stabilize the high molecular weight complex of proteins in the melanosome membrane that includes tyrosinase, tyrosinase-related protein 1, and dopachrome tautomerase (20). Finally, more recently it has been proposed that P protein regulates melanosomal pH and may also be involved in trafficking of proteins to the membrane during melanosome biogenesis and assembly. Polymorphisms in human P gene have been identified (21). Those polymorphisms have been identified with differing frequency in different ethnic groups (21). The functional significance of such mutations and whether they are involved in regulating normal pigment variation between ethnic groups still remains unknown.

FUNCTION OF MELANOSOMES AND MELANIN

Epidermal content of melanin, packaging and distribution of melanosomes can impact on photoprotection. Many studies have demonstrated that melanin confers protection from UV light (22).

In 1968, Mitchell observed that the Australoid subjects with non-aggregated, large melanosomes were protected from UV light-induced skin malignancies. On the other hand, Australian and European subjects had a high incidence of skin cancer (23).

Olson et al. demonstrated a racial differential in the MED. Individuals with darkly pigmented black skin had an average MED 15 to 33 times greater than that of individuals with white skin (17).

Although melanin confers a protection from UV radiation, Kotrajaras and Klingman reported that pigmented skin can also experience significant photodamage, manifested by epidermal atypia and atrophy, dermal collagen and elastin damage, and marked hyperpigmentation (24).

RACIAL DIFFERENCES IN SKIN CANCER INCIDENCE

DNA damage induced by UV radiation is a critical primary event in skin photocarcinogenesis. Constitutive skin pigmentation dramatically affects the incidence of skin cancer, and photoprotective function of melanin in the skin is highly significant (25).

The incidence of skin cancer among people with pigmented skin is relatively low. In white subjects either chronic or episodic high-intensity exposures are thought to be a major etiologic factor in the development of basal cell carcinoma, squamous cell carcinoma, and melanoma (26).

The melanin content and melanosomal dispersion pattern in people with phototype V and VI is thought to be responsible for providing protection from the carcinogenic effects of UV radiation (27).

The development of melanoma is inversely correlated with the degree of pigmentation of skin that is exposed to the sun. In white subjects it has been found that there is an increased susceptibility to melanoma compared with Hispanic, Asian, and black subjects.

In Hispanic, Asian, and black subjects, melanoma arises more often on nonsun-exposed sites with less pigment such as the palms, soles, and subungueal areas while in white subjects, melanoma occurs primarily on sun exposed or intermittently sun-exposed skin. When individuals with pigmented skin give rise to melanoma, they are more likely to develop an acral lentiginous melanoma (28).

Tadokoro et al. in 2003 first reported observations on the effects of melanin on UV responses in different racial groups. They compared levels of DNA damage and their removal as well as melanin content in the skin of human subjects representing six ethnic origins and different phototypes and

UV sensitivities. Their observations highlighted that DNA damage in all subjects was greater immediately following UV exposure and was gradually repaired thereafter. Furthermore, although DNA damage was more severe in the light skin, UV-sensitive skin types, even the darkest, developed significant DNA damage (25).

RACIAL DIFFERENCES IN PHOTOAGING

People with dark skin usually "photoage better" than those with light skin. Individuals with black skin are thought to evidence firmer and smoother skin than individuals with lighter skin at the same age. Furthermore, the melanin content and melanosomal dispersion pattern is thought to confer protection from the accelerated aging induced by exposure to UV radiation.

Photoaging among black subjects does occur but it is more common in individuals with relatively fair skin and also photoaging tends to occur at a later age in black subjects than in white subjects.

Inconsistent pigmentation (hypopigmentation or hyperpigmentation) is a sign of photoaging in people with pigmented skin. These findings are consistent with the study conducted by Klingman et al. on Asian women with an average skin phototype of IV. Signs of photoaging including epidermal atrophy, cell atypia, and poor polarity and disorder differentiation have been observed. In conclusion, deeply or darkly pigmented skin can still experience photodamage as evidenced by pigmentation disorders and other signs of epidermal and dermal damage (29,24).

REFERENCES

1. Coon CS. The Origin of Races. New York: Alfred A. Knopf, 1962.
2. Fitzpatrick TB. The validity and practicality of sun reactive skin type I through IV. Arch Dermatol 1988; 124:869–871.
3. Pathak MA, Nghiem P, Fitzpatrick TB. Acute and chronic effects of the sun. In: Freedberg IM, Eisen AZ, Wolff K, et al., eds. Fitzpatrick's Dermatology in General Medicine, Vol. 1. New York: McGraw-Hill, 1999:1598–1608.
4. Pathak MA, Fitzpatrick TB. Preventive treatment of sunburn, dermatoheliosis and skin cancer with sun protective agents. In: Freedberg IM, Eisen AZ, Wolff K, et al., eds. Fitzpatrick's Dermatology in General Medicine, Vol. 1. New York: McGraw-Hill, 1999:2742–2746.
5. Youn JI, Oh JK, Kim BK, et al. Relationship between skin phototype and MED in Korean, brown skin. Photodermatol Photoimmunol 1997; 13:208–211.
6. Roh KY, Kim D, Ha SJ, Ro YJ, Kim JW, Lee HJ. Pigmentation in Koreans: study of the differences from Caucasian in age, gender and seasonal variation. Br J Dermatol 2001; 144:94–99.
7. Leenutaphong V. Relationship between skin and cutaneous response to UV radiation in Thai. Photodermatol Photoimmunol 1995; 11:198–203.

8. Lock-Andersen J, Wulf HC. Seasonal variation of skin pigmentation. Acta Derm Venereol 1997; 77:185–194.

9. Lock-Andersen J, Knudstorp ND, Wulf HC. Facultative skin pigmentation in Caucasians: an objective biological indicator of lifetime exposure to ultraviolet radiation? Br J Dermatol 1998; 138:826–832.

10. Lock-Andersen J, Drzewiecki KT, Wulf HC. The measurement of constitutive and facultative skin pigmentation and estimation of sun exposure in Caucasians with basal cell carcinoma and cutaneous malignant melanoma. Br J Dermatol 1998; 139:610–617.

11. Jimbow K, Quevedo WC, Fitzpatrick TB, Szabo G. Some aspects of melanin biology. J Invest Dermatol 1976; 67:72–89.

12. Toda K, Pathak MA, Parrish A, Fitzpatrick TB. Alteration of racial differences in melanosome distribution in human epidermis after exposure to ultraviolet light. Nat New Biol 1972; 236:143–144.

13. Staricco RJ, Pinkus H. Quantitative and qualitative data on the pigment cells of adult human epidermis. J Invest Dermatol 1957; 28:33–45.

14. Rawles ME. Origin of melanophores and their role in development of color patterns in vertebrates. Physiol Res 1948; 28:383.

15. Montagna W, Carlisle K. The architecture of black and white facial skin. J Am Acad Dermatol 1991; 24:927–929.

16. Szabo G, Gerald AB, Pathak MA, Fitzpatrick TB. Racial differences in the fate of melanosomes in human epidermis. Nature 1969; 222:1081–1082.

17. Olson RL, Gaylor J, Everett MA. Skin color, melanin, and erythema. Arch Dermatol 1973; 108:541–544.

18. Iwata M, Corn T, Iwata S, Everett MA, Fuller BB. The relationship between tyrosinase activity and skin colour in human foreskin. J Invest Dermatol 1990; 95:9–15.

19. Fuller BB, Spaulding DT, Smith DR. Regulation of the catalytic activity of pre-exisiting tyrosinase in black and caucasian human melanocyte and cell cultures. Exp Cell Res 2001; 262:197–208.

20. Puri N, Gardner JM, Brilliant MH. Aberrant pH of melanosomes in pinkeyed dilution (p) mutant melanocytes. J Invest Dermatol 2000; 115:607–613.

21. Brilliant MH. The mouse p(pink-eyed dilution) and human P genes, oculo-cutaneous albinism type 2 (OCA2) and melanosomal pH. Pigm Cell Res 2001; 14:86–93.

22. Kaidbey KH, Agin PP, Sayre RM, Kligman A. Photoprotection by melanin—a comparison of black and Caucasian skin. J Am Acad Dermatol 1979; 1: 249–260.

23. Mitchell R. The skin of Australian arborigines: a light and electron microscopi-cal study. Australas J Dermatol 1968; 9:314.

24. Kotrajaras R, Klingman AM. The effect of topical tretinoin on photodamaged facial skin: Thai experience. Br J Dermatol 1993; 129:302–309.

25. Tadokoro T, Kobayashi NM, Zmudzka BZ, et al. UV induced DNA damage and melanin content in human skin differing in racial ethnic origin. FASEB J 2003; 17:1177–1179.

26. Taberi DP, Narukar V, Moy RL. Skin cancer. In: Johnson BL, Moy RL, White GM, eds. Ethnic Skin: Medical and Surgical. St. Louis, Missouri: Mosby, 1998.

Photore

27. Crombie IK. Racial differences in melanoma incidence. Br J Cancer 1979; 40:185.
28. Cress RD, Holly EA. Incidence of cutaneous melanoma among non Hispanic whites, Hispanics, Asians and blacks: an analysis of California Cancer Registry data; 1988–93. Cancer Causes Control 1997; 8:246–252.
29. Halder RM. The role of retinoids in the management of cutaneous conditions in Blacks. J Am Acad Dermatol 1998; 39:S98–S103.

5

Hair Anthropology

Leszek J. Wolfram, E. Dika, and Howard I. Maibach
Department of Dermatology, University of California at San Francisco School of Medicine, San Francisco, California, U.S.A.

INTRODUCTION

The hair, the skin color, together with other phenotypic traits have long been used as criteria to divide man into racial groups. Linaeus, a botanist, classified the human race by skin color into *Europaeus albus*, *Afer niger*, *Asiaticus luridus*, and *Americanus rutus* (1). Blumenback later divided mankind into five groups: Caucasian (white), Mongolian (yellow/white), Malayan (brown), Ethiopian (black), and American (red). Blumenback noted also that there were so many intermediate gradations in skin color, body habitus, and so forth that the differences between all races appeared of little consequence (2).

Anthropologists today largely discard classifications based on skin color, but they do accept Coon's classification based on geographic origin (Table 1) (3).

These days most of them believe that adaptive phenotypes in different human populations do not imply that the traits are in fact of genetic origin and thereby "racial" (4).

Racial variation is developed through natural selection processes; different biologic traits in the races developed because these traits facilitated adaptation to a particular environment.

Changes in international demographics lead to less differences among populations. Furthermore, variation between individual members of a racial

Table 1 Classification of Modern Races

Caucasoid	Europeans, Ainus from North Japan, the Middle East, North Africa, India
Mongoloid	East Asians, Indonesians, Polynesians, Micronesians, Amerindians, Eskimos
Australoid	Australian Aborigens, Melanesians, Papuans, Tribal Indians, Negritos
Congoid	Negros Pygmies of Africa
Capoid	African bushmen, Hottentots

Source: From Refs. 2 and 3.

or ethnic group may at times assume greater importance than inter-racial variation in its impact on health and disease.

Hence, phenotypic differences between human beings exist.

Categorizing hair types into three major groups—African, Asian, and Caucasian—makes it easier to recognize characteristics specific to each hair type. In this chapter, curliness, color, and cross-section parameters of ethnic hair and its pathological presentations will be discussed.

SCALP HAIR

All hair regardless of its ethnic origins exhibits common characteristics of morphology, chemical composition, and molecular structure. This section of the review is intended to provide a summary of the salient elements of hair structure and chemistry, and their fundamental interplay that contributes to the properties of the hair fiber and its unique response to external stimuli.

Hair follicles, tens of thousands of which are deeply invaginated in the scalp tissue, are the essential growth structures of hair. At the base of each follicle cells proliferate and as they stream upwards, they undergo profound and progressive biochemical change, transforming soft cytoplasm into hard and fibrous material known as hair.

Human head hair grows steadily, approximately 1 cm per month and continuously for three years (anagen phase) before entering a brief, transient stage (catagen) and a two months resting stage (telogen) during which the old hair is shed. With the onset of the new anagen phase the hair regrows from the same follicle. At the growth cycles are asynchronous between the various follicles, hairs are not shed simultaneously, as they are in many animals. At any given time some hairs are growing, some resting, and some being shed—a process facilitated by brushing, combing, or washing. The number of hairs growing on human scalp averages 100,000 and thus a daily count of 100 or so of shed hairs is expected. Occasionally, however, inordinately large number of hairs may enter synchronously the telogen phase,

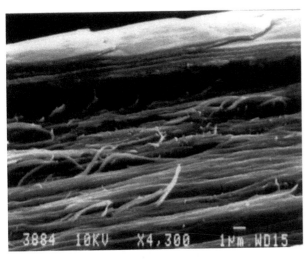

Figure 1   Scanning electron micrograph of longitudinal hair section.

resulting in significant hair loss (telogen effluvium). The occurrence of the latter can be diagnostically assessed by a trichogram test, which measures the anagen/telogen ratio in plucked hairs. Witzel and Braun-Falco (5) found that in healthy scalps the anagen/telogen ratios for men and women yield the values of 5.53 and 7.73, respectively. Significant downtrend from these values might be indicative of physiological disorder of the hair follicles.

Scalp hair is typically 50–80 μm in diameter and its exterior consists of a layer of flat, imbricated cuticle cells pointing out from root to tip. Enveloped by the overlapping cuticle sheath is the fibrous hair cortex that constitutes the bulk of the fiber (Fig. 1). During the process of keratinization, the plasma membranes of cortical cells are modified and form a strongly adhesive layer between the adjacent cells. This is the only continuous phase in the fiber that fuses the cortical cells and provides adhesion between the cortex and the surrounding cuticles. Dispersed throughout the structure of the cortex are the melanin pigment particles. Their number, chemical characteristics, and distribution pattern determine the color of hair. In many (but not all) hairs, vacuolated medulla cells are present in the central region of the fiber.

The Cuticle

Within the follicle, the hair cuticles originate as a single cell layer. The cells flatten as they ascend the follicle and in the fully keratinized hair they are in the form of square sheets 0.5 μm thick and 50 μm in length. Their proximal portions are firmly attached to the cortex and the distal edges protrude towards the tip of the fiber (Fig. 2). Extensive overlapping of the cells

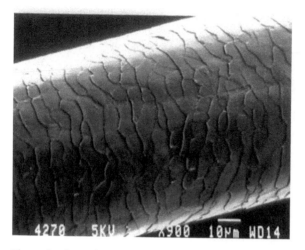

Figure 2 Scanning electron micrograph of the hair surface.

(up to 5/6 of their length) and a slight tilt away from the fiber axis give the hair surface a ratchet-like appearance. These imbrications are highly functional. By interlocking with the pointing downward cuticles of the inner root sheath, they contribute to the follicular anchorage of the growing hair. Pulling out a hair "by its roots" results in tearing away at the inner root sheath and brings about dislodgement of individual cells, which then coil on themselves (Fig. 3). The imbricated surface also serves as a self-cleansing feature. As the hairs grow and move relative to each other, the outward

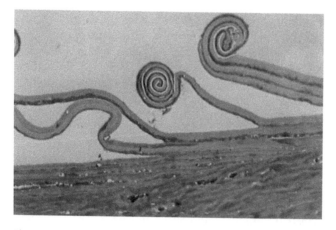

Figure 3 Transmission electron micrograph of the longitudinal section of hair that was pulled out of the follicle.

pointing cuticular edges facilitate removal of trapped dirt particles and desquamating scalp cells. In the course of the process of maturation and keratinization, a stratified, lamellar structure develops within each cuticle cell. The outer surface of each cell is enveloped by a continuous membrane termed epicuticle. A thin lipid film of 18-methyleicosanoic acid is grafted onto the epicuticle providing the hair surface with the attributes of low friction and hydrophobicity. Below the epicuticle lies the major component of the cuticle cell—exocuticle. The proteins of the exocuticle are densely cross-linked by disulfide bonds of cystine. In contrast, the abutting, lower layer of endocuticle is poor in cystine, highly water swellable, and mechanically weak. It is noteworthy how well the cuticle sheath is adapted to meet the environmental challenge. A water-repellent surface facilitates drying of hair and the cuticular imbrications keep the fibers and scalp clean. The tough exocuticle provides a measure of protection against physical assaults, while soft endocuticle cushions impacts. It is worth pointing out that examination of hair cross-sections suggests concentric multilayer cuticular bands surrounding the fiber. This is only a perception created by the extensive overlap of single cuticle cells. Also, as the thickness of the cuticles is invariant with the hair diameter, it follows that the cuticle/cortex ratio will increase with the decreasing diameter of the fiber.

The Cortex

This morphologically dominant and mechanically most important component of hair is made up of elongated, interdigitated, spindle-like cells approximately 100 μm long and 5 μm across the maximum width. The cells are fused tightly and oriented parallel to the axis of the fiber. Each cell is packed with fine, axially oriented filaments (microfibrils) that consist of highly organized helical proteins responsible for the diagnostic X-ray diffraction pattern of α-keratins. The microfibrils are grouped into larger assemblies termed macrofibrils. By using specific staining techniques of electron microscopy, the structural resolution of these fibrillar assemblies has been attained. The results indicate that each macrofibril represents a structural composite consisting of rods of microfibrils embedded in cystine-rich matrix (Fig. 4). There are some variations in the packing mode within the macrofibrils and in the macrofibrillar arrangements within the cortical cells. Two different packing dispositions have been designated as paracortex and orthocortex, their structural differences having been demonstrated (6) by both electron microscopy and Methylene Blue staining technique (optical microscopy). Thus, the crimp in Merino wool is caused by the asymmetric distribution of the para- and orthocortex along the fiber length, with the para component always on the inside of the crimp and the ortho on the outside. There have been suggestions (7) that a similar bilateral distribution of the ortho and para cells might be responsible for curliness of

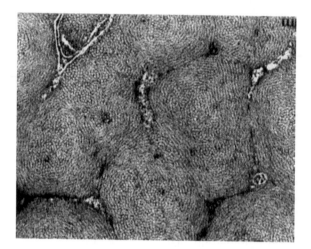

Figure 4 Transmission electron micrograph of hair microfibrils.

human hair. Methylene Blue staining of curly albino African hair by one of the authors (L.J.W.) revealed no such bilateral disposition.

Chemical Composition

The bulk of hair is proteinaceous in nature with the structural lipids and mineral residues representing only a minor fraction. The amino acid make-up of the hair is given in Table 2, which summarizes the results of amino acid analyses of human hair that have appeared over the past 30 years. Viewed from the perspective of biological variability, dietary habits, sampling techniques, environmental effects, and diversity of texture, it is remarkable how uniformly the data cut across ethnic groups. Although there is considerable variation within each set of data, the ranges overlap and there are no obvious contrasts between hairs of different ethnicity. The macromolecular structure of keratin fibers derives its stability from a variety of interchain and intrachain interactions that hold the protein chains together. The interactions range from covalent bonds to weaker interactions, such as hydrogen bonds, coulombic interactions (salt links), van der Waals forces, and (in presence of water) hydrophobic bonds. Although relatively weak and readily broken by water, the hydrogen bonds are the most numerous (approx. 4.6 mM/g) and are essential elements in α-helical conformation. Central to the stability of keratin is the disulfide bond of cystine, which displays both a high degree of inertness and selective reactivity. It is the latter that has been the key to solubilization of keratin, laying the groundwork for the resolution of its molecular structure. Two major fractions of the solubilized keratin have been isolated: one of low sulfur content and high molecular weight and the other with high sulfur content and low

Table 2 Ranges of Amino Acid Composition of Human Hair of Various Racial Origin–(μM/g)

Amino acid	African	Brown Caucasian	Oriental
Alanine	370–509	345–475	370–415
Arginine	482–540	466–534	492–510
Aspartic acid	436–452	407–455	456–500
Cysteic acid	10–30	22–58	35–41
Cystine	1310–1420	1268–1608	1175–1357
Glutamic acid	915–1017	868–1053	1026–1082
Glycine	467–542	450–544	454–498
Histidine	60–85	56–70	57–63
Isoleucine	224–282	188–255	205–244
Leucine	484–573	442–558	515–546
Lysine	198–236	178–220	182–196
Methionine	6–42	8–54	21–37
Phenylalanine	139–181	124–150	129–143
Proline	642–697	588–753	615–683
Serine	672–1130	851–1076	986–1101
Threonine	580–618	542–654	568–593
Tyrosine	179–202	126–194	131–170
Valine	442–573	405–542	421–493

Source: From Refs. 8–11.

molecular weight. The low sulfur proteins yielded a keratin diffraction pattern that was not found in the sulfur-rich fractions. The differences in the chemical composition and physical characters of the proteins were major factors in assigning them as integral elements of the filament/matrix structure put forward by Birbeck and Mercer (12). Thus, the low sulfur, high molecular weight helical proteins form the backbone of filaments, whereas the high sulfur proteins with no defined crystallographic orientation form the matrix. Two general approaches to solubilization have been developed. One relies on the reductive cleavage of disulfide bonds, the other on their oxidative fission. On the whole, the fractionation of the solubilized keratin into component fractions yields similar results. The oxidatively solubilized proteins have been termed α, β, and γ keratoses originating from helical (low sulfur), membrane-derived, and high sulfur proteins, respectively. Table 3 summarizes the fractionation results of oxidatively solubilized hair of different ethnic origin. Clearly, the fractionation pattern is very similar with no indication of significant differences in the filament and matrix texture between the hair types.

High-pressure differential scanning calorimetry has been widely employed to evaluate and monitor the structural integrity of keratin fibers (13,14). The fibers are exposed in a closed system and in presence of

Table 3 Keratose Fractions of Solubilized Hair (wt %)

Keratin	Keratose (%)		
	α	β	γ
Caucasian hair	43	15	33
African hair	43	15	33
Oriental hair	42	14	34
Merino wool	56	10	25

water to a progressive rise in temperature, and the denaturation enthalpy (related to thermal stability of helical component-fibrils) as well as the denaturation temperature (functionality of matrix proteins) are evaluated. In a recent high-pressure differential scanning calorimetry study, samples of Caucasian, Oriental, and African American hair have been evaluated in such a manner (15). The results collated in Table 4 suggest that there is little difference, if any, between the fibers. The data complement quite well those obtained from fractionation experiments, thus augmenting a view that the fundamental structural integrity of hair is race-invariant.

Physical Properties

Hair appearance provides instantly a recognition of the interplay of diverse physical parameters. The obvious attributes, such as hair geometry, color, luster, etc., intertwine with the spatial arrangement of fiber arrays and yield a judgment on aesthetics of appearance.

There has been a tendency to group the physical attributes of hair into two general categories. The first one deals with the properties that are material specific, such as hair shape, color, fiber diameter, tensile strength, friction, etc. The other focuses on characteristics of hair assemblies and entails their response to combing, styling, wetting, etc. Although the intrinsic properties of single fibers are likely to have a dominant role in the behavior of hair assemblies, the latter by the sheer multiplicity of hair-to-hair contacts can significantly modulate such behavior.

Table 4 Denaturation Enthalpies and Temperatures for Hair Samples of Different Ethnic Origins

Hair type	Denaturation temperature (°C)	Denaturation enthalpy
Oriental	150.1	19.2
Caucasian	153.5	21.2
African	153.0	19.5

Hair Geometry

Apart from its color, the shape of hair is the most obvious appearance characteristic. The shape of hairs varies from perfectly straight, and via incremental increase in curvature and its spatial disposition, to tight helical coils and kinks. In terms of uniformity of geometry, the Asian hair is almost invariably straight whereas the African hair is invariably curly. The Caucasian hair is the least uniform in this respect, displaying variation of geometrical form from straight to wavy. Overall, both the straight Oriental hair and the curly African hair seem to be dominant over either curly or straight Caucasian hair.

The cause for hair curliness has long been debated and hypotheses linking it either to the cross-sectional parameters (16) or to para–ortho cortex disposition (12) within the hair shaft have been advanced. Examining the follicular biopsies of African Americans, Price and Wofram noticed their curly shape but followed the matter no further. Recent studies by Lindelof et al. (17) and Barnard (18) left little doubt that the shape of hair was inherent in the hair follicle. Thus, straight follicle delivers straight hair and curly or helical follicles produce the curly hair.

The external shape of hair is only one aspect of hair geometry. The others are the fiber thickness and cross-sectional parameters. Because the hair fibers are seldom round, the descriptor of "hair diameter" is somewhat misleading unless accompanied by information of fiber ellipticity. Table 5 lists the results of such combined measurements obtained on Caucasian, Asian, and African American hair (15). The fibers clipped closely to the scalp were donated by individuals (20 in each case) and were measured at 65% relative humidity. The "equivalent diameter" descriptor d was calculated from or $d = (A \times B)^{1/2}$, where A stands for the long axis of hair cross-section and B stands for the short axis. The "ellipticity" (E) determined from $E = A/B$ is now widely used in fiber metrics, replacing the older term "index." The trait that distinguishes the African hair fiber from others is not only the high ellipticity factor but also its broad range, particularly when compared with highly uniform Asian hair. This may be caused by twists that are frequently observed along the length of the fiber.

Table 5 Cross-Sectional Parameters of Hair

Hair type	Ellipticity (range)	Equivalent diameter (μm)	
		Range	Mean
Caucasian	1.43–1.56	67–78	72
Asian	1.21–1.36	69–86	77
African	1.67–2.01	54–85	66

Hair Color

Variation in skin and hair color between different ethnicities is a striking human characteristic.

The color of intact hair is derived mainly from the secretory products of melanocytes. These products consist of a range of melanin pigments having different structures and composition. The two most important and chemically distinct classes of melanin are eumelanin (black pigment) and pheomelanin (red pigment). The relative production of these two types, at least in the mouse, is controlled by the extension (E) locus and agouti (A) locus that regulate the relative amount of these two forms of melanin. The locus E encodes the MC1 receptors and the A locus encodes the agouti peptide that is an antagonist at the MC1 receptor. The significance of these agouti and MC1 receptors in pigmentation was initially found in mice, but has now been shown to have similar role in other mammals like cattle, fox, horses, pigs, sheep, and dogs. The role of agouti in man is, however, at least in terms of pigmentation, not fully understood. It shows a high degree of polymorphism (19). More than 40 different alleles of the human MC1 receptor have been identified. Particular variants of MCR1 receptor gene, such as Arg 151Cys, Arg 160Trp, Asp 294His, have been associated with red hair, fair skin, and inability to tan; some authors found that the frequency of these alleles is also higher, as expected, in persons with melanoma or other forms of skin tumor.

There is also substantial evidence suggesting that all pigments are biogenetically related, arising from a common metabolic pathway in which dopaquinone is the key intermediate. A link between eumelanin and pheomelanin accounting for the possibility of intermeshing of pigmentary pathways has been suggested by Prota (20). In terms of hair color, such intermeshing could possibly account for the warm tones seen frequently in brown hair. Figure 5, which displays spectral reflectance curves of black (Oriental), brown, and red hair, illustrates this point. The brown hair shows spectral characteristics that appear intermediate to the fully eumelanic (black) and fully pheomelanic (red) fibers.

The pigmentary activity of the hair bulb differs markedly from that of the superficial epidermis. Thus, in white Caucasians black hair may grow on almost colorless skin, and in the process of hair graying the melanocytes of the hair follicle may cease to function, whereas those of surrounding epidermis retain their ability to produce melanin. It is noteworthy that the hair bulb melanocytes are able to synthesize melanin only in the anagen stage of hair growth.

All pigmented hair lightens when exposed to sunlight, the effect being particularly noticeable at low latitudes and high humidity environments. The mechanism of this photobleaching process involves interaction of melanin with molecular oxygen to generate highly reactive species such as superoxide anion O_2^-, which dismutates in the presence of moisture to yield hydrogen

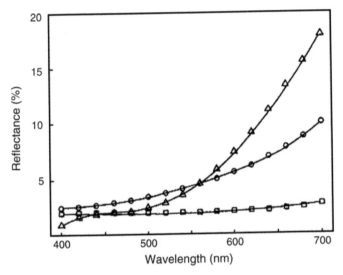

Figure 5 Reflectance spectra of natural red (Δ), brown (O), and black (□) hair.

peroxide that is the active bleaching agent (21). It is noteworthy that eumelanic hair lightens much more than hair with pheomelanin pigment, a phenomenon related most probably to resistance of the latter to oxidative degradation.

Mechanical Properties

All animal fibers with α-keratin structure developed as an outer covering to protect animals during exposure to a wide range of environmental conditions. Such fibers are pliable, and resilient, and recover from repeated mechanical deformations with little loss of their physical properties. Human scalp hair displays all these valuable characteristics. A layer of overlapping cuticle cells lessens the effects of external impacts, whereas the fibrous cortex contributes to mechanical stability. In the area of fiber evaluation, tensile measurements play an important role by providing information not only of the strength and extensibility of hair but also of the molecular mechanism involved in such mechanical deformations. This testing mode is relatively well comprehended by the public, for whom fiber strength is tantamount to its "wellness."

The tensile properties are a function of the integrity of the corticular structure in general and of the filament matrix composite in particular. The high sensitivity of the composite to moisture underscores the necessity of making measurements under well-controlled conditions of humidity. Also, any imperfections of the hair structure, whether innate or environmentally induced, are likely to affect the results.

Table 6 presents compilation of results of tensile testing on Caucasian, Asian, and African hair conducted at different laboratories. The "strength" values are presented in term of "stress" that accounts for the varying diameters of the tested hair, thus making the results directly comparable. The obvious discrepancies are striking. Although the tensile properties of the Asian and Caucasian hair are comparable and matched by two samples of African hair, the other two are considerably weaker and more brittle. This raises an important question: Which samples are truly representative of the African hair or are all samples representative of some population segments? Note that although testing of Oriental and Caucasian hair is carried out on both the commercial samples and the hair provided by the donors, the results are comparable. The supply of commercial Afro hair is very limited, which forces the researchers to sample the hair from individuals. Although care is taken to ensure "harvesting" the hair with no cosmetic "history" this cannot be always verified, as the latter is rich and widespread in the case of African hair. In testing such hair, one of the authors (L.J.W.) has often encountered fibers with an axial twist resulting in narrow segments. Such segments proved to be weak points, and, on extension, fibers broke invariably in those locations.

It seems appropriate at this point to bring up the issue of hair care practices and associated with them often the problem of hair damage. The demand for hair aesthetics is universal and cuts across all ethnic barriers. Significant numbers of people are clearly dissatisfied with the hair they grow and want to change its appearance. Not surprisingly, the straight hair is waved, the curls are straightened, the color is modulated or gotten rid of altogether. While some changes can be accomplished simply by styling, others require chemical modification of hair that causes significant alteration of the original structure. On the whole, the hair tolerance to most of such modifications is high, and when carried out judiciously they do not lead to hair breakage, although they leave the hair more sensitive to daily rituals such as washing and brushing. Unfortunately, the African hair, due to its tight curliness, requires somewhat more drastic approaches to styling than any other hair type. Whether it is alkaline relaxing or repeated hot combing, it leaves the hair more fragile and requires of the consumer the utmost of care to maintain its healthy appearance. Even when intact, the African hair demonstrates its potential for breakage. Let us consider such a simple daily practice as combing. Pulling a comb through the hair separates the hair strands, a process that generates some resistance that can be readily measured. Fig. 6 is a depiction of comparative effort to comb a tress of straight (Caucasian or Oriental) and curly African hair. The comb tresses were identical in weight and length. Not only is the African hair more difficult to comb (by factor of 10) but also its combing pattern is qualitatively different. In the case of straight hair, the engagement of the comb causes some parallelism of individual hair strands and results in

Table 6 Mechanical Properties of Hair[a]

Hair type	Breaking stress (MPa)								Breaking extension (%)							
	Dry (65% RH)				In H$_2$O				Dry (65% RH)				In H$_2$O			
	A	B	C	D	A	B	C	D	A	B	C	D	A	B	C	D
Caucasian	188	178	184	180	165	155	162	–	44	46	49	38	62	49	61	–
Asian	190	185	–	–	158	165	–	–	46	47	–	–	62	48	–	–
African	191	180	148	112	156	160	94	–	42	41	39	29	54	48	42	–

[a] A, B, C, and D denote different locations where the tests were conducted.

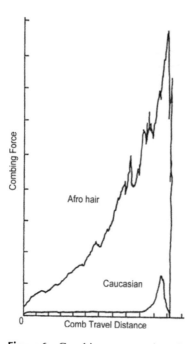

Figure 6 Graphic representation of work required to comb African and Caucasian hair.

a clear pathway ahead of the teeth of the comb. Thus, the comb moves through the hair mass with relatively little effort; it is only at the tip of the tress that the resistance of a multitude of individual hair crossovers has to be overcome and the combing force sharply increases. On the contrary, insertion of comb into highly curved African hair does not induce hair parallelism and thus creates no clear pathway. The engagement and motion of the comb lead to a displacement and intensification of individual curl entanglements, which are reflected in an immediate and progressive rise in the combing force. The curly geometry of African hair has an interesting consequence in the case of wet combing. Unlike straight hair, which is more difficult to comb wet than dry, wet combing of African hair is easier than dry combing (22).

HAIR DENSITY

Few studies have been developed in order to quantify the normal hair density among humans, and even fewer studies in comparing the ethnic differences (23). A retrospective study performed by Sperling (24), analyzing 4 mm punch biopsy specimens taken from 22 African Americans and 12 Caucasian patients showed that the hair density is significantly lower in African Americans than in age-matched Caucasians. Caucasian subjects had an average of 35.5 total hairs including 30.4 terminal hairs per 4 mm biopsy versus 21.4 total hair follicles including 18.4 terminal follicles in

African American subjects (24). Bernstein and Rassman, while reporting on hair transplants, noted that the scalp follicular density in African Americans is lower than in Caucasians, 1.6 versus 2.0 hairs/mm^2, a ratio of 4:5 (25).

Loussouarn, in 2001, analyzed the literature data about hair growth, and hair density in Africans. A phototrichogram technique was used in a hair area of 1 cm^2. They compared the differences of hair density between men and women of their population with unpublished data obtained in a Caucasian population. The population size, gender, distribution, and age were comparable (26). They showed a lower hair density in African subjects and a much lower growth rate, confirming the preceding studies.

BODY AND FACIAL HAIR

Human genital hairs, in Caucasians, are usually lighter than scalp hairs and have a reddish tint. Axillary hairs are also reddish when compared with scalp hairs. A brown-haired individual's beard is often lighter than the scalp hairs.

Hair color darkens with age. This phenomenon is predominant in blond, red, and light-brown-haired people, and it takes place between the ages of 13 and 20 years. Hormonal factors have been evoked. Graying is an obvious sign of aging at 34 ± 8 years in Caucasians (27).

General observations suggest the natural levels of pilosity in different races, where it seems that mongoloids such as the Chinese and Japanese have very little body hair and Northern Europeans have more. Groups termed Euro-Americans were compared with East Asians by Ewing, confirming this generalization in both genders. Sex-matched androgen estimations were the same, and consistent with an end-organ difference (28).

Even when different ethnic groups have the same underlying diagnosis, their levels of hirsutism may differ. Only one out of nine Japanese with polycystic ovarian syndrome had hirsutism compared with 63% of Northern Europeans with the same diagnosis. When 25 Japanese women with polycystic ovarian syndrome were compared with 25 Italian and 25 Hispanic American women with the same disease, the Japanese were significantly less hirsute and less obese (29–32).

Afro-Caribbeans are usually considered to have less body hair than Northern Europeans; however, a detailed study reveals little information. A report from the U.S. Health Examination Survey commented that Afro-Caribbeans developed secondary sexual hair earlier than their white counterparts but no comparison of hair distribution was made (33).

When facial hair was examined in adult white and black Americans, no difference was found until the age of 40 years (34). At that point, the hair on the face of white Americans continued to increase, whereas that on black Americans leveled off.

Comparison between Europeans were made in demobilized soldiers after World War I. Current statistical methods and ethnic categories were not used at that time and the result allowed the observation that "Russian Jews" and those from "Italian provinces" had a high proportion of men considered of high pilosity, compared with "English and German protestants" (35).

Pathologies and Ethnic Hair

Hair loss is a common problem that challenges the patient and clinician with a host of cosmetic, psychological, and medical issues. Alopecia occurs in both men and women and in all racial and ethnic populations, but the etiology varies considerably from group to group. There are no large-scale studies in the literature that compare the incidence of different alopecias among ethnic groups. However, it is widely reported that in African people, many forms of alopecia are associated with hair-care practices (e.g., traction alopecia, trichorrhexis nodosa, and central centrifugal cicatricial alopecia) (36,37). The use of thermal or chemical hair straightening, and hair braiding or weaving are examples of styling techniques that place African Americans at high risk for various "traumatic" alopecias. Halder reported alopecias as the fifth most common dermatoses in African Americans, with chemical and traction alopecia cited as the predominant types (38). There are no recent epidemiologic data addressing the true incidence of alopecia in black people. Although the exact cause of these alopecias is unknown, a multifactorial etiology including both genetic and environmental factors is suspected. A careful history and physical examination, together with an acute sensitivity to the patient's perceptions (e.g., self-esteem and social problems), are critical in determining the best therapy course. Therapeutic options for these patients range from alteration of current hair grooming practices or products, to use of specific medical treatments, to hair replacement surgery (39,40).

ACQUIRED TRICHORRHEXIS NODOSA

One of the most common, identifiable forms of hair-shaft damage is acquired trichorrhexis nodosa. Easily broken hairs upon minimal manipulation of the hair shaft typify this condition clinically. For instance, a pull test may cause a significant number of hairs to break off mid-shaft. Macroscopically, these hair shafts may contain small white nodes at irregular intervals. Microscopically, these nodes often produce a bristle-like projection that becomes the site of hair-shaft breakage. Although some patients with this condition have an underlying congenital weakness of the hair shaft related to keratin formation (e.g., argininosuccinic aciduria), trichorrhexis nodosa is more commonly acquired, and results from physical or chemical trauma. Excessive brushing, "stressed" hairstyles (e.g., braids), heat application, and scratching associated with seborrheic dermatitis can all contribute to the damage, as can manipulations involving shampooing, perming, and straightening. Presumably, the decreased tensile strength of chemically treated hair in African Americans, heat exposure, and other drying agents play a role in the development of breakage. The involved hairs often break a few centimeters from the scalp in areas stressed by combing, braiding, or sleeping (41).

TRACTION FOLLICULITIS AND TRACTION ALOPECIA

Traction folliculitis occurs primarily in children. Clinically, it is characterized by erythema and scaling, papules, or pustules. It is imperative that tinea capitis first be ruled out by fungal culture. Cultures of pustules seen with uncomplicated traction folliculitis have consistently yielded no growth or normal bacterial flora (42). The hair dressing used or other factors may play a role in the development of folliculitis (43).

In traction alopecia related to braids or ponytails, hair loss usually occurs in the temporal areas anterior and superior to the ears, but the frontal and occipital areas are occasionally affected. If the traction is continued long term, a permanent cicatricial alopecia may develop; this appears to require three to five years to develop and is usually evident by early adolescence in children so affected. Frontal and temporal alopecia that appears in adulthood occurs almost exclusively from hair rollers. One will usually see rather dense growth of intermediate hairs at the periphery and sparse vellus hair in the center of the affected areas. Sponge rollers are the worst offenders. Biopsy of areas of traction alopecia in the early stages generally reveals a subacute perifollicular inflammation with occasional overlying parakeratosis. Long-standing cases show a normal overlying epidermis but absent or very sparse small follicles (44).

Traction alopecia can be prevented. All health care professionals and cosmeticians need to be aware of this condition and must educate the parent or individuals grooming the affected person's hair not to pull it so tight; loosely wrapping the hair on the rollers and/or using paper wrappers with sponge rollers will decrease the traction.

Even if traction alopecia is obvious, however, topical minoxidil in 1% to 2% concentration has caused some improvement in a few patients.

Earles (45) has used hair transplants and rotational flaps to correct traction alopecia surgically, but the scarring associated with the latter procedure in particular may be unacceptable. If superinfection is suspected, as evidence by crusting and inflammation, a 10-day course of systemic antibiotics directed at pathogenic *Staphylococci* is recommended.

SEBORRHEIC DERMATITIS

Seborrheic dermatitis may be aggravated by some of the ingredients in hair products that are commonly used by African Americans. Lanolin is by far the one ingredient most likely to aggravate the condition, but soybean oil, wheat germ oil, lecithin, castor oil, petrolatum, and squalene may also cause problems. In many cases, simply avoiding products with these ingredients will alleviate the problem. Moisturizers that generally can be used without problems in patients with seborrheic dermatitis include glycerine and propylene glycol for natural styles or curls, and white petrolatum, jojoba oil, or some of the simpler pomade formulations for hot-pressed or chemically relaxed hair.

Because daily shampooing is too drying for African American hair or too impractical for most African American females with hot-pressed hair, African Americans with seborrheic dermatitis can reasonably only be asked to shampoo once a week.

CENTRAL CENTRIFUGAL CICATRICIAL ALOPECIA

Clinically, central centrifugal cicatricial alopecia is characterized by a well-defined area of hair loss over the top of the head. There is obvious loss of follicular orifices on clinical inspection of involved areas, with clusters of hair generally scattered in the area of scarring alopecia. The hair loss can be profound and nearly total in the involved area. Polytrichia is mentioned as a feature of this condition, but this finding may be a more common natural occurrence in African Americans than is generally recognized.

The predilection for the top of the head in central centrifugal cicatricial alopecia has not been explained. This condition includes that formerly termed "hot comb alopecia"; in that condition, the localization of hair loss has been hypothesized to be secondary to the petrolatum running down the hair shaft and onto the scalp (46,47). On the sides and back of the head, the petrolatum would tend to run down toward the scalp margins where the hair shafts are extended horizontally away from the scalp.

However, the direct causal relationship of this clinical condition and hot combs has been questioned. Sperling and Sau (46) described a similar clinical scarring alopecia in African American women who had not used, or infrequently use, hot combs and thus proposed the term follicular degeneration syndrome to replace the term hot comb alopecia. In their study, they noted that the earliest observable histologic abnormality present in all patients was premature degeneration of the inner root sheath of certain follicles scattered amid histologically normal hairs. They also noted a cicatricial alopecia on the crown of the scalp of African American men who had no history of prior use of chemical or physical modalities to straighten or style the hair, and with similar histologic findings to that seen in affected women.

At a recent conference on cicatricial alopecia, a working classification of the various permanent and destructive types of alopecia was proposed (48).

The term central centrifugal cicatricial alopecia was chosen to describe this condition of central scarring hair loss in African Americans; it is clinically distinct in its well-developed stages, poorly recognized in its very early stages, and without a definitively proven relationship to hair care products. Histologically, biopsies of affected scalp are usually diagnosed by histopathologists as "pseudopelade," although this condition is very distinct clinically from pseudopelade of Brocq.

PSEUDOFOLLICULITIS BARBAE AND FOLLICULITIS BARBAE

Pseudofolliculitis barbae consists clinically of perifollicular and follicular papules and papulopustules in shaved areas of those people with inherently kinky or curly hair.

The culprit is the curved follicle and consequently the curved hair shaft, which grows back into the skin surface or pierces the follicular wall when the hair is cut very short.

Severe scarring may result. Shaving is the usual precipitating stimulus of the condition, and pseudofolliculitis barbae has been noted in 45% to 83% of black men secondary to societal standards for a clean-shaven face (38).

Extrafollicular penetration occurs when the hair shaft completes an arc with the sharp-pointed cut hair tip invaginating the epidermis 1 to 2 mm from the follicular opening as it grows back toward the skin. Transfollicular penetration occurs when the skin is pulled taut prior to shaving, causing the pointed tip to retract under the skin as tension is released. This can also occur with electrolysis or when hairs are plucked with tweezers and break off short within the follicle (48).

It may create a marked inflammatory response and a foreign body-type reaction. The extrafollicular form of pseudofolliculitis barbae is the more difficult of the two to manage. Growing a beard is the only certain cure, but many men with this condition feel that they must conform to the practice of being clean shaven, especially in certain professions (members of military services, etc.).

For those individuals who can tolerate them, depilatories are highly effective in controlling pseudofolliculitis barbae. In general, depilatory lotions act more slowly than pastes and creams but are less irritating and can be used more often (49).

Electrolysis or laser hair removal are particularly useful in women with pseudofolliculitis barbae (50), while eflornithine cream is a potential therapeutic aid. Recently a treatment with topical glycolic acid has also been evaluated (51).

FOLLICULITIS KELOIDALIS

Originally described in 1869 by Kaposi, and also termed acne keloidalis or dermatitis capillitii, folliculitis keloidalis is a chronic inflammatory and potentially scarring process that occurs primarily over the posterior neck and scalp, mainly in African American men. The lesions are usually distributed in areas where a razor or liner is used to shape the hairline, thus causing folliculitis and pseudofolliculitis in susceptible individuals. The early soft papules become firmer with time, and susceptible individuals can form keloidal papules and plaques. With the close-cut hair styles currently preferred by young African American men, there has been an increase in the incidence of these problems (52).

Histologically, early papules represent terminal hairs engulfed in a mixed inflammatory infiltrate at the infundibulum and midisthmus levels, which later develop into a chronic granulomatous infiltrate in the lower follicle. Sebaceous gland atrophy is present, as well as a mixed plasma cell–lympocytic perivascular infiltrate. With time, the smoldering granulomatous inflammation leads to scar formation (53).

In order for any treatment of folliculitis keloidalis to be effective, one must avoid all the predisposing factors that can lead to follicular damage. Patients should be advised not to allow their necks to be lined with either a razor or a liner; the hair should be left at least 2 or 3 mm above the skin surface.

Where active folliculitis exists, a topical or systemic antibiotic is required. Tetracycline 0.5 to 1 g, doxycycline 100 to 200 mg, minocycline 100 mg, and erythromycin 0.5 to 1 g per day have been effective. Topical erythromycin, clindamycin, and mupirocin have also been proved to be effective in milder cases.

The therapy may be continued as long as the problem persists (53).

DISSECTING CELLULITIS (PERIFOLLICULITIS CAPITIS ABSCENDENS ET SUFFODIENS)

Managing patients with dissecting cellulitis effectively is difficult. The etiology has not been delineated, but the condition is considered to be a part of the follicular occlusion triad that also includes acne conglobata and hidroadenitis suppurativa. All three of these conditions may exist at the same time in susceptible individuals and are most common in African American males (54). Dissecting cellulitis is characterized by multiple large abscesses, chronic draining sinuses, follicular occlusion, and cicatricial alopecia. Hypertrophic scars and, at times, keloids may develop. Lesions often coalesce to form massive carbuncles. Cultures are usually negative or grow out normal bacterial flora or *Staphylococcus aureus*. In recent years, most of the cultures prepared by the author have grown out coagulase-negative *Staphylococcus* organisms (54).

Systemic antibiotics, systemic corticosteroids, and extensive surgical removal have all been used in the past with varying degrees of success (55). Oral isotretinoin has been reported to be effective (56). Other therapies, such as oral zinc therapy, have been reported (57).

REFERENCES

1. Ehrlich PR, Raven PH. Differentiation of population. Science 1969; 165: 1228–1232.
2. Coon CS. The Origin of Races. New York: Alfred A. Knopf, 1962.

3. Coon CS, Garn SM, Birdsell JB. Races: a Study of the Problems of Race Formation in Man. Springfield, IL: Charles C Thomas, 1950.
4. Molnar S. Races, Types, and Ethnic Groups: the Problem of Human Variation. Englewood Cliffs. NJ: Prentice-Hall, Inc., 1975.
5. Witzel M, Braun-Falco O. The hair follicle status of the human scalp under physiological conditions. Arch Klin Exp Dermatol 1963; 216:221.
6. Horio M, Kondo T. Crimping of wool fibres. Text Res J 1953; 23:373.
7. Swift JA. Fundamentals of Hair Science. Weymouth, Dorset, U.K.: Micelle Press, 1998.
8. Somonds DH. The Amino acid composition of keratins. Parts V: a comparison of the chemical composition of merino wools of differing crimp with that of other animal fibers text. Res J 1958; 28:314.
9. Menkart J, Wolfram LJ, Mao I. Caucasian hair, Negro hair and wool: similarities and differences. J Soc Cosmet Chem 1966; 17:769.
10. Robbins C, Kelly C. Amino acid analysis of cosmetically altered hair. J Soc Cosmet Chem 1969; 20:555.
11. Wolfram LJ, Lindermann KO. Some observations on the hair cuticle. J Soc Cosmet Chem 1971; 22:839.
12. Birbeck MS, Mercer EH. The electron microscopy of the human hair follicle. Introduction and the hair cortex. J Biophys Biochem Cytol 1957; 3:203.
13. Spei M, Holzen R. Thermoanalytical investigation of keratin. Colloid Polym Sci 1987; 265:96.
14. Wortmann F-J, Deutz H. Characterizing keratins using HPDSC. J Appl Polym Sci 1993; 48:13.
15. Quadflieg J. Fundamental properties of African hair. PhD dissertation at DWI, Aachen, Germany, 2004.
16. Dawber RPR, Messenger AG. Hair follicle structure and the physical properties of hair. In: Dawber RPR, ed. Diseases of the Hair and Scalp. Oxford, U.K.: Blackwell Science, 1997:23.
17. Lindelof B, Forslind B, Hedblad M-A, Kavius U. Human hair form. Arch Dermatol 1988; 124:1359.
18. Bernard B. Hair shape of curly hair. J Am Acad Dermatol 2003; 48:S120.
19. Rees JL. Genetics of hair and skin color. Annu Rev Genet 2003; 37:67–90.
20. Prota G. Recent advances in the chemistry of melanogenesis in mammals. J Invest Dermatol 1980; 75:122.
21. Wolfram LJ, Albrecht L. Chemical- and photo-bleaching of brown and red hair. J Soc Cosmet Chem 1987; 38:179.
22. Epps J, Wolfram LJ. Characterization of black hair. J Soc Cosmet Chem 1983; 34:213.
23. Maibach HI. Anthropology of hair. In: Behrman HT, ed. The Scalp in Health and Disease. St Louis, CV: Mosby Co., 1952.
24. Sperling LC. Hair density in African Americans. Arch Dermatol 1999; 135: 656–658.
25. Bernstein RM, Rassman WR. The aesthetics of follicular transplantation. Dermatol Surg 1997; 23:785–799.
26. Loussouarn G. African hair growth parameters. Br J Dermatol 2001; 145: 294–297.

27. Rook A, Dawber R. Disease of the Hair and Scalp. 2. Blackwell Scientific Publications, 1982:10–47.
28. Ewing JA, Rouse B. Hirsutism, race, and testosterone levels: comparison of East Asians and Euroamericans. Hum Biol 1978; 50:209–215.
29. Kurachi K, Mizuutami MS, Matsunato K. Plasma testosterone and urinary steroids in Japanese women with polycystic ovaries. Acta Endocrinol 1971; 68:293–302.
30. Conway GS, Honour JW, Jacobs MS. Heterogeneity of the polycystic ovary syndrome: clinical, endocrine, and ultrasound features in 556 point. Clin Endocrinol 1989; 30:459–470.
31. Carmina E, Koyama T, Chang L, Stanczyk FZ, Lobo RA. Does ethnicity influence the prevalence of adrenal hyperandrogenism and insulin resistance in polycystic ovary syndrome? Am J Obstet Gynecol 1992; 167:1807–1812.
32. Cela E, Robertson C, Rush K, Kousta E, et al. Prevalence of polycystic ovaries in women with androgenetic alopecia. Eur J Endocrinol 2003; 149:439–442.
33. Harlan WR, Harlan EA, Grillo GP. Secondary sex characteristics of girls 12–17 years of age. The U.S. Health Examination Survey. J Pediatrics 1980; 96:1074–1078.
34. Trotter M. A study of facial hair on the white and negro races. St Louis, Missouri. Washington Univ Stud Ser 1922; 9:273–279.
35. Danforth CH, Trotter M. The distribuition of hair in white subjects. Am J Phys Anthropol 1922; 5:259–265.
36. Richards MG, Oresajo OC, Halder MR. Structure and function of ethnic skin and hair. Dermatol Clin 2003; 21:595–600.
37. Wilborn SW. Disorders of hair growth in African Americans. In: Olsen AE, ed. Disorders of Hair Growth: Diagnosis and Treatment. McGraw-Hill Companies, Inc., 2003:497–517.
38. Halder RM. Pseudofolliculitis barbae and related disorders. Dermatol Clin 1988; 6(3):407–412.
39. McMicheal JA. Ethnic hair update: past and present. J Am Acad Dermatol 2003; 48:S127–S133.
40. Franbourg A, Hallegot P, Baltenneck F, Toutain C, Leroy F. Current research on ethnic hair. J Am Acad Dermatol 2003; 48:S115–S119.
41. Kamath YK, Hornby SB, Weigmann HD. Effect of chemical and humectant treatment on the mechanical and fractographic behaviour of Negroid hair. J Soc Cosmet Chem 1985; 36:39–52.
42. Wickett RR. Permanent waving and straightening of hair. Cutis 1987; 39: 496–497.
43. Cannel DW. Permanent waving and hair straightening. Clin Dermatol 1988; 6:71–82.
44. Brooks G, Burmeister F. Black hair care ingredients. Cosmet Toilet 1988; 103:93–96.
45. Earles RM. Surgical correction of traumatic alopecia marginalis or traction alopecia in black women. J Dermatol Surg Oncol 1986; 12:78–81.
46. Sperling LC, Sau P. The follicular degeneration syndrome in black patients. "Hot comb alopecia" revisited and revised. Arch Dermatol 1992; 130:763–769.
47. Olsen EA, Bergfeld WF, Cotsarelis G, Price VH, Shapiro J, et al. Summary of North American Hair Research Society (NAHRS)-sponsored workshop on cicatricial alopecia. Duke University Medical Center, February 10–11, 2001. J Am Acad Dermatol 2003; 48:103–110.

48. Strauss JS, Kligman AM. Pseudofolliculitis of the beard. Arch dermatol 1956; 74:533–542.
49. Kligman AM, Millls OH. Pseudofolliculitis of the beard and topically applied tretinoin. Arch Dermatol 1973; 107:551–552.
50. Kauver ANB. Treatment of pseudofolliculitis barbae with a pulsed infrared laser. Arch Dermatol 2000; 136:1343–1346.
51. Perricone NV. Treatment of psudofolliculitis barbae with topical glycolic acid: a report of two studies. Cutis 1993; 52:232–235.
52. Dinehart SM, Herzberg AJ, Kerns BJ, Pollack SV. Acne keloidalis: a review. J Dermatol Surg Oncol 1989; 15:642–647.
53. Kantor GR, Ratz JL, Wheeland RG. Treatment of acne keloidalis nuchae with carbon dioxide laser. J Am Acad Dermatol 1986; 14:263–267.
54. Glenn MJ, Bennett RG, Kelly AP. Acne keloidalis nuchae: treatment with excision and second-intention healing. J Am Acad Dermatol 1995; 33:243–246.
55. Moyer DG, Williams RM. Perifolliculitis capitis abscendens and suffodiens. Arch Dermatol Syphilol 1956; 73:256–263.
56. Shewach-Millet M, Fiv R, Shapiro D. Perifolliculitis capitis abscendens et suffondiens treated with isotretinoin. J Am Acad Dermatol 1986; 15:1291–1292.
57. Berne B, Venge P, Ohman S. Perifolliculitis capitis abscendens et suffondiens (Hoffman). Complete healing associated with oral zinc therapy. Arch Dermatol 1985; 121:1028–1030.

6

The Transverse Dimensions of Human Head Hair

J. Alan Swift

Department of Textiles and Paper, University of Manchester, Manchester, U.K.

INTRODUCTION

Awareness is universal that the natural external form of the hair on the head, and the average thicknesses of the individual fibers, varies between individuals and most noticeably between human races (i.e., those whose ancestors originated from distinctly separate locations around the world). Hairdressers are particularly aware of these differences and temper their approach to cutting and styling accordingly. The hair toiletries industry, in supplying over-the-counter products for use by individuals and in supplying materials specifically for use by the hairdresser, formulate ranges of products to cater to these different hair types. An underlying interest amongst scientists supporting this industry is to understand the factors controlling hair form and, in the longer term, to find out what might be done to influence them. This includes investigations of the genetic, biological, and chemical processes in the follicle that might dictate normal hair form. Studies of the mechanical behavior of individual fibers and of hair arrays are also underway, as well as investigations of toiletry products best suited to the given natural form or even, such as in styling, waving and straightening processes, to a change in overall form. Of considerable interest in many of these investigations is knowledge of the cross-sectional dimensions of individual hairs and how this might be related not only to its overall form but also to its mechanical behavior. This chapter is therefore devoted to the definition of hair "diameter," considerations on the effects of cross-sectional dimensions upon the hair's mechanical properties, and descriptions of the various methods for measuring these dimensions. Finally, lists of published cross-sectional dimensions are presented for hairs of different racial origin, and the origins of natural curliness and ellipticity of fiber section are considered.

RACE AND ETHNICITY

In this highly contentious, and often emotive, subject the distinctions in terminology and understanding have been considered at great length (1–5). The term "ethnic" relates to the characteristics of a human group having racial, religious, social, political, linguistic, and certain other traits. On the other hand, and according to common parlance, "race" singularly defines a group of people of common ancestry distinguished from others by physical characteristics such as those being considered in the present chapter. Originally each group developed in isolation by continental or geographic separation but in many of today's societies, because of racial intermarriage, it is often difficult to classify individuals. Despite this underlying problem, hair type is still one of the major characteristics by which we commonly discriminate between members of the different groups; other characteristics being color of eyes and skin, stature, etc. While race cannot be defined according to discrete genetic groupings, genetic information has been used to group individuals into clusters that do equate with ancestral geographic origin (6). Unfortunately such genetic classifications were not available when the measurements to be presented and discussed in this paper were carried out. Therefore, in the absence of suitable all-embracing classification, this author prefers to continue to use the long-established, albeit highly limited, broad divisions of racial type with descriptions of hair type as follows (7):

Mongoloid—coarse, usually black and straight-haired people originating from the Far East such as those predominantly living in, for example, Japan, China, Korea, and Thailand.

Caucasoid—finer, lighter colored and gently curly-haired people originating from Northern Europe and now also living in North America and Australasia.

Negroid—coarse, usually black and extremely curly-haired people originating from Central Africa but forming significant populations in for example the Caribbean and the United States. This type of hair is often described as being woolly in overall geometric form.

One is aware that one of the major factors discriminating between hairs of these three major types is that of overall geometric form, ranging from the straight hairs of the Mongoloid group through the slightly curly hairs of the Caucasoid group to the intensely curly hairs of the Negroid group. Given the desire of some for their natural hair form to be changed for cosmetic purposes to that of one of the other groupings, interest is in the follicular processes controlling natural curliness and how they might be modified. The genes controlling hair form remain to be identified. Perhaps, genetic manipulation one day might offer the means for effecting changes in hair form that are less drastic than the temporarily effective chemical treatments used today.

HAIR DIAMETER—SOME DEFINITIONS

In transverse section, human head hairs are for the most part elliptical in shape, with a degree of ellipticity that, as we will see later, varies according to racial origin. It is quite inappropriate to refer to each fiber, except by qualification, as being defined by a singular physical diameter. More appropriately, and with the assumption that hairs are elliptical in section, it is convenient to define each by its major and minor axial diameters, D_{maj} and D_{min}, respectively. Alternatively, one might refer to just one of the diameters and the degree of ellipticity of the fiber, $E = D_{maj}/D_{min}$. One notes in passing that the transverse cross-sectional area, A, of each hair is $\pi \cdot D_{maj} \cdot D_{min}/4$ or $\pi \cdot D_{maj}^2/4 \cdot E$ or $\pi \cdot D_{min}^2 \cdot E/4$.

A useful concept on occasions is to refer to a hair's equivalent circular diameter, D_{eq}. This is the diameter of a hypothetical equivalent fiber of circular cross-section having the same cross-sectional area as the hair in question. In passing it is worth noting for hairs of elliptical section that $D_{eq} = (D_{maj} \cdot D_{min})^{1/2}$. In this context, the author (Swift JA. 2005, unpublished data) has determined, by the mass per unit length (MPUL) method discussed later, an average D_{eq} for white British subjects of $69.45 \pm 11.24\,\mu m$ (two adjacent segments from each of 10 root-end untreated hairs from each of 10 subjects).

THE EFFECT OF A HAIR'S TRANSVERSE DIMENSIONS UPON ITS MECHANICAL BEHAVIOR

Load-extension experiments are frequently used to investigate variations in the material properties of hairs, such as those brought about by cosmetic treatment or that might occur naturally between the hairs of different racial groups. A defining material parameter is the modulus of extension. This is, for that particular part of the load-extension curve, the load per unit cross-sectional area per proportional increase in length produced by that load. To date, no significant difference has been established between the modulus of extension for different racial groups of untreated, undamaged hair. Thus, irrespective of racial origin, the intrinsic material properties of all hairs with respect to their stretching behavior are seemingly the same. For any given undamaged hair, the load to extend it (or tensile stiffness) is dependent only upon its cross-sectional area.

It is in bending (flexing) behavior where a hair's transverse dimensions have an extraordinary influence and discriminate between major racial groups (8). Interestingly, our tactile and visual perceptions of the coarseness or fineness of hair seem more likely to be influenced by the difficulty or ease with which the hair can be flexed than by its tensile mechanical behavior. Under a given set of conditions for untreated, undamaged hairs, their bulk moduli are identical. On this basis, the force (F) to flex a hair through a given distance at a given distance from a fixed fulcrum is proportional to the product of the hair's major axial diameter and the third power of its minor axial dimension, i.e.,

$$F \propto D_{maj} \cdot D_{min^3}$$

The minor axial diameter thus has a dominant influence on the hair's ability to be flexed. This means, for example, that for hairs of the same cross-sectional area, those with the greatest degree of ellipticity will flex more easily and will be perceived as being finer and softer than the others. As an aside, and given that all undamaged hairs at their root ends possess a cuticle of constant thickness (9), the cuticle is predicted to bear a very high proportion of the force to flex the fiber (10).

Using transverse hair dimension data published by Vernall in 1961 (11) for four human races, Swift (8) calculated stiffness indices based upon $D_{maj} \cdot D_{min}^3$ and showed that these were in reasonable accord with common perceptions of the head hair's textural behavior among these different races.

METHODS FOR MEASURING HAIR TRANSVERSE DIMENSIONS

Some of the instrumental approaches that have been used for measuring the transverse dimensions of human hair are listed in Table 1, together with their relative limitations and accuracies. In passing it is worth mentioning two valuable techniques used for preparing hair specimens for microscopy. One is the simple hand-held Hardy microtome (31) by which transverse sections of hair can be quickly cut with a single-edged razor blade. The other method is that of Teasdale et al. (21) and is particularly useful for preparing specimens for measurement in the scanning electron microscope. In it a bundle of hairs is threaded through a short tube of electrical "shrink-wrap" (of the type used for the insulated binding of wires together in electronic circuits). When this is gently heated, the tube shrinks and in doing so compresses the hair bundle to produce a stiff rod. Thick transverse sections can be readily cut by hand from this rod with the aid of a razor blade.

Given the recent application of the laser-scan micrometer (LSM) to the measurement task and its extraordinarily high level of accuracy, this method is specifically highlighted in the following section.

Table 1 Methods Used for Measuring the Transverse Dimensions of Human Hair

Method title	Accuracy (µm)	Notes and limitations	References
Micrometer screw gauge	3	Hair rotates between jaws and delivers only D_{min}. Mechanical distortion is a problem	Swift JA. 2005, unpublished data
LM from sections (LMS)	1	Section distortion and focus can be a problem	11–15
perpendicular projection (LMP)	1	Rotate hair on long axis to gain D_{min} and D_{maj}	14, 16–20
SEM	0.2	Measurements made by imaging the surface of conductively coated hair sections	Swift JA. 2005, unpublished data; 21–23
Vibroscope	0.5	Measure resonant frequency for transverse vibration of weighted hair of known length. Knowing mass density of hair (1.31 g/cm^3) then equation for vibration of flexible strings enables calculation of cross-sectional area and hence D_{eq}. Time consuming; not recommended	24
Laser diffraction	0.1	Hair in collimated laser beam yields diffraction intensity maxima on screen. Measure distance between first maxima either side of central axis. Fraunhofer diffraction equation enables calculation of projected fiber width. Rotation of hair gives D_{min} and D_{maj}. Accurate but not as convenient as laser-scan micrometer method. r.h. sensitive.	25–28
MPUL		Measure mass and length of hair segment. Using hair mass density, calculate D_{eq}. Works well for segments of 10 mm length and mass measured with Cahn microbalance	Swift JA. 2005, unpublished data; 29
LSM	0.1	Hair is rotated as projected width in laser beam is measured. Delivers D_{min} and D_{maj}. Supremely accurate and reproducible. Sensitive to r.h.	Swift JA. 2005, unpublished data; 30

Abbreviations: LM, light microscope; SEM, scanning electron microscope; MPUL, mass per unit length; LSM, laser-scan micrometer; LMS, light microscope sections; LMP, light microscope projection; r.h, relative humidity.

The Laser-Scan Micrometer

In 1985, Busch and Schumann (32) reported the use of an LSM for measuring the transverse dimensions of human hair. Since then the instrument, on account of its very high accuracy and versatility, has become a relatively common part of the human hair researcher's armory.

Within the typical basic LSM, such as the LSM-3105 manufactured by the Mitutoyo Company, a beam from a 1 mW visible semiconductor laser (670 nm) is reflected off a polygonal mirror rotating at constant high speed. For each presented facet of the mirror, the beam, after passing through a collimating lens, perpendicularly traverses the object to be measured at constant speed. Beyond the object, and after passing through a convergent lens, the laser beam is brought to focus on a point photoelectric detector. The projected width of an object is measured according to the accurate timing of the detector dark period during the laser traverse across the object, as against the timing for another separate object of accurately calibrated projection width (usually a wire).

The basic LSM is adapted so that a single hair, mounted perpendicular to the direction of the laser beam traverse, is rotated at constant speed. The instrument delivers a train of consecutive projection width measurements for computer input and analysis typically at a rate of 40 Hz. In the case of a hair rotated at constant speed (say 0.25 Hz), the measurements are temporally of sinusoidal form. It is a simple matter with the input of these data to a computer to detect the maxima and minima from the data train representing the D_{maj} and D_{min} values for that particular hair. Other parameters might also be calculated at the same time such as the cross-sectional area (A) of the fiber or its equivalent circular diameter (D_{eq}), based upon the elliptical assumption.

Using the Mitutoyo LSM-3105, this author found for the same hair rotated at the constant speed of 0.25 Hz, and making 100 separate measurements in quick succession, an average D_{maj} of 100.22 μm (±0.097 μm) and a corresponding D_{min} of 59.85 μm (±0.106 μm). In a further adaptation, a single hair that after removal from the instrument could be repositioned within three seconds at exactly the same point in the measuring beam, was rotated by hand. One hundred such repetitive measurements yielded an average D_{maj} of 98.62 μm (±0.213 μm) and a D_{min} of 63.15 μm (±0.080 μm). By measuring hairs before and after coating with a thin reflective layer of silver, the author also established that the correct projected diameters of hairs were obtained irrespective of their underlying color in the range from blonde to jet black. These experiments attested to the very high accuracy of the LSM approach and its potential for evaluating the effects of a range of experimental treatments on a hair's transverse dimensions. Furthermore, the instrument is well placed for assessing the transverse dimension of head hairs of a range of racial origins, but as yet the scientific community awaits publication of an exhaustive study in this area.

Errors of the Elliptical Assumption

It is clear when one examines cross-sections of hairs in the microscope that, while the majority appear to be elliptical in form, a small proportion (variable but in the region of 5%) are kidney shaped, i.e. they possess perimeters that are not everywhere of convex form. In such cases where only the two diameter measures, D_{maj} and D_{min}, are used for calculating cross-sectional area according to the analytical equation for the ellipse in which the area is $\pi/4 \cdot D_{maj} \cdot D_{min}$, unknown but potentially significant errors might be introduced. Under such circumstances, and where absolute accuracy might be essential, it would be necessary to use one of the other methods listed here (such as MPUL or sections under the microscope). The LSM offers some potential for assessing the extent to which each given hair is analytically elliptical in form. For this the fiber should be rotated at a slow enough constant speed as to obtain the order of say 100 consecutive measurements of projected diameter for each 360° of rotation. An alternative fiber cross-sectional area is obtained for each complete revolution as the sum of the areas of all the triangular elements subtending 360/100° at the center of the fiber. This is then compared with the area defined by $\pi/4 \cdot D_{maj} \cdot D_{min}$ derived from the same data set. The author is not aware of any definitive publications reporting tests of the elliptical assumption by this approach.

PUBLISHED INFORMATION OF THE TRANSVERSE DIMENSIONS OF HAIRS BY RACE

Table 2 contains a selection of transverse measurements of human head hairs made by various authors. In it the designation of race was taken from the original publications. For completion, and where the type of measurement has permitted this to be done, the author has used the basic data to provide additional information. Thus, corresponding values were calculated for the equivalent circular diameter, D_{eq} (noting in passing that this is directly proportional to the cross-sectional area of each fiber). A bending stiffness parameter was also calculated on the basis of $D_{maj} \cdot D_{min}^{3} \cdot 10^{-7}$. To the extent that a wide variety of methods have been used, some caution is necessary in making comparisons of D_{maj} and D_{min} measurements between authors. On the other hand, the axial ratios D_{maj}/D_{min}, which are of our particular interest, will make possible valid comparisons between authors. It is unfortunate that authors of the primary date presented in Table 2 have not carried out measurements of the corresponding degrees of curliness of the hairs. Despite this, our common knowledge of the different racial groups listed leads us to a good assessment of the likely levels of curliness of the hairs, with extremes between subjects of African origin and those from Far Eastern countries such as Japan.

Table 2 Transverse Measurements of Human Head Hairs by Various Authors and Methods

Authors	Method type	Race type[a]	D_{maj}[b] (μm)	D_{min}[b] (μm)	Nhair[c]	Npeop[d]	D_{eq}[b,e] (μm)	D_{maj}/D_{min}[e]	Stiff[f]
Steggerda and Seibert (15)	LMS	Maya	79.93 (15.9)	64.90 (11.0)	986	10	72.02	1.23	2.18
		Hopi	83.70 (20.7)	65.31 (13.0)	617	10	73.94	1.28	2.33
		Navajo	78.76 (19.4)	61.95 (13.4)	1002	10	69.85	1.27	1.87
		Zuni	84.33 (21.7)	62.81 (12.6)	643	10	72.78	1.34	2.09
		Dutch	63.93 (16.1)	47.28 (9.6)	858	10	54.98	1.35	0.68
		Negro	90.62 (20.6)	51.7 (11.7)	873	10	68.45	1.75	1.25
Vernall (11)	LMS	Chinese	94.28 (8.57)	76.79 (7.15)	580	20	86.06	1.28	4.27
		Western European	81.94 (7.81)	56.74 (5.73)	609	21	69.42	1.44	1.50
		Asiatic Indian	92.94 (7.28)	66.49 (6.50)	754	26	79.74	1.40	2.73
Keis et al. (30)	LSM	Negroid	98.23 (7.58)	58.52 (6.63)	551	19	76.93	1.69	1.97
		Piedmont	88.56	65.12	25	1	75.94	1.36	2.45
		L. brown European	83.48	57.18	25	1	69.09	1.46	1.56
		D. brown European	99.15	65.22	25	1	80.42	1.52	2.75
		Indian	101.77	70.68	25	1	84.81	1.44	3.59
		Japanese	112.43	84.53	25	1	91.94	1.33	6.79
		Chinese	84.89	73.18	25	1	78.82	1.16	3.33
		African American	81.91	64.75	25	1	81.91	1.60	2.22

Study	Method	Ethnicity							
Hess and Seegmiller (12)	LMS	Caucasian	—	—	50	1	44.84	—	—
Tolygesi et al. (18)	LMP	Caucasian	110.8 (11.0)	67.8 (23.8)	12	2	86.7	1.60	3.45
		Chinese	106.4 (18.3)	82.8 (10.2)	12	2	93.86	1.30	6.04
		Negro	118.8 (15.2)	66.1 (15.1)	12	2	88.6	1.90	3.43
Teasdale et al. (23)	SEM	European	84.5 (10.8)	55.4 (6.2)	1605	20	68.42, (69.6)[g]	1.54	1.44
		Japanese	103.1 (14.0)	76.8 (8.8)	886	10	88.75, (89.8)[g]	1.36	4.67
Syed et al. (33)	LMP	Caucasian	83.14 (8.16)	64.52 (2.34)	10	>1	73.24	1.29	2.23
		African American	98.89 (11.66)	54.10 (5.20)	10	>1	73.14	1.83	1.56
Kamath et al. (34)	—	Caucasian	—	—	—	—	—	1.17	—
		Negroid	—	—	—	—	—	1.90	—
Menkart et al. (35)	—	Caucasian	—	—	—	—	—	1.41	—
		Negro	—	—	—	—	—	1.78	—
Franbourg et al. (36)	LSM	Caucasian	80 (1)	60 (1)	11	1?	69.3	1.32	1.73
		Asian	86 (1)	70 (1)	4	1?	77.6	1.22	2.95
		African	98 (2)	55 (1)	14	1?	73.4	1.75	1.63
Wolfram (37)	—	Caucasian	88.18[h]	58.79[h]	—	20	72h	1.43–1.56	1.79
		Asian	87.29	67.93	—	20	77	1.21–1.36	2.81
		African	89.52	48.66	—	20	66	1.67–2.01	1.03

(Continued)

Table 2 Transverse Measurements of Human Head Hairs by Various Authors and Methods (*Continued*)

Authors	Method type	Race type[a]	D_{maj}[b] (µm)	D_{min}[b] (µm)	Nhair[c]	Npeop[d]	D_{eq}[b,e] (µm)	D_{maj}/D_{min}[e]	Stiff[f]
Trotter and Duggins (14)	LM	White	77.18[i],	50.12[i],	100,	16,	62.2[i];	1.54[i];	0.97,
		American children	80.38[j]	52.88[j]	100	16	65.2[j]	1.52[j]	1.19
Swift (2005, unpublished data)	LSM	European	84.50	57.37	1400	140	69.58	1.49	1.59
		Mongoloid	98.31	75.49	500	50	86.15	1.30	4.23
		African	109.65	63.10	150	15	83.18	1.74	2.75
	MPUL	White British	—	—	200	10	69.45	—	—

[a] Race type as given in the original publication.
[b] Figures in parenthesis are standard deviations.
[c] Total number of hairs considered.
[d] Total number of subjects.
[e] In some cases calculated by the author from the D_{maj} and D_{min} data.
[f] Bending stiffness calculated on the basis of $D_{maj} \times D_{min}^3 \times 10^{-7}$.
[g] Calculated from cross-sectional area measurements.
[h] D_{maj}, D_{min} and bending stiffness calculated on the basis that mean ellipticity was at middle of the range.
[i] Measured from sections.
[j] Measured by fiber rotation.
Abbreviations: LM, light microscope; LSM, laser-scan micrometer; MPUL, mass per unit length; SEM, scanning electron microscope; LMS, light microscope sections; LMP, light microscope projection.

An inescapable conclusion from the accumulated information in Table 2, which confirms earlier individual studies (38), is that the eccentricity of hair cross-sectional shape (D_{maj}/D_{min}) is for the most part directly related to the degrees of hair natural curliness of the different racial groups. Thus, we find eccentricities of greater than 1.6 firmly associated with curly haired Afro subjects and of less than about 1.3 being mainly associated with the stick-straight hair of peoples from the Far East. Races with hairs of intermediate levels of curliness tend to be found between these two extremes of eccentricity. The theoretical index of bending stiffness presented in the last column of Table 2 shows a very wide range of values spanning almost one order of magnitude. Despite the larger major axial diameters occurring mainly among the hairs of Afro groups, these tend to have bending stiffnesses of intermediate values, by far the greatest stiffness being reserved for the Far Eastern groups (consistent with common tactile and visual perceptions). This reinforces earlier statements (8) of the extraordinary influence of a hair's minor axial diameter upon its flexural rigidity.

It is unfortunate that the information provided in Table 2 lacks the comprehensiveness for other useful relationships to be eked out. For future studies of a similar kind, the exclusive use of the LSM is highly recommended and corresponding measurements of curliness be made. The hair must be carefully cleaned and measurements ought to be carried out at a standard level of relative humidity and temperature. Also to be considered are the possibility of variations in diameter along the hair's length (13,16,17), the age and sex of each subject (13), and their nutritional status (19,20). An additional requirement for experimental consistency would be information above the particular sites on the scalp from which the hairs were derived.

THE ORIGINS OF HAIR CURLINESS AND OF THE CURLINESS/ELLIPTICITY RELATIONSHIP

It is of considerable interest to know why a firm direct relationship would seem to exist between the amount of natural curliness of a hair and the degree of eccentricity of its transverse section. It is often argued that hairs are curly because they are formed within a longitudinally curved follicle, but this in itself does not necessarily argue for ellipticity of the fiber section. There can be little doubt that mitosis within the matrix cells of the follicle provides the pressure for propelling the cells of the forming hair towards the skin surface within the constraints of the surrounding structures. The hair proper is formed within the constraining influence of the early hardening cells of the inner root sheath that acts as a mold within which the final fiber is shaped. Some believe that mitotic pressure is asymmetrically distributed in this early contact with the hardened sheath and that this causes the follicle to become curved. Indeed, in this respect, Bernard (39) has observed an intrinsic asymmetry of cellular differentiation in the hair follicle. On the other hand, at the stage before the cells destined to become the final hair have hardened, hydraulically there would be an equalization of pressure across the transverse section at this point. It may be that the constraint offered by the inner root sheath is asymmetrically distributed and that the cross-section becomes distorted. On the other hand, for a hair of elliptical section to develop would require the strength of the inner root sheath to be systematically weaker in the direction of the major elliptic axis than in the minor elliptic axis and that seems most unlikely. Thus, this line of thought argues neither for the development of ellipticity nor for curliness.

A possibility to be considered is that both ellipticity and curvature arise from a unidirectional lateral force being applied to the hardened inner root sheath. An interesting analogy here is that of a garden watering hose. Under the application of a unidirectional transverse force of increasing magnitude the hose not only becomes increasingly curved but its initial circular section also becomes increasingly elliptical. A similar process applied to the follicular sheaths would thus provide for the final hardening of the hair shaft to be longitudinally curled and with ellipticity of section. The origin of such a lateral force remains a matter of speculation but could arise from the activity of the arrector pili muscle.

REFERENCES

1. Jones CP. Race, racism and the practice of epidemiology. Am J Epidemiol 2001; 154:299.
2. Kaplin JB, Bennett T. Use of race and ethnicity in biomedical publication. J Am Med Assoc 2003; 289:2709.
3. Kaufman JS, Cooper RS. Considerations for use of racial/ethnic classification in etiologic research. Am J Epidemiol 2001; 154:291.
4. McKenzie K, Crowcroft NS. Describing race, ethnicity and culture in medical research. Br Med J 1996; 312:1054.
5. Senior PA, Bhopal R. Ethnicity as a variable in epidemiological research. Br Med J 1994; 309:327.
6. Bamshad MJ, Olsen SE. Does race exist? Sci Am 2003; 289:50.
7. Trotter M. A review of the classification of hair. Am J Phys Anthropol 1938; 24:105.
8. Swift JA. Some simple theoretical considerations on the bending stiffness of human hair. Int J Cosmet Sci 1995; 17:245.
9. Wolfram LJ, Lindemann MKO. Some observations on the hair cuticle. J Soc Cosmet Chem 1971; 22:839.
10. Swift JA. The cuticle controls bending stiffness of hair. J Cosmet Sci 2000; 51:37.
11. Vernall DG. A study of the size and shape of cross-sections of hair from four races of man. Am J Phys Anthropol 1961; 19:345.
12. Hess WM, Seegmiller RE. Computerised analysis of resin-embedded hair. Trans Am Microsc Soc 1988; 107:421.

13. Seibert HC, Steggerda M. The size and shape of human head hair along its length. J Hered 1942; 33:302.
14. Trotter M, Duggins OH. Age changes in head hair from birth to maturity. Am J Phys Anthropol 1948; 6:489.
15. Steggerda M, Seibert HC. Size and shape of head hair from six racial groups. J Hered 1941; 32:315.
16. Hutchinson PE, Thompson JR. The cross-sectional size and shape of human terminal scalp hair. Br J Dermatol 1997; 136:159.
17. Jackson D, Church RE, Ebling FJ. Hair diameter in female baldness. Br J Dermatol 1972; 87:361.
18. Tolygesi E, Coble DW, Fang FS, et al. A comparative study of beard and scalp hair. J Soc Cosmet Chem 1983; 34:361.
19. Vandiviere HM, Dale TA, Driess RB, et al. Hair shaft diameter as an index of protein-calorie malnutrition. Arch Environ Health 1971; 23:61.
20. Sims RT. The measurement of hair growth as an index of protein synthesis in malnutrition. Br J Nutr 1968; 22:229.
21. Teasdale D, Philippen H, Blankenburg G. Cross-sectional parameters of human hair. Part 1. Principles and measurement methods. Ärzt Kosmetol 1981; 11:161.
22. Teasdale D, Schlüter R, Blankenburg G. Cross-sectional parameters of human hair. Part 2. Application of the methods and statistical analysis. Ärzt Kosmetol 1981; 11:252.
23. Teasdale D, Philippen H, Schlüter R, et al. Cross-sectional parameters of human hair. Part 3. Measurements of European and Japanese hair types. Ärzt Kosmetol 1982; 12:425.
24. Montgomery DJ, Milloway WT. The vibroscopic method for determination of fibre cross-sectional area. Textile Res J 1952; 22:729.
25. Li C-T, Tietz JV. Improved accuracy of the laser diffraction technique for diameter measurement of small fibres. J Mater Sci 1990; 25:4694.
26. Curry SM, Schawlow AL. Measuring the diameter of a hair by diffraction. Am J Phys 1974; 45:412.
27. Macdonald J, O'Leary SV. Measuring the diameter of a hair with a steel rule. Am J Phys 1994; 62:763.
28. Burras E, Fookson A, Breuer M. Precise measurement of humidity effects on human scalp hair diameter. In: Orfanos CE, Montagna W, Stüttgen E, eds. Hair Research. Berlin: Springer Verlag, 1981:634.
29. Scala J, Hollies NRS, Sucher KP. Effect of daily gelatine ingestion on human scalp hair. Nutr Rep Int 1976; 13:579.
30. Keis K, Ramaprasad KR, Kamath YK. Studies on light scattering from ethnic hair fibres. J Cosmet Sci 2004; 55:49.
31. Hardy JI. A Practical Laboratory Method of Thin Cross Sections of Fibers. In: Circular 378. Washington, D.C.: U.S. Dept. Agric., 1935.
32. Busch P, Schumann H. Automated and computerised studies of the dimensions and tensile properties of human hair. Ärtz Kosmetol 1985; 15:347.
33. Syed AN, Kuhadja A, Ayoub H, et al. African American hair; its physical properties and differences relative to Caucasian hair. In: Hair Care: Cosmetics and Toiletries. Illinois: Carol Stream, 1996:37.

34. Kamath YK, Hornby SB, Weigmann H-D. Effect of chemical and humectant treatments on the mechanical and fractographic behaviour of Negroid hair. J Soc Cosmet Chem 1985; 36:39.
35. Menkart J, Wolfram LJ, Mao I. Caucasian hair, Negro hair and wool: similarities and differences. J Soc Cosmet Chem 1966; 17:769.
36. Franbourg A, Hallegot P, Ballenneck F, Leroy F. Current research on ethnic hair. J Am Acad Dermatol 2003; 48:S115.
37. Wolfram LJ. Human hair: a unique physicochemical composite. J Am Acad Dermatol 2003; 48:S106.
38. Hayashi S, Okumura T, Ishida A. Preliminary study on racial difference in scalp hair. In: Kobari T, Montagna W, eds. Biology and Disease of the Hair. Baltimore, Maryland: University Park Press, 1975:555.
39. Bernard BA. Hair shape of curly hair. J Am Acad Dermatol 2003; 48:S120.

7

Influence of Ethnic Origin of Hair on Water-Keratin Interaction

Alain Franbourg
L'Oréal Recherche, Centre Charles Zviak, Clichy, France

Frédéric Leroy
L'Oréal Recherche, Aulnay, France

Marielle Escoubés
Laboratoires des Biomatériaux et Polymères, CNRS-Lyon, Lyon, France

Jean-Luc Lévêque
L'Oréal Recherche, Centre Charles Zviak, Clichy, France

INTRODUCTION

There have been many published studies of the equilibrium between water vapor and keratin. Many of these studies concern the kinetics of thermodynamic equilibrium, the quantities of water bound at equilibrium, and the energy of interaction of water molecules at keratin-binding sites. Based on the studies, different states of binding of the molecule with keratin have been described: at very low relative humidity (partial water vapor pressure <0.2), the water molecules penetrate the structure, thanks to their strong polarity and small size, and they bind with high energy of absorption to COO^- and NH^{3+} sites. At higher humidity levels, the water binds to the peptide group and condenses with itself (1).

The mobility of molecules, or of the proteins plasticized by water, has also been extensively studied using spectroscopic methods: nuclear magnetic resonance, IR (2–4) and dielectric relaxation methods (5,6). By studying mechanical properties as a function of time after change in the water equilibrium, it was possible to analyze the distribution of water in the amorphous and crystalline zones of hair keratin (7). The effects of hydration on the molecular structure of keratin have also been studied using X-ray diffraction (8).

The equilibrium between liquid water and keratin fibers has been the subject of far fewer studies. These studies using gravimetric methods (determination of absorption) or methods to measure diametral swelling demonstrated the role of the reduction level (cystin/cystein ratio) on the degree of swelling and that of "sensitization" of fibers (e.g., oxidation in an alkaline medium) on the kinetics of swelling (9).

Such studies were conducted more often in wool fibers and occasionally on hair from Caucasian subjects (in most cases) or Asian subjects. The case of African and of African American hair does not appear to have been investigated, despite the known difficulties in their cosmetic management and especially the problem of the breakage of fibers during combing (10). Broadly speaking, the importance of hydration to all properties of keratin fibers has been very extensively documented.

The present study deals specifically with the influence of the ethnic origin of hair (Caucasian, African American, or Asian) on hydration parameters in the vapor phase and in water. This question has not as yet been systematically studied, although a lower degree of hydration of African American hair has been described by one author (11).

MATERIALS AND METHODS

Hair Samples

Hairs were taken at the root from three different subjects of each ethnic origin. The hairs underwent no treatment modifying the chemical and/or physical structure of the keratin present. The hair samples were taken wet after applying a shampoo and then dried at 60°C for 10 minutes. Before any measurements were made, the lock of hair was washed a second time with a standard shampoo.

Water Vapor Sorption Analysis

Measurements were made using equipment already described (12), comprising a controlled microbalance and microcalorimeter thermostatically maintained at a constant temperature (22°C) and connected symmetrically to a standard sorption/desorption apparatus. The Setaram B92 microbalance was used to record variations in the mass of the sample by means of an electromagnetic system with automatic resetting (sensitivity: 1 μg). The thermocouple located in the differential isotherm microcalorimeter was used to measure the difference in temperature between the sample and the reference standard during all thermal phenomena occurring within the sample. Precision was 10% and reproducibility of the tests was better than 5%.

The tests were performed as follows: two identical samples (microbalance and microcalorimeter) were desorbed for at least 12 hours in a vacuum chamber at 10^{-4} Torr. A water evaporator was used to establish a specified partial water vapor pressure P/P_0 within the apparatus. This evaporator allowed the pressure to be increased in steps by changing the temperature in the water bath (between $-10°C$ and $22°C$).

For each increase in partial pressure, weight gain at equilibrium M_∞ was recorded; a hydration isotherm was drawn and the energy associated with this increase in mass calculated, allowing determination of the mean molar energy of interaction of the water ΔH in kJ/mol and plotting of the energy curve. Finally, we analyzed the change in mass increase as a function of time and used the results to determine the kinetic laws governing hydration of keratins. There are two possible cases: diffusion controls the phenomenon of sorption, giving a kinetic profile of sorption obeying Fick's law, which for a cylinder (infinite length and radius a) is given by:

$$\frac{\partial C}{\partial t} = \frac{1}{r}\frac{\partial}{\partial r}\left(rD\frac{\partial c}{\partial r}\right) \tag{1}$$

Cranck (13) showed that for a cylindrical solid in an infinite reservoir, this law could be simplified and approximated by the following equation:

$$\frac{M_t}{M_\infty} = 2\left[\frac{2}{\sqrt{\pi}}\left(\frac{Dt}{r^2}\right)^{1/2} - \frac{1}{2}\frac{Dt}{r^2} - \frac{1}{6\sqrt{\pi}}\left(\frac{Dt}{r^2}\right)^{3/2} + \cdots\right] \tag{2}$$

If water diffusion occurs too rapidly to regulate hydration, access of adsorption sites by water involves the crossing of barriers, the kinetics of which follows an exponential first-order process:

$$\frac{M_t}{M_\infty} = 1 - \exp(-k \cdot t) \tag{3}$$

Water Swelling of Hair

The measuring instrument used to determine radial swelling of fibers was developed in our laboratories (Fig. 1A). The principle of measurement is based on continuous determination of diameter during penetration of water into the fiber. The diameter of the hair is measured using a sensor to detect displacement; it exerts a very low pressure on a section of hair several millimetees long. The diameter is first measured and then a drop of water is carefully applied. The change in diameter subsequent to swelling is then recorded directly as a function of time. Analysis of the curves (Fig. 1B) allows determination of two parameters: final swelling (in percent), which is obtained by measuring the mean value in the asymptotic part of the curve and swelling rate (% per minute), which is determined by measuring the slope over the first 10 seconds of the curve.

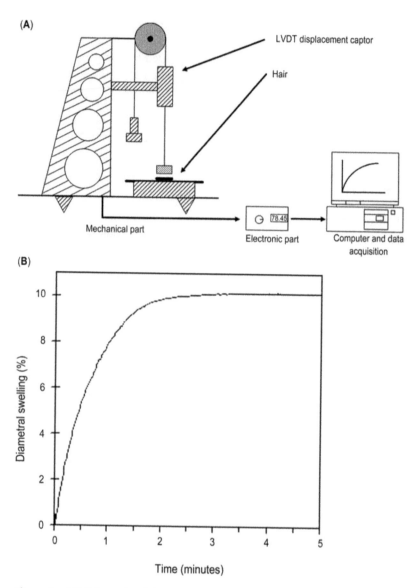

Figure 1 (**A**) Schematic of the device developed for measuring the swelling of hair in water. (**B**) Typical swelling curve of a hair in water. The swelling rate is obtained from the slope of the tangent at $T = 0$.

Statistics

Statistical analysis was performed by means of the SPSS package (SPSS Inc., Chicago, Illinois) for variance analysis. Because experimental data were not homogenous, we used the Hochberg and Tamhane procedure for multiple comparisons (14). $p < 0.05$ is considered as the limit.

EXPERIMENTAL RESULTS

Sorption Isotherms

The values for water content (expressed as the percentage of dry weight for the three types of samples) obtained after equilibrium, at the different water vapor pressures, are shown in Figure 2.

The isotherms for the three hair types are sigmoidal, with a concave section at low pressures and an exponential increase at high pressures; in all cases, there was good definition of the equilibrium values, even at saturation pressure.

The key point concerning comparison of the three hair types is that the Caucasian and Asian samples had the same hydration isotherms while the African American samples had a statistically significantly lower isotherm. These differences (approximately 15% at high partial pressures) cannot be ascribed to measurement uncertainties in view of the precision and reproducibility of the experiment.

Measurement of Enthalpy

The mean energies of interaction obtained for four ranges of incremental partial pressures are shown in Table 1.

Our results confirmed those of previously published studies concerning Caucasian hair keratin. Energy values decrease as partial pressure and water content increase: an energy of the order of 14 to 15 kcal/mol was noted for weight gain of less than 6% to 7%, thus confirming a marked interaction

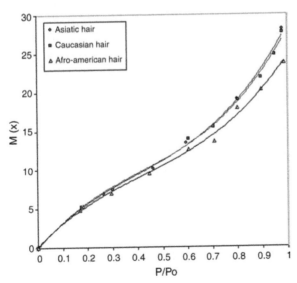

Figure 2 Sorption isotherms for the three types of hair. Isotherm of African American hair is lower than the other two.

Table 1 Hydration Energies for the Three Hair Types at Different Increments of Partial Pressure

P/P_0	$\Delta M/M$ (%)	ΔH (kcal/mol)		
		Caucasian	Asian	African American
0.00–0.17	5.5	14.7	15.2	–
0.00–0.30	7.0	13.9	13.9	13.8
0.30–0.60	5.5–13.0	12.5	10.8	11.5
0.60–0.95	13.0–25.0	7.0	7.0	6.8

between the primary water molecules and the keratin sites. These values are characteristic of the so-called monolayer sorption in the Brunauer–Emmett–Teller model. The sorption energy curve thus decreases rapidly to around 7 kcal/mol at partial pressures greater than the mean value for the ambient atmosphere.

The differences between the three types of hair are not significant.

Sorption Kinetics

The kinetic data for hydration of the three hair types were analyzed for partial pressures of 0.16, 0.30, 0.60, 0.80, and 0.98. The curves in Figure 3 show the experimental values obtained for each hair types at low (0.16), medium (0.3), and high (0.8) partial pressure. For each curve, the laws that best apply to the data are also indicated, i.e., Fick's diffusion law [Eq. (2)] and the first-order law [Eq. (3)].

It is clear that the kinetic mechanism varies for all hair types as a function of the degree of hydration. For the lowest partial pressure value of 0.16 (corresponding to a weight gain $\leq$5–6%), transport of water throughout the hair was regulated by diffusion. For partial pressures of 0.6 and higher, the first-order law was fully consistent with the data. To our knowledge, there is no allusion to this change in regulatory kinetic mechanism during the course of hydration of hair in any previous study.

Regarding the comparison between the three hair types, it is interesting to note that the behavior of the Asian hair samples was different to that of the other two types; this was particularly evident during the tests at high partial pressure ($P/P_0 = 0.8$). $P/P_0 = 0.8$ and 0.98 are given in Table 2. For example, at $P/P_0 = 0.98$, the rate constant $k \times 10^4$ seconds decreased as follows: *African American (27.6) = Caucasian (29.2) > Asian (12.2)* with the Asian hair samples giving a particularly low value (less than half of the value for the other two types).

Swelling in Water

The swelling curves for the three types of hair appear on Figure 4. The values of the two parameters (swelling rate and swelling maximum) and

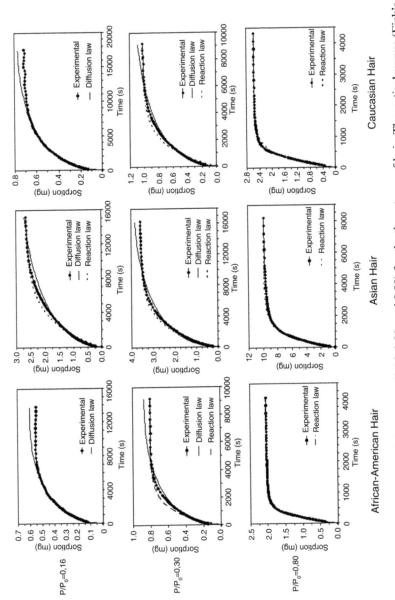

Figure 3 Sorption kinetics at three partial pressures (0.16, 0.30, and 0.80) for the three types of hair. Theoretical curves (Fick's law and Reaction law) are also plotted.

Table 2   Rate Constant Values ($k \times 10^4$ in sec) Obtained for the Different Types of Hair

	African American	Caucasian	Asian
$P/P_0 = 0.80$	35.1	28.3	14.1
$P/P_0 = 0.98$	27.6	29.2	12.2

Note: Sorption of water by Asian hair is roughly two times slower than by the two other types of hair.

statistics appear respectively in Table 3. These data and statistical analyses showed that the maximal radial swelling in water is significantly lower in African American hair than in Caucasian ($p < 0.001$) and Asian hair ($p < 0.01$), with no difference between Asian and Caucasian. Furthermore, a faster rate of swelling is noted for Caucasian hair compared to Asian hair ($p < 0.04$).

DISCUSSION

The above studies demonstrated differences in hydration as a function of ethnic type in terms of both equilibrium and kinetics: sorption by African American hair is lower at equilibrium in both the vapor phase and in water. The rate constant for Asian hair is very clearly lower than the two other hair types of hair at partial pressures greater than 0.6. Regarding kinetic characteristics, all hair types exhibited a change in kinetic mechanism as a function of the degree of hydration involving a transition from a diffusion law to a first-order law as the vapor pressure increased. The present results concern both equilibrium points in water and the kinetic profiles at equilibrium.

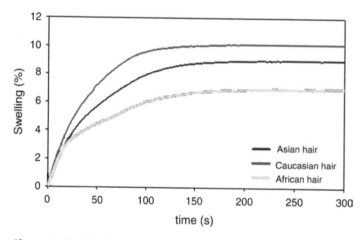

Figure 4   Swelling in water for the three types of hair. Swelling maximum and swelling rate are extracted from these curves (Table 3).

Table 3 Experimental Results for the Maximum Swelling (%) and the Swelling Rate (%/min) of the Three Types of Hair

	Maximum swelling (%)	Swelling rate (%/min)
African American	7.1 ± 2.1	11.1 ± 6.2
Caucasian	9.9 ± 1.2	14.1 ± 3.1
Asian	9.0 ± 0.7	10.9 ± 2.3

Note: Results expressed as mean ± standard deviation.

Equilibrium in Water

Compared with Caucasian and Asian hair samples, the sorption values recorded for hair of African American origin were approximately 10% lower at medium partial pressures, 15% towards saturation pressure, and 21% to 28% in liquid water.

It is difficult to account for these results on the basis of previously published studies on the differences in the biochemical properties between these different hair types (15,16). The same is also true of the structural organization of keratin in these various hair types reported in a recent study involving X-ray diffraction (17). The differences in properties described in the literature, particularly regarding mechanical properties, are generally ascribed to the shape or diameter of the hair fibers rather than to any intrinsic differences in the actual nature of the keratin itself (10,11). More precisely, the proteins and the amino acids of which keratin is composed are the same. For instance cystein, which together with salt bridges and hydrogen bonds, is responsible for crosslinking of the structure thereby restricting swelling, exhibited no difference in concentration between the three sample types. It is consequently very difficult to explain these results in terms of differences in protein structure between the different types of hair.

This aspect of the result is further underlined by the results obtained by means of calorimetry. The energy of interaction noted was approximately 14.5 kcal/mol at low partial pressures (corresponding to a water content of 6%), decreasing to around 7 kcal/mol at high partial pressures corresponding to water content values higher than 20%. These values, which are consistent with those given in the literature, showed no difference according to the ethnic origin of the hair samples and suggest that the nature of adsorption sites for water molecules is broadly equivalent for all three hair types analyzed.

Causative factors may thus be sought among the other components of hair likely to modify the equilibrium with water, in particular lipids, salts, and trace elements. Regarding lipids, a recent study has shown that certain lipids are distributed differently in the various compartments of the hair shaft (cuticle, cortex, and medulla) according to ethnic type (18). This study suggests that lipids could affect accessibility of water molecules to some adsorption sites in the case of African American hair.

Equilibrium Kinetics

Two main results were obtained with the experiments carried out in the vapor phase: there is a change in the kinetic mechanism during the course of hydration of the fibers, and for medium to high partial pressures, the rate constant is two times lower for Asian hair than for African American and Caucasian hair.

Concerning the first point, it is well known that within keratins, stratum corneum or hair, the water diffusion coefficient increases with hydration. It is thus possible that diffusion that initially regulates the overall kinetics begins to occur too rapidly and that first-order kinetics subsequently becomes the preponderant phenomenon. A precise study of any change in the kinetic profile would require a precise measurement of the coefficient of diffusion as a function of the equilibrium partial pressure. Such a measurement is dependent on a very precise determination of hair diameter which is difficult to obtain, particularly in the case of African American hair.

In the aqueous phase, these kinetic results were confirmed only for Asian hair, which swells at a statistically significantly lower rate than Caucasian hair. The kinetic profile of African American hair also appears lower, but the difference in this case is not statistically significant. Measurements on this type of hair are less precise because of the more marked ellipticity.

These differences concerning equilibrium kinetics cannot be interpreted on the basis of current knowledge about the relative composition of these three types of fibers; for example, little is known about the nature, concentration, and localization of the different types of lipids present in hair.

CONCLUSION

This study is the first to show differences in hydration between hair types as a function of ethnic origin: African American, Caucasian, and Asian. The first difference concerns African American hair, which equilibrates at 10% to 15% less water according to relative humidity and exhibits less swelling in water. The second difference concerns Asian hair, for which the kinetic data were very different from that seen with African American and Caucasian hair. In the range of high humidity values, where kinetics were of first order, the rate constant was approximately two times lower.

These differences cannot be explained by the different shapes or diameters of the fibers but are more probably due to differences in the biochemical composition of the fibers that have not yet been investigated with adequate precision. Further studies are required in order to understand the specific characteristics of each hair type. There is no doubt that the formulation of cosmetic products that are better adapted to the characteristics of each type hair will benefit from these new studies.

REFERENCES

1. Morton WE, Hearle JW. Physical Properties of Keratin Fibers. 3rd ed. Textile Institute, 1993:147.
2. Hansen JR, Yellin W. NMR and infra-red spectroscopic studies of Stratum Corneum hydration. In: Jellinek, ed. Water Structure and the Water-Polymer Interface. London: Plenum, 1972.
3. Clifford J, Sheard B. Nuclear magnetic resonance investigation of the state of water in human hair. Biopolymers 1966; 4:1057.
4. Lynch LJ, Marsden KH. An NMR study of keratin hydration. J Chem Phys 1969; 56:5681.
5. Algie JE, Gamble RA. Dielectric properties of wool and horn containing absorbed water. Kolloid Z. Z. Polym 1973; 251:554.
6. Lévêque JL, Garson JC, Pissis P, Boudouris G. Free water in keratin? A depolarisation thermal current study. Biopolymers 1981; 20:2469.
7. Feughelman M. A two-phase structure for keratin fibers. Text Res J 1959; 29:223.
8. Franbourg A, Leroy F. Synchrotron light: a powerful tool for the analysis of human hair damage, 11th DWI Symposium Hair 96", Rostock, 1996.
9. Klemm E. Proc Sci Sect Toilet Goods Assoc 1965; 43:7.
10. Kamath YK, Hornby SB. Mechanical and fractographic behavior of Negroid hair. J Soc Cosmet Chem 1984; 35:21.
11. Syed AN, Kuhadja A, Ayoub H, Ahmad K. African American hair. Cosmet Toiletries 1995; 1(10):20.
12. Lévêque JL, Escoubes M, Rasseneur L. Water-keratin interaction in human stratum corneum. Bioeng Skin 1987; 3:227.
13. Cranck J. The Mathematics of Diffusion. New York: Oxford University Press, 1955:70.
14. Hochberg Y, Tamhane AC. Multiple Comparisons Procedures. New York: John Wiley and Sons, 1987.
15. Nappe C, Kermici M. Electrophoretic analysis of alkylated proteins of human hair from various ethnic groups. J Soc Cosmet Chem 1989; 40:91.
16. Dekio S, Jidoi J. Hair low sulfur protein composition does not differ electrophoretically among different races. J Dermatol 1988; 15:393.
17. Franbourg A, Hallegot P, Baltenneck F, Toutain C, Leroy F. Current research on ethnic hair. J Am Acad Dermatol 2003; 48:6S–115S.
18. Kreplak L, Briki F, Duvault Y, et al. Profiling lipids across Caucasian and African American hair transverse cuts, using synchrotron infra red microspectrometry. Int J Cosmet Sci 2001; 23:369.

8

The Age-Dependent Changes in Skin Condition in Ethnic Populations from Around the World

Greg G. Hillebrand, Mark J. Levine[†], and Kukizo Miyamoto

*The Procter & Gamble Company, Cincinnati, Ohio, U.S.A.,
and Kobe, Japan*

INTRODUCTION

Understanding the ethnic differences in the visual and biophysical properties of skin has been the focus of several research studies and several reviews cover this subject (1–7). However, caution needs to be exercised when making general conclusions from observational studies of ethnic differences. When a difference is observed, the basis for that difference might be attributed to endogenous (genetic) and exogenous (environmental) factors. Defining which factor(s) is responsible for a given difference is difficult. First, there is difficulty in designing experiments that control for known and potentially confounding variables such as gender, age, season of year, body site, geography (place of residence), and lifestyle (socioeconomic level, diet, etc.). Second, within each ethnic group, a specific skin parameter will span a large range thereby requiring large base sizes to ensure that study sampling accurately reflects the population means. Finally, the methods used and the way measurements are done can greatly influence results and conclusions.

[†] Deceased.

One of the most researched areas, yet controversial, concerns ethnic differences in skin sensitivity to topical agents or environmental stress. Toward this end, researchers have focused on the structural elements of the stratum corneum (8–11), its permeability (12–15) and sensitivity to irritants (14–20). Robinson (2) summarized these studies in a review on the differences in susceptibility to skin irritation based on population. Most of the experimental data using objective methods such as the appearance of erythema, decreased skin permeability by trans-epidermal water loss (TEWL), or increased blood flow by laser Doppler flowmetry, support the notion that Caucasian skin is more susceptible to the skin irritation effects of chemicals compared to black or Hispanic skin. Robinson (1) did not observe a difference in susceptibility to skin irritation between East Asians (Chinese) and Caucasians.

Several observational studies have focused on the ethnic differences in the skin's biophysical properties. Differences have been noted in, for example, skin resistance, conductance, capacitance, mechanical properties, and pH (13,21,22). Skin color is the most obvious visible skin feature that distinguishes one population from another. Color is related to the number, size, type, and distribution of cytoplasmic pigment granules called melanosomes, which contain melanin (23). The role melanin plays in protecting skin from solar-induced damage accounts for the increased susceptibility of light-skinned people to get skin cancer (24). Racial differences in constitutive pigmentation (25) are also likely related to racial differences in the incidence of pigmentation disorders (26) and the visible signs of skin aging such as skin wrinkling (27). It is generally believed that darker skin types are less prone to the damaging effects of acute and chronic ultraviolet (UV) radiation exposure (27,28). For acute protection, Kollias (29) measured the minimum erythema dose (MED) in heavily pigmented (skin type V) versus fair-skinned Caucasians (skin types I and II). The MED of skin type V was about two times that of skin types I and II, in close agreement with the ratio of pigment in the two groups. For chronic protection, the association between skin type and the visible signs of skin aging, for example, wrinkles and hyperpigmentation, is less well quantified. Certainly a person's lifetime accumulation of UV exposure is a huge factor in determining several skin characteristics. Within a given racial or ethnic population, place of residence can be an important confounding variable. For example, Japanese women who have lived all their lives in northern Japan have several significant differences in skin condition versus women living in southern Japan (30,31).

It is worthwhile to pause and discuss the words "racial" and "ethnicity" for the two should not be used interchangeably as they often are. Anthropologists generally recognize three primary racial groups in the human population: the Caucasoid, the Negroid and the Mongoloid. Ethnicity on the other hand is quite different. An ethnic population can be defined based on, for example, a common language, geography, nationality, culture, or history. Race clearly helps define an ethnic group, but an ethnic group is not defined solely by race. Thus, there are hundreds and hundreds of ethnic groups in the world yet there are only three primary races. Some researchers use the term "ethnic skin" to define any skin that is "non-white," a practice that can cause considerable confusion. When discussing differences in skin condition between different populations, it is important to clearly define both ethnicity and race. Generalizations about the skin characteristics of a given ethnic population need to be considered in the context of how, when, and where the data were collected. "black" is not an accurate descriptor. Ethnic descriptors, such as "African Americans living in Los Angeles," are more helpful when communicating results.

Our aim is to discuss the age-dependent changes in skin characteristics in various ethnic populations we observed in a relatively large base size study across a wide age range of female subjects (32). We also discuss an analysis of the host and environmental factors significantly associated with specific skin parameters to try and explain the basis for the differences in skin condition.

CONSIDERATIONS FOR CLINICAL DESIGN, EXECUTION, AND ANALYSIS

Several precautions should be considered when designing and executing large clinical surveys of skin condition among ethnic groups. In our experience, potential pitfalls abound so taking time to identify opportunities for artifacts is time well spent, especially given the high cost associated with studies of this type. Ideally, skin measurements should be collected at the same time (season) of the year and all data should be collected in a short period of time to prevent seasonal effects. Inclusion or exclusion criteria should be well defined and strictly adhered to. Depending on the study objectives, subject participation may require that they have lived in the vicinity of the study location all of their lives to prevent latitudinal (lifetime UV exposure) effects (30,31). Subjects declaring themselves "mixed race" should be noted. All subjects should be prepared for skin measurements in exactly the same manner. That is, they should all cleanse their skin with the same skin care cleanser and should have "equilibrated" in the same way before any skin measurement. Ideally, measurements should be conducted in a room with controlled temperature and humidity. If such a room is not available, ambient room conditions should be at least controlled for temperature. Methods must be identical throughout the study and instruments should have a standard operating procedure that includes calibration to insure consistent and accurate measurements day to day. Ideally, all measurements should be conducted by the same person to prevent operator error. If this is not possible, then operators should all be trained and qualified by the same trainer. Besides these areas of attention, there are less understood factors that may profoundly affect skin condition that might affect the study results such as diet (33) and socioeconomic factors (34). The myriad of factors that can affect skin condition means that small base size surveys are highly prone to sampling error. For this reason, studies

Table 1 Number of Subjects by Ethnicity and City

Ethnicity	City	n
Caucasian	Los Angeles	439
Caucasian	London	469
Caucasian	Rome	445
Asian-Indian	London	474
African American	Los Angeles	435
Latino/Hispanic	Los Angeles	310
East Asian[a]	Los Angeles	207
Japanese	Akita	381
Japanese	Kagoshima	300

[a]Chinese, Japanese, Korean.

should include a sufficient sampling of subjects to yield an accurate estimate of the true population mean. For the work discussed here, Table 1 shows the number of subjects surveyed in each of the ethnic populations by city. The age range spanned from 10 to 70 years old with about equal weighting for each decade of life (our target was 75 individuals per decade but this was not achievable for certain ethnic populations because of recruiting difficulties). Table 2 shows the methods used for each of the skin measurements.

Measurements of wrinkles, pigmented spots, pores, sebum secretion, lightness, hydration, and pH were subjected to an analysis of variance (ANOVA), which accounted for variability due to age-category (10–19, 20–29, 30–39, 40–49, 50–59, 60–69), ethnic group, and the interaction of age-category with ethnic group. Least squares means for each combination of age-category by ethnic group are calculated and displayed in the histograms. Pair-wise comparisons of the ethnic groups compare the six age-group means for each skin parameter in a 6° of freedom contrast.

Table 2 Methods and Measurements

Measurement	Skin site	Method
Wrinkling	Left face	Imaging
Hyperpigmented spots	Left face	Imaging
Pores	Left face	Imaging
Hydration	Left cheek/left vental forearm/left calf	Corneometer
Sebum excretion	Middle forehead	Sebumeter
Color	Left cheek/left upper inner arm	Chromameter
pH	Left cheek/ left vental forearm/left calf	pH meter

DIFFERENCES IN FACIAL WRINKLING

Clinical imaging is a fast and accurate "no touch" method that has found tremendous utility for the noninvasive and objective measurement of skin topography. Traditional 2-D imaging relies on the generation of shadows thrown across skin wrinkles under controlled tangential illumination followed by the quantification of those shadows via sophisticated image analysis algorithms. More recently, relatively low cost 3-D imaging systems are available to measure skin smoothness and wrinkle depth with micrometer precision and millisecond capture times. We used 2-D imaging to quantify facial skin wrinkling over a wide age range in several ethnic populations (32). Images were collected using a facial imaging system (Fig. 1A and B) that employed a commercially available high resolution digital camera mounted into a standardized illumination box fitted with head positioning aids. The captured image is shown in Figure 1C. The

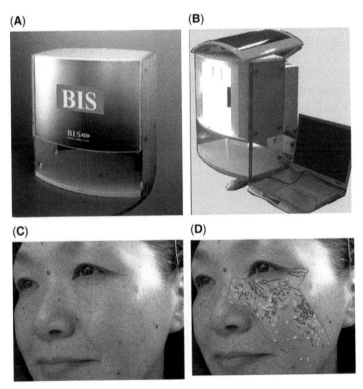

Figure 1 (**A**) The Beauty Imaging System (BIS), (**B**) BIS with door open and computer, (**C**) example of BIS Image and (**D**) image in C showing masked region of interest (medium gray) and image analysis overlay of detected wrinkles or fine lines (dark gray) and hyperpigmented spots (white) in the region of interest.

region of interest (ROI) on each image was defined ("masked") in the same way for all images using predefined landmarks on the face (e.g., left and right corners of eye, bridge of nose, corner of mouth). The ROI was analyzed using customized software that automatically identifies and quantifies wrinkles or fine lines. We also used these images to quantify hyperpigmented spots (both red and brown pigmented spots) and pores. Figure 1D shows the same image as in Figure 1C with an image analysis overlay for wrinkles and hyperpigmented spots in the ROI. The absolute amount of wrinkling and hyperpigmentation was normalized to the size of the ROI. In this way, the severity of a skin feature can be compared from one subject to the next; subjects with large heads (and therefore large ROIs) can be compared to subjects with small heads (and correspondingly small ROIs). These normalized data are defined as "wrinkle area fraction," "hyperpigmented spot count fraction," and "pore count fraction."

Figure 2 shows the mean wrinkle area fraction by age group for four ethnic populations living in Los Angeles, California, U.S.A.: East Asians, Latinos, African Americans, and White Caucasians. As expected, facial wrinkling increased with increasing age in all groups. Wrinkling increased in the order East Asians < Latinos = African Americans < Caucasians. Skin lightness (L^* value) was measured with the Minolta Chomameter on the forehead (facultative skin color) and upper inner arm (constitutive skin color) of these same subjects. Mean forehead L^* value increased in the order African American < Latino = East Asian < Caucasian. Importantly, mean ethnic group facultative or constitutive skin color lightness did not predict the propensity for facial skin wrinkling. We expected, based on skin lightness, that the African Americans would show the least skin wrinkling. While

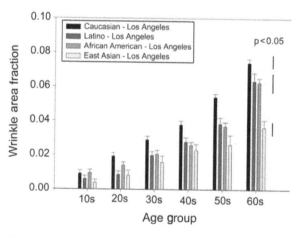

Figure 2 Facial wrinkling by age group in ethnic groups living in Los Angeles. Error bars: standard error.

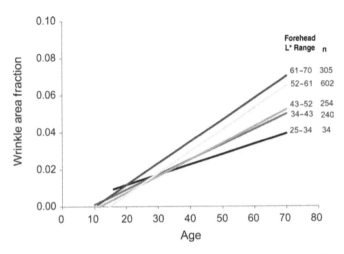

Figure 3 Regression lines for facial wrinkling versus age by forehead L* range.

the mean facial wrinkle area fraction for African Americans was significantly less than Caucasians, it was the East Asians who exhibited the lowest wrinkle area fraction at any given age (Fig. 2). However, skin color for a given population spans a wide range. For example, the African Americans living in Los Angeles showed L* values ranging from as low as 26 to as high as 63. Figure 3 shows the wrinkle data of Figure 2 segmented by forehead L* value range *without* regard to ethnic population. The group of individuals with the highest forehead L* values had the most facial wrinkling. Conversely, the group of individuals with the lowest L* values showed the least facial wrinkling.

In the Los Angeles study, the inclusion or exclusion criteria for subject participation had no restrictions for lifetime place of residence. That is, participation in the study did not require subjects to have lived all their lives in southern California (because of the difficulty in subject recruiting). Had such a restriction been employed, the differences in skin condition observed between ethnic populations might have been even more marked. This is because lifetime place of residence influences many of the visible and biophysical skin parameters within a given ethnic population. The skin of Japanese women living all their lives in northern Akita Japan was compared to a peer population of Japanese women who had lived all their lives in southern Kagoshima Japan (30). Kagoshima is estimated to receive 1.5 times more UVB radiation than Akita and it was hypothesized that the visible signs of photodamaged would be more pronounced in the Kagoshima women. Japan makes an attractive venue for studies of this type because its homogeneous population base helps to minimize confounding effects of racial or ethnic influences on skin sensitivity to sunlight. Figure 4 shows

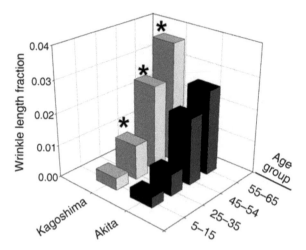

Figure 4 Wrinkle length fraction by age group and study location. Kagoshima bars marked by asterisk (∗) are significantly different ($p < 0.05$) than the corresponding Akita age group.

that Kagoshima subjects exhibited significantly more facial skin wrinkling than their age-matched Akita counterparts.

The differences observed in facial wrinkling between the women of northern versus southern Japan were likely due, in part, to differences

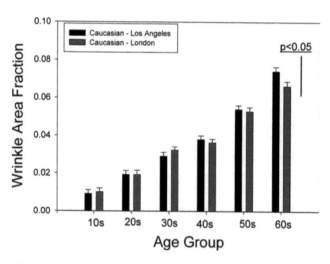

Figure 5 Facial wrinkling by age group in Caucasians living in Los Angeles and London. Error bars: standard error.

in lifetime sun exposure. However, when we compared facial wrinkling in Caucasian women living in Los Angeles versus London, we were somewhat surprised to find little difference in facial wrinkling (Fig. 5). In a similar intraracial comparison, East Asians (principally, women of Japanese, Korean and Chinese ancestry) living in Los Angeles showed no significant difference in facial skin wrinkling compared to Japanese women living in Akita Japan (32). The low level of facial wrinkling for East Asians living in Los Angeles and Japanese living in Akita suggests that oriental skin may be somewhat resistant to skin wrinkling. It is likely that population differences in other genetic factors besides skin pigmentation, such as population differences in DNA repair, are important in determining the propensity to develop skin wrinkles associated with chronic sun exposure (35).

DIFFERENCES IN HYPERPIGMENTATION

We used digital imaging followed by image analysis to quantify facial hyperpigmentation. Hyperpigmentation is expressed here as the number of spots in the area measured (spot count fraction) as show in Figure 1D. Figure 6 shows facial hyperpigmented spot count fraction by race and age group for (1) subjects living in Los Angeles and (2) all subjects surveyed from around the world. For the Los Angeles groups, facial hyperpigmentation increased with increasing age in the order East Asian = Latino < Caucasian < African American. Comparing all ethnic groups, the Japanese and East Asians showed the least facial hyperpigmentation while African Americans, Caucasians from Los Angeles, and Caucasians from London showed the most.

It was surprising to find that African Americans had the highest hyperpigmented spot count fraction versus the other ethnic groups. As with wrinkling, the propensity to develop hyperpigmented regions on the face was not predicted by skin color lightness. The Asian-Indians living in London, while having relatively dark skin tone, showed relatively low hyperpigmented spot count fraction values, on par with the East Asians and Japanese.

DIFFERENCES IN SKIN HYDRATION

The Corneometer CM 825PC (Courage-Khazaka) was used to measure the skin electrical capacitance, a measure of stratum corneum hydration, on the left upper cheek area, the left ventral forearm and the left outer calf. Measurements, not exactly at the same location, were made in triplicate and the average of these three measurements was calculated and used for group statistics.

Figure 7 shows Corneometer readings on the cheek (Fig. 7A), forearm (Fig. 7B), and calf (Fig. 7C) by age and ethnic group for subjects living in

(A)

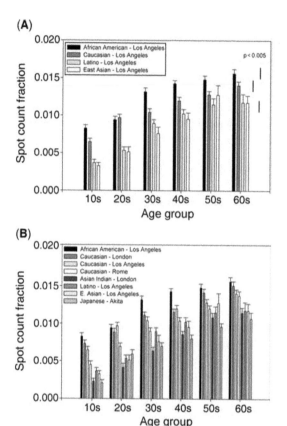

Figure 6 Facial hyperpigmented spots by age group in (**A**) ethnic groups living in Los Angeles and (**B**) all ethnic groups and cities. Error bars: standard error.

Los Angeles. The relative difference between ethnic groups in stratum corneum capacitance was dependent on skin site measured and age group being compared. On the cheek, African Americans, Latinos, and East Asians had significantly higher stratum corneum capacitance than Caucasians ($p < 0.001$). Warrier et al. also observed lower capacitance values in Caucasians versus African Americans (13). It was interesting to observe that skin hydration, measured with the Corneometer, increased with increasing age on both the cheek and forearm. It is generally assumed that skin dryness increases with age. Our results suggest that stratum corneum hydration (capacitance) goes up, not down with age, at least on the cheek and forearm. On the other hand, sebum excretion declines significantly after the third or fourth decade (see below). The perception of facial skin dryness in mature skin may be more related to lower surface sebum as opposed to less hydration.

(A)

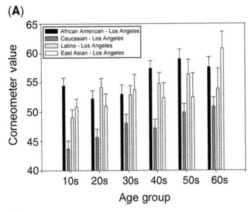

(B)

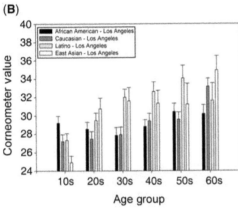

(C)

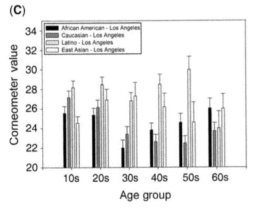

Figure 7 Stratum corneum hydration on the **(A)** cheek, **(B)** forearm, and **(C)** calf by age and ethnic group in Los Angeles. Error bars: standard error.

DIFFERENCES IN OTHER SKIN PARAMETERS

pH

The Skin pH Meter pH 900 (Courage-Khazaka) was used to measure skin surface pH on the left cheek, left ventral forearm, and left outer calf in the four ethnic populations surveyed in Los Angeles. Skin measurements were made in duplicate, not exactly at the same location, for each skin site and the average of the duplicate measurements were used for group statistics. Figure 8 shows skin pH on the cheek (Fig. 8A), forearm (Fig. 8B), and calf (Fig. 8C) by age and ethnicity. There was no obvious trend for skin pH to change with age. Nor was there a statistically significant difference between the ethnic groups in skin pH. We noted, however, that skin pH values varied over a wide pH range from subject to subject (from below 4.0 to above 7.5). However, the intrasubject variability from skin site to skin site was remarkably small. For example, subjects with low pH values on the arm also had low pH values on the calf and cheek. Subjects with high pH values on the arm also had corresponding high pH values on the calf and cheek. Statistically, for 86% of the 1391 Los Angeles subjects surveyed, an individual's forearm skin pH was less than 0.5 pH units different from the same individual's cheek skin pH. For 68% of the 1391 subjects surveyed, there was less than 0.25 pH units difference between the forearm skin pH and the cheek skin pH. The narrow range of skin pH values within any one individual suggests that skin pH is controlled at a more "systemic" level or by homeostatic mechanisms, not by the presence or absence of surface lipids and sweat.

Sebum Excretion

Thirty minutes after cleansing to remove all surface sebum (detergent scrub, rinse, 70% ethanol swab), skin surface sebum on the forehead was measured with the Sebumeter SM 810 (Courage-Khazaka). Figure 9 shows the level of sebum excretion on the forehead by age and ethnic group for subjects living in Los Angeles. Sebum excretion increases during the early decades, peaking in the 30s and 40s and declines substantially in the later decades. African Americans showed significantly more sebum excretion than East Asians and Hispanics. Hispanics had the lowest sebum secretion, significantly less than both the Caucasians and the African Americans.

Pore Count

The number of visible facial pores was quantified using digital imaging followed by image analysis of the facial cheek area depicted in Figure 1D. Figure 10 shows facial pore count fraction by race and age group for the four ethnic groups living in Los Angeles. The number of visible pores increases with increasing age though age 40, thereafter decreasing slightly.

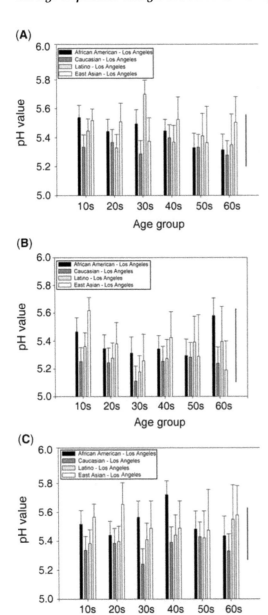

Figure 8 Skin pH on the (**A**) cheek, (**B**) forearm, and (**C**) calf by age and ethnic group in Los Angeles. Error bars: standard error.

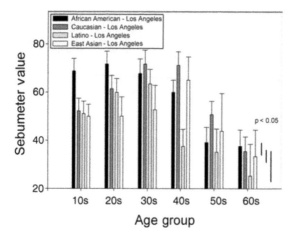

Figure 9 Sebum excretion on the forehead by age and ethnic group in Los Angeles. Error bars: standard error.

African Americans show substantially more visible pores than any of the other ethnic groups. There was a clear negative relationship between skin color lightness and pore count fraction; lighter skin African Americans had low pore count fraction while darker skin African Americans had higher pore count fractions (data not shown). Visual inspection of the images confirmed the image analysis data. It may be that pores, like skin shine, are more apparent on darker skin.

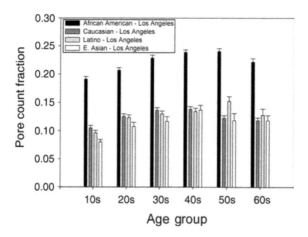

Figure 10 Facial pores by age group in ethnic groups living in Los Angeles. Error bars: standard error.

Table 3 Host and Environmental Factors Significantly Associated $(+/-, p < 0.05)$ with Facial Wrinkling, Hyperpigmentation, and Pores for Ethnic Groups Living in Los Angeles

Group	Wrinkling	Hyperpigmentation	Pores
African American	Blistering < 20 (+) Blistering > 20 (+)	BMI (+)	None
Caucasian	Pregnancy (+) Education (−)	BMI (+) Smoking (+)	BMI (+)
Latino	Menopausal (+) HRT (+) Pregnancy (+)	Blistering > 20 (+) BMI (+) Sleep (+)	Smoking (+)
East Asian	BMI (+) Pregnancy (+)		Education (+)

Abbreviations: Blistering <20, number of blistering sunburns before age 20; Blistering >20, number of blistering sunburns after age 20; BMI, body mass index; Pregnancy, number of full term pregnancies; Education, years of education; Smoking, number of years smoking; HRT, number of years taking hormone replacement therapy for menopause; Menopausal, number of years being menopausal; Sleep, average hours of sleep per day.

Other Factors

Subjects answered a structured questionnaire that collected data on potential host and environmental factors that might be associated with facial skin aging. Associations made in this manner must be considered with caution and should be followed up with controlled clinical studies to confirm the association. It was interesting to find that having a higher body mass index was significantly associated with hyperpigmentation in three out of the four ethnic groups studied (Table 3). Having more full term pregnancies was associated with having more facial wrinkling in three out of four ethnic groups.

DISCUSSION

In this survey, we collected quantitative data on several skin parameters in women from various ethnic groups across a wide age range (10–70 years old). Several aspects about our study design deviate from the ideal. Ideally, all data would be collected in a short period of time to prevent seasonal effects. While all of our data were collected in the fall or winter months, there was a long time from the start (October in London) to the finish (March in Los Angeles) of the study. Ideally, subjects would have lived in the vicinity of the study location all of their lives to prevent latitudinal effects (30,31). Except for the subjects who lived all their lives in and around Akita and Kagoshima, Japan, we did not exclude subjects who had lived outside of Los Angeles, London or Rome. For example, many of the

Asian-Indians living in London had lived for several decades in India. Ideally, the same study personnel would conduct all measurements for a given method to prevent operator error. We tried to minimize operator error by (i) having a single person train all study personnel, (ii) using the same protocols at all study sites, and (iii) using the same model of instruments (and in some cases, the same instrument) at all study sites.

By focusing on the differences in the group means for a given skin parameter, it is easy to lose sight of the fact that most of the skin parameters measured in this study span a huge range of values within any given ethnic group. The fact is that the distribution of values for one ethnic group overlaps tremendously with the distribution of values for another ethnic group. While the group means might be statistically and significantly different, ethnic groups generally share more in common than is depicted by the group means in the histograms.

In memory of our good friend and statistician, Mark Levine.

REFERENCES

1. Robinson MK. Racial differences in acute and cumulative skin irritation responses between Caucasian and Asian populations. Contact Dermatitis 2000; 42:134–143.
2. Robinson MK. Population differences in skin structure and physiology and the susceptibility to irritant and allergic contact dermatitis: implications for skin safety testing and risk assessment. Contact Dermatitis 1999; 41:65–79.
3. Berardesca E, Maibach HI. Racial differences in skin pathophysiology. J Am Acad Dermatol 1996; 34:667–672.
4. Berardesca E, Maibach HI. Racial differences in skin function: an update. Cosmetics Toiletries Mag 1995; 110:31–32.
5. Hood HL, Wickett RR. Racial differences in epidermal structure and function. Cosmetics Toiletries Mag 1992; 107:47–48.
6. Wesley N. Racial (Ethnic) differences in skin properties. Am J Clin Dematol 2003; 4:843–860.
7. Berardesca E, Maibach H. Ethnic skin: Overview of structure and function. J Am Acad Dermatol 2003; 48:S139–S142.
8. Corcuff P, Lotte C, Rougier A, Maibach HI. Racial differences in corneocytes. Acta Derm Benereol (Stockh) 1991; 71:146–148.
9. Thomson ML. Relative efficiency of pigment and horny layer thickness in protecting the skin of Europeans and Africans against solar ultraviolet radiation. J Physiol 1955; 127:236–246.
10. Weigand DA, Haygood C, Gaylor JR. Cell layers and density of Negro and Caucasian stratum corneum. J Invest Dermatol 1974; 62:563–568.
11. Whitmore SE, Sago NJ. Caliper-measured skin thickness is similar in white and black women. J Amer Acad Derm 2000; 42:76–79.
12. Reed JT, Ghadially R, Elias PM. Skin type, but neither race nor gender, influence epidermal permeability barrier function. Arch Dermatol 1995; 131:1134–1138.

13. Warrier AG, Kligman AM, Harper RA, Bowman J, Wickett RR. A comparison of black and white skin using noninvasive methods. J Soc Cosmet Chem 1996; 47:229–240.
14. Kompaore F, Tsuruta H. In vivo differences between Asian, Black and White in the stratum corneum barrier function. Int Arch Occup Environ Health 1993; 65:S223–S225.
15. Kompaore F, Marty JP, Dupont CH. In vivo evaluation of the stratum corneum barrier function in Black, Caucasians and Asians with two non-invasive methods. Skin Pharm 1993; 6:200–207.
16. Maibach HI, Berardesca E. Racial and skin color differences in skin sensitivity: implications for skin care products. Cosmetics Toiletries Mag 1990; 105:35–36.
17. Berardesca E, Maibach HI. Racial differences in sodium lauryl sulphate induced cutaneous irritation: black and white. Contact Dermatitis 1988; 18:65–70.
18. Berardesca E, Maibach HI. Racial differences in pharmacodynamic responses to nicotinates in vivo in human skin: Black and White. Arch Derm Venereol 1990; 70:63–66.
19. Basketter DA, Griffiths HA, Wang XM, Wilhelm KP, McFadden J. Individual, ethnic and seasonal variability in irritant susceptibility of skin: The implications for predictive human patch test. Contact Dermatitis 1996; 35:208–213.
20. Dickel H, Taylor JS, Evey P, Merk HF. Comparison of patch test results with a standard series among white and black racial groups. Am J Contact Dermatitis 2001; 12:77–82.
21. Johnson LC, Corah NL. Racial differences in skin resistance. Science 1963; 139:766–767.
22. Takahashi M, Watanabe H, Kumagai H, Nakayama Y. Physiological and morphological changes in facial skin with aging (II): A study on racial differences. J Soc Cosmet Chem Japan 1989; 23:22–30.
23. Kollias N. The physical basis of skin color and its evaluation. Clinics in Derm 1995; 13:361–367.
24. Kollias N, Sayre RM, Zeise L, Chedekel MR. Photoprotection by melanin. J Photochem Photobiol B 1991; 9:135–160.
25. Roh K, Kim D, Ha S, Ro Y, Kim J, Lee H. Pigmentation in Koreans: study of the differences from Caucasians in age, gender and seasonal variations. Brit J Derm 2001; 144:94–99.
26. Jimbow M, Jimbow K. Pigmentary disorders in oriental skin. Clin Dermatol 1989; 7:11–27.
27. Goh SH. The treatment of visible signs of senescence: the Asian experience. Brit J Derm 1990; 122(S35):105–109.
28. Marks R. Aging and photodamage. In: Sun Damaged Skin. London: Martin Dunitz, 1992:5–7.
29. Kollias N, Malallah YH, Al-Ajmi H, Baqer A, Johnson BE, Gonzales S. Erythema and melanogenesis action spectra in heavily-pigmented individuals as compared to fair-skinned Caucasians. Photodermatol Photoimmunol Photomed 1996; 12:183–188.
30. Hillebrand GG, Schnell B, Miyamoto K, Ichihashi M, Shinkura R, Akiba S. The age-dependent changes in skin condition in Japanese females living in northern vs. southern Japan. Int Fed Soc Cos Chem Mag 2001; 4:89–96.

31. Akiba S, Shinkura R, Miyamoto K, Hillebrand G, Yamaguchi N, Ichihashi M. Influence of chronic UV exposure and lifestyle on facial skin photo-aging—results from a pilot study. J Epidemiol 1999; 9:S136–S142.
32. Hillebrand GG, Levine MJ, Miyamoto K. The age-dependent changes in skin condition in African Americans, Caucasians, East Asians, Indian Asians and Latinos. Int Fed Soc Cos Chem Mag 2001; 4(4):259–266.
33. Purba MB, Kouris-Blazos A, Wattanapenpaiboon N, et al. Skin wrinkling: can food make a difference? J Am Col Nutri 2001; 20:71–80
34. Malvy D, Guinot C, Preziosi P, et al. Epidemiologic determinants of skin photoaging: Baseline data of the SU.VI.MAX cohort. J Am Acad Dermatol 2000; 42:47–55.
35. McCredie M. Cancer epidemiology in migrant populations. Recent results in cancer research 1998; 154:298–305.

(A) **(B)**

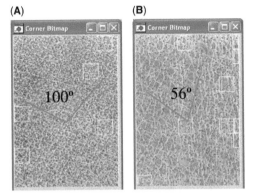

Figure 12.4 Skin micro relief obtained on the ventral forearm from **(A)** a 30-year-old woman and **(B)** a 78-year-old woman. (*See p. 158*)

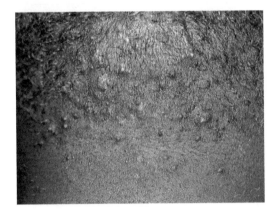

Figure 14.1 Acne keloid. (*See p. 182*)

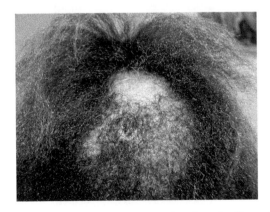

Figure 14.2 Centrifugal central scarring alopecia. (*See p. 183*)

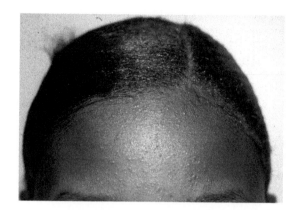

Figure 14.3 Pomade acne. (*See p. 186*)

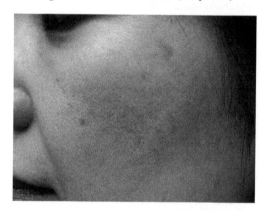

Figure 14.4 Facial lentigo on Asian skin. (*See p. 187*)

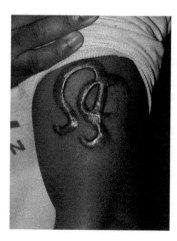

Figure 14.5 Fraternity keloid. (*See p. 187*)

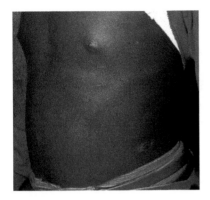

Figure 14.7 Scale highlights lesions of pityriasis rosea. (*See p. 189*)

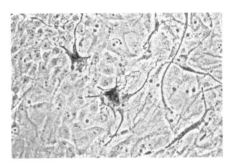

Figure 17.1 Cell coculture of melanocytes and keratinocytes. (*See p. 225*)

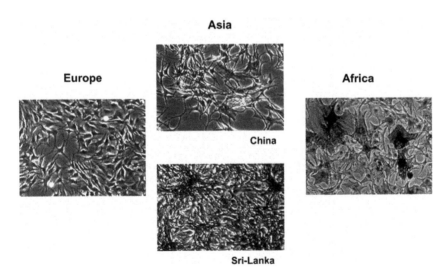

Figure 17.2 Morphology of melanocytes in monoculture according to their ethnical origin. (*See p. 225*)

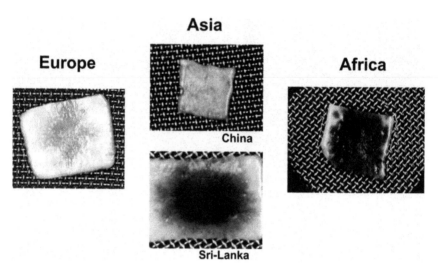

Figure 17.3 Pigmented reconstructed skin according to melanocyte ethnical origin. (*See p. 226*)

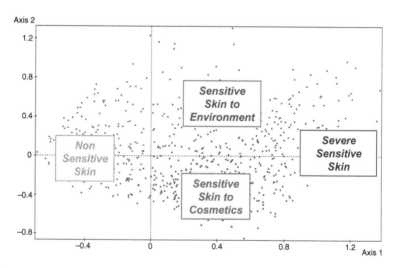

Figure 18.2 Projection of the subjects according to their severity and type of sensitive skin. (*See p. 237*)

9

Update on Racial Differences in Susceptibility to Skin Irritation and Allergy

Michael K. Robinson

The Procter & Gamble Company, Cincinnati, Ohio, U.S.A.

INTRODUCTION

The critical assessment of differences in susceptibility to irritant and allergic skin reactions has to be based upon the collective evidence from many studies on epidemiology and direct testing in small base size populations. Results from individual studies can be misleading. As illustrated schematically in Fig. 1, a significant difference in response between two distinct sample populations in any given study could be a true reflection of the populations at large, or simply an artefact of sampling bias. This has important implications for dermatotoxicological safety testing and risk assessment. Consistent and biologically relevant population differences (based on race, gender, age, etc.) would necessitate the identification and testing of the most sensitive population in order to safeguard all consumers. However, a lack of consistent or biologically relevant population differences would indicate that testing of any population would be adequate to protect other equally sensitive populations.

Several years ago, a fairly comprehensive review of the literature was compiled on population differences in skin biology and reactivity and the implications for skin safety testing and risk assessment (1). It was noted, at the time, that the only compelling data suggestive of true racial differences

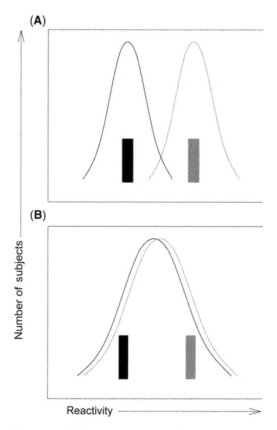

Figure 1 (**A**) Two study populations, designated by gray and black bars, are drawn from two overall populations with different mean reactivity levels. The reactivity of the test samples reflects the true difference in reactivity of the populations from which the samples were drawn. (**B**) Two study populations with the same differential reactivity shown in (**A**), were drawn from two overall populations with nearly identical mean reactivity. Here, the sample populations were drawn from opposite reactivity extremes of the overall populations. As a result, the difference in reactivity of the study populations is not a true reflection of the overall population reactivity.

in susceptibility to skin irritation or skin allergy indicated a reduced suscep-tibility among black vs. Caucasian subjects (2–5); most likely due to a less penetrable stratum corneum (6). Speculation about increased skin reactivity among Asian versus Caucasian subjects (7,8) was difficult to confirm exper-imentally due to little comparative data and conflicting results from the few published studies available at the time (9–12). From the stand point of skin safety testing and risk assessment, it was suggested that the common practice of skin testing in predominantly Caucasian female subjects was a fairly conservative approach in that, Caucasian females have been generally shown to be among the more reactive human sub-population. It was recognized that special population-specific testing might be appropriate under certain circumstances (limited geographical marketing, regulatory requirements, etc.), but that there was little scientific justification to mandate testing in specific populations based on the available data (1).

During the past six years, further studies have been conducted that shed some additional light on the subject of racial differences in skin sensitivity. Most of the recent work has focused on studies of skin irritation susceptibility, but a few studies have also touched on differences in susceptibility to allergic contact dermatitis, atopic dermatitis, and sensory irritation or the self perception of sensitive skin. This new information is summarized in the sections below, with additional perspective concerning possible implications for skin safety test methods and risk assessment.

RACIAL DIFFERENCES IN SUSCEPTIBILITY TO SKIN IRRITATION

As noted above, the pre-1999 literature on racial susceptibility to chemically-induced skin irritation was mixed. The notion that Caucasians are more sensitive than blacks was supported by consistent findings among a couple of historical studies providing direct comparison testing (2,3) as well as the additional evidence of a better skin barrier and reduced chemical penetration through the stratum corneum among black subjects (6,13). These findings have recently been extended through the use of confocal microscopy, which showed increased severity of microscopic histopathology changes with irritant exposures among Caucasian versus black subjects (14).

The further notion that Asian skin is more sensitive than Caucasian skin was much more speculative. Some of the speculation was based on largely anecdotal evidence related to sensitivity to sensory skin symptoms (7,8). Objective comparative test results were limited to non-concurrent comparisons of cosmetic or drug tolerance profiles between Asian and Caucasian subject populations (10,15) and a rather sparsely documented study of cumulative irritation patch test results between Japanese and Caucasian subjects (9). More direct studies of chemically-induced skin irritation, using a short term acute irritation test protocol (16), showed no evidence of increased skin sensitivity between Asian and Caucasian subjects (11,12).

To try and enhance the existing dataset on Caucasian versus Asian susceptibility to skin irritation, a combined acute and cumulative skin irritation patch test study was conducted among Caucasian, Japanese, and Chinese test subjects recruited together and tested concurrently at the same location (17). The Asian subjects recruited for this study were all native born Japanese or Chinese, who had immigrated to the United States for employment or educational reasons. An initial study of 28 Caucasian subjects and 20 Japanese subjects showed some evidence of increased reactivity in the Japanese subjects. In an acute (up to 4-hour exposure) patch test protocol

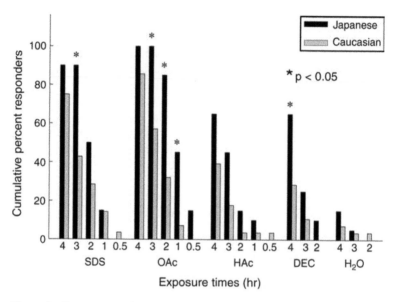

Figure 2   Separate panels of Caucasian (N = 28) and Japanese (N = 20) test subjects were exposed to the following test materials: 20% sodium dodecyl sulfate (SDS), 100% octanoic acid (OAC), 10% acetic acid (HAC), 100% decanol (DEC), water (H_2O). The test procedure used was a graduated exposure (up to 4-hr) acute irritation occluded patch test as previously described (12,16). Based on the cumulative response incidences at each time point examined, there were 5 exposure times with 3 of the test materials (indicated by ∗) at which the Caucasian population response was significantly less than the Japanese population response. Several additional exposure time/test material combinations showed directionally reduced Caucasian population responses. *Source*: From M.K. Robinson, Contact Dermatitis 42: 134–143, 2000; by permission.

(12,16), the Japanese subjects were consistently more reactive to a number of test materials (surfactant, organic acids, fatty alcohol, water) at various exposure durations. Several of these differences achieved statistical significance (Fig. 2). In a concurrent protocol (using 14 repeat 24-hour exposures) to test cumulative skin irritation to several low concentrations of surfactant [sodium dodecyl sulfate (SDS)], the irritation profile was the same for all, but the lowest SDS concentration, where, again, the Japanese subjects were more reactive (Fig. 3). For subjects that showed the most severe responses in the cumulative irritation test, the time to recover was the same for both the Caucasians and Japanese.

Since the results from this study were contrary to our earlier findings among Chinese subjects (12), we repeated this exact combined acute and cumulative skin irritation test protocol among Caucasian, Japanese, and Chinese subjects. In contrast to the results of our Caucasian/Japanese study, this

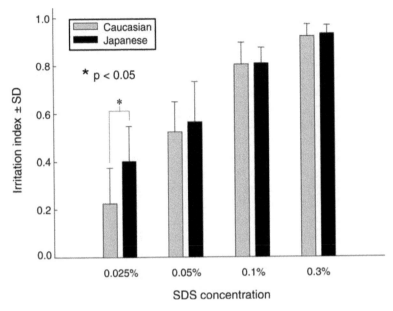

Figure 3 The same test populations shown in Figure 2 were concurrently exposed (different test site) to 14 consecutive 24-hr occluded patches of a series of sodium dodecyl sulfate (SDS) concentrations (0.025%–0.3%). Once a subject received a skin irritation grade of ≥3 (moderate response on 0–6 severity scale), no additional patches were applied and a grade of 3 was carried out for the remainder of the 14 days for data calculation purposes. An irritation index was calculated for each subject, for each SDS concentration, by summing their skin grades for all 14 time points and dividing by 42 (maximum grade possible if cutoff grade of 3 were assigned for all 14 time points). As indicated, the Caucasian population had a significantly lower cumulative irritation response to the lowest (0.025%) SDS concentration tested. *Source*: From M.K. Robinson, Contact Dermatitis 42:134–143, 2000; by permission.

3-way comparison study showed virtually identical skin reactivity profiles in the acute irritation protocol for all three subject populations. In the cumulative irritation protocol, the Chinese subjects actually showed slightly reduced skin reactivity compared to either the Caucasian or Japanese subjects. These findings served to reinforce the notion that, while it may be possible to detect population differences in skin irritation reactivity within individual small base sized studies, it can be difficult to confirm these differences in repeat studies. This may well be due to the inherent variability in human skin reactivity to irritants within and between test subjects (18,19).

A similar approach (although different protocols) was used by Foy and colleagues to study the susceptibility to skin irritation among Caucasian versus Japanese female subjects in a single acute 24 hour and four repeat cumulative exposure (one 24-hour and three 18-hour exposures) formats

(20). Like the first study summarized above, they observed a trend towards increased reactivity to various surfactant chemicals (acute protocol) and cosmetic formulations (cumulative protocol) among the Japanese subjects. Also, pigmentation changes associated with the acute surfactant reactions took longer to resolve in the Japanese subjects. Aramaki and colleagues also tested surfactant irritation in Caucasian and Japanese women using various instrumental measures of color change and barrier function (21). They used 24-hour acute exposures to low concentrations of SDS. Little difference was found in SDS-induced changes in comparative transepidermal water loss, stratum corneum hydration, sebum secretion, or erythema. A slight increase in pigmentation was seen in the Japanese subjects.

When all of these study results are examined in totality, there is a suggestion of at least a slight increase in reactivity in Japanese versus Caucasian subjects, even if individual study results tend to produce conflicting conclusions. In order to try and look more "globally" at Asian versus Caucasian differences in irritant skin reactivity, we recently collated our results of racial comparison studies across several years of testing to see if any composite trends would emerge (22). The results of four studies conducted at a single clinical laboratory over a 4-year period (including Caucasian, Japanese, and Chinese test subjects) were compiled. Over 100 subjects from each racial population were included in the composite analysis of the results of acute irritation testing of three chemicals (20% SDS, 10% acetic acid, and 100% decanol) that had been included in all four studies. For each chemical, there was a directional or significant increase in the reactivity among the combined Asian population (Fig. 4). These collective results thus provide support for the notion of at least a slightly increased sensitivity among Asian versus Caucasian subjects.

RACIAL DIFFERENCES IN SUSCEPTIBILITY TO ALLERGIC CONTACT DERMATITIS (SKIN SENSITIZATION)

Similar to the differences in susceptibility to skin irritation, the most direct assessment of differences in susceptibility to allergic skin reactions requires comparative experimental skin sensitization testing. This type of testing is ethically problematic as it induces a permanent change in immune reactivity to chemicals that test subjects might later encounter in the marketplace. Thus, only two experimental sensitization studies of racial differences in skin susceptibility exist in the historical dermatology literature (4,5). Both studies compared black and Caucasian subjects and, in both, there was greater susceptibility among the Caucasian subjects, a likely reflection of reduced chemical penetration through the stratum corneum of black subjects and, thus, reduced allergen exposure.

Another approach to the study of susceptibility to skin allergy relies on patch test surveys of clinics comparing response profiles across different

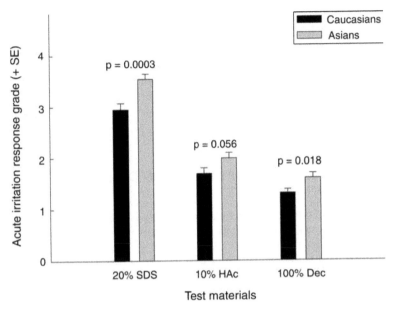

Figure 4 Acute skin irritation responses were compiled for Caucasian and Asian (combined Chinese and Japanese) test subjects across 4 studies conducted between July 1995 and March 1999 at a single test facility. The individual studies were published separately (12,17). The number of test subjects [for the 3 test materials: 20% sodium dodecly sulfate (SDS), 10% acetic acid (HAC), and 100% decanol (DEC)] were: SDS (115 Asian, 107 Caucasian), HAC (117 Asian, 109 Caucasian), and DEC (117 Asian, 108 Caucasian). The time-to-respond for each subject in each study was converted to an acute skin irritation response grade as previously described (12). The mean grades ($\pm$ SE) were determined and compared by t-test. *Source*: From M.K. Robinson, Contact Dermatitis 46:86–93, 2002; by permission.

ethnic populations. Earlier (23) and more recent (24,25) studies have shown similar overall response rates among black and Caucasian patients. Differences have been noted in rates of sensitization to specific allergens; however, there is no ability to discern whether this reflects differences in true susceptibility or simply differences in exposure patterns across the different populations. There have been no reported studies of direct experimental susceptibility or epidemiological profiles of response rates between Caucasian and Asian populations.

RACIAL DIFFERENCES IN ATOPIC DERMATITIS

Another manifestation of skin allergy is atopic dermatitis (26). This differs from allergic contact dermatitis, in that it is commonly a manifestation of immediate-type allergic hypersensitivity (IgE-mediated); whereas allergic contact dermatitis is representative of delayed-type hypersensitivity (T–cell mediated). Also, atopic dermatitis is predominantly found among children and adolescents. As in the case of allergic contact dermatitis, population comparisons based on epidemiologic profiles can be difficult; there is no straight forward way to separate indigenous susceptibility from other etiological factors (exposures, diet, etc.). Still, a recent review (27) has highlighted some differences in susceptibility between Caucasians and either Asian or black populations, with the Caucasian population showing the lesser prevalence.

RACIAL DIFFERENCES IN SENSORY IRRITATION OR SELF-ASSESSED SKIN SENSITIVITY

As noted above, there has been speculation in the past of increased sensory skin reactivity (e.g., sting, burn, itch) among Asian versus Caucasian subjects (7). Unfortunately, the peer-reviewed literature has little to offer towards confirming or refuting this conjecture. Our prior screening of Asian and Caucasian subjects using a modified 5% and 10% lactic acid stinging test (28), showed a similar incidence of "stingers" among Asian (41%) and Caucasian (52%) subjects recruited into an acute irritation patch test study (12). There was also no correlation between reactivity in the stinging test and subsequent erythematous reactivity to topical irritant challenge in either population. A very recent study of thermal pain sensitivity among Asian ethnic sub-populations (Chinese, Malay, Indian) also showed no differences (29). Clearly, these results are not supportive of any generally increased sensory irritation reactivity among Asian subjects.

A somewhat different approach was taken by Jourdain and colleagues in an attempt to gain a more widespread perspective on the question of racial variations in the self-assessed perception of skin sensitivity (30). They phone-surveyed approximately 200 women across four ethnic groups (black, Asian, Caucasian, and Hispanic) residing in the metropolitan area around San Francisco, California. The majority of subjects (52%) considered themselves to have sensitive facial skin. In terms of overall prevalence, there were no significant differences between any of the ethnic groups surveyed. Some specific differences were noted between the populations. These were most commonly related to the causal or triggering factors associated with the facial skin sensitivity (i.e., cosmetics, environmental insults, food, and alcohol) and, to a smaller degree, the type of symptoms elicited (e.g., itch). Overall, there were far more similarities than differences among all these survey subjects.

SUMMARY

As noted earlier, a general caution needs to be applied to any population comparison study reporting differences in skin biology, reactivity, or symptoms.

The caution simply relates to the fact that known intra-individual differences in skin reactivity (19) and the potential breadth of reactivity across large population clusters, makes it difficult to draw definitive conclusions from studies on limited numbers of subjects. With regard to racial differences in skin reactivity, there has been a prevailing tendency to regard blacks as a less sensitive population than other ethnic groups because of lesser penetrability of the stratum corneum (13). Historically consistent findings of reduced irritant and induced allergic skin reactivity among black subjects versus Caucasians tend to support this notion; although, this is not true universally, as other studies have indicated a general similarity in irritant reactivity among blacks, Caucasians and Asians (31,32).

Direct comparison testing of skin irritation susceptibility between Caucasian and Asian subjects has continued to produce a mixed collection of results since this topic was reviewed previously (1). Increased reactivity among Asian subjects and no difference in reactivity have been reported (17,20), even with repeated testing in the same laboratory (17). The compilation of results across multiple years of testing does provide some additional support for a slightly increased reactivity among Asians in acute irritation testing (22). However, it needs to be emphasized that the magnitude of the measured differences, though statistically significant, were quite small and unlikely to be of much biological relevance–particularly when considered in the context of actual risk of marketplace-relevant skin irritation (33). Differences in neurosensory skin reactivity might be a more meaningful index, if it were to translate into true differences in product acceptability profiles among ethnically diverse consumer populations. Even here, the speculation (7) has been difficult to confirm by direct testing (12) or survey (30).

Understanding both individual and population variation in skin reactivity will continue to be an important consideration as it relates to product and ingredient skin safety testing and risk assessment. As noted above, small differences in reactivity detected within and across studies, may not equate to any real difference in risk of adverse skin responses in the market and should not be used as justification for mandating population-specific safety testing. This is particularly true when other available data (use test, exposure, habits and practices, etc.) support adequate margins of safety (22). Current well devised and documented skin safety testing and risk assessment procedures (34–41) have a proven track record of protecting consumer populations across the globe and such procedures are flexible enough to consider and account for population differences (racial, age, gender, sensitive skin, etc.) whenever they are deemed relevant.

REFERENCES

1. Robinson MK. Population differences in skin structure and physiology and the susceptibility to irritant and allergic contact dermatitis: implications for skin safety testing and risk assessment. Contact Dermatitis 1999; 41:65.

2. Marshall EK, Lynch V, Smith HW. On dichlorethylsulphide (mustard gas) variations in susceptibility of the skin to dichlorethylsulphide. J Pharm Exp Therap 1919; 12:291.

3. Weigand DA. Gaylor JR. Irritant reaction in Negro and Caucasian skin. South Med J 1974; 67:548.

4. Rostenberg A, Kanof NM. Studies in eczematous sensitizations a comparison between the sensitizing capacities of two allergens and between two different strengths of the same allergen and the effect of repeating the sensitizing dose. J Invest Dermatol 1941; 4:505.

5. Kligman AM. The identification of contact allergens by human assay. 3. The maximization test: a procedure for screening and rating contact sensitizers. J Invest Dermatol 1966; 47:393.

6. Kompaore F, Tsuruta H. In vivo differences between Asian, Black and White in the stratum corneum barrier function. Int Arch Occup Environ Health 1993; 65:S223.

7. Asian skin "more prone" to burning, stinging, redness from H&BA products. F-D-C reports: The Rose Sheet, 1998.

8. Christensen M, Kligman AM. An improved procedure for conducting lactic acid stinging tests on facial skin. J Soc Cosmet Chem 1996; 47:1.

9. Rapaport MJ. Patch testing in Japanese subjects. Contact Dermatitis 1984; 11:93.

10. Ishihara M, Takase Y, Hayakawa R, et al. Skin problems caused by cosmetics and quasidrugs: Report by six university hospitals to Ministry of Health and Welfare. Skin Research (Hifu) 1986; 28:80.

11. Basketter DA, Griffiths HA, Wang XM, et al. Individual, ethnic and seasonal variability in irritant susceptibility of skin: The implications for a predictive human patch test. Contact Dermatitis 1996; 35:208.

12. Robinson MK, Perkins MA, Basketter DA. Application of a 4-h human patch test method for comparative and investigative assessment of skin irritation. Contact Dermatitis 1998; 38:194.

13. Weigand DA, Haygood C, Gaylor JR. Cell layers and density of Negro and Caucasian stratum corneum. J Invest Dermatol 1974; 62:563.

14. Hicks SP, Swindells KJ, Middelkamp-Hup MA, et al. Confocal histopathology of irritant contact dermatitis in vivo and the impact of skin color (black vs. white). J Am Acad Dermatol 2003; 48:727.

15. Tadaki T, Watanabe M, Kumasaka K, et al. The effect of topical tretinoin on the photodamaged skin of the Japanese. Tohoku J Exp Med 1993; 169:131.

16. Basketter DA, Whittle E, Griffiths HA, et al. The identification and classification of skin irritation hazard by a human patch test. Food Chem Toxicol 1994; 32:769.

17. Robinson MK. Racial differences in acute and cumulative skin irritation responses between Caucasian and Asian populations. Contact Dermatitis 2000; 42:134.

18. Judge MR, Griffiths HA, Basketter DA, et al. Variation in response of human skin to irritant challenge. Contact Dermatitis 1996; 34:115.

19. Robinson MK. Intra-individual variations in acute and cumulative skin irritation responses. Contact Dermatitis 2001; 45:75.

20. Foy V, Weinkauf R, Whittle E, et al. Ethnic variation in the skin irritation response. Contact Dermatitis 2001; 45:346.
21. Aramaki J, Kawana S, Effendy I, et al. Differences of skin irritation between Japanese and European women. British Journal of Dermatology 2002; 146:1052.
22. Robinson MK. Population differences in acute skin irritation responses—race, sex, age, sensitive skin and repeat subject comparisons. Contact Dermatitis 2002; 46:86.
23. North American Contact Dermatitis Group: Epidemiology of contact dermatitis in North America: 1972. Arch Dermatol 1973; 108:537.
24. Dickel H, Taylor JS, Evey P, et al. Comparison of patch test results with a standard series among white and black racial groups. Am J Contact Dermatitis 2001; 12:77.
25. DeLeo VA. Taylor SC, Belsito DV, et al. The effect of race and ethnicity on patch test results. J Am Acad Dermatol 2002; 46:S107.
26. Hanifin JM. Atopic Dermatitis. In: Middleton E, Reed C. E, Ellis EF, Adkinson NF, Yuninger JW, and Busse WW. Allergy Principles and Practice. 1993; 1581–1604. St. Louis, MO, Mosby.
27. Mar A, Marks R. The descriptive epidemiology of atopic dermatitis in the community. Australasian Journal of Dermatology 1999; 40:73.
28. Christensen M, Kligman AM. An improved procedure for conducting lactic acid stinging tests on facial skin. Journal of Cosmetic Science 1996; 47:1.
29. Yosipovitch G, Meredith G, Chan YH, et al. Do ethnicity and gender have an impact on pain thresholds in minor dermatologic procedures? A study on thermal pain perception thresholds in Asian ethnic groups. Skin Research and Technology 2004; 10:38.
30. Jourdain R, De Lacharriere O, Bastien P, et al. Ethnic variations in self-perceived sensitive skin: epidemiological survey. Contact Dermatitis 2002; 46:162.
31. Gean CJ, Tur E, Maibach HI, et al. Cutaneous responses to topical methyl nicotinate in black, oriental, and caucasian subjects. Arch Dermatol Res 1989; 281:95.
32. McFadden JP, Wakelin SH, Basketter DA. Acute irritation thresholds in subjects with Type I-Type VI skin. Contact Dermatitis 1998; 38:147.
33. Modjtahedi SP, Maibach HI. Ethnicity as a possible endogenous factor in irritant contact dermatitis: comparing the irritant response among Caucasians, blacks, and Asians. Contact Dermatitis 2002; 47:272.
34. Robinson MK, Stotts J, Danneman PJ, et al. A risk assessment process for allergic contact sensitization. Food Chem Toxicol 1989; 27:479.
35. Gerberick GF, Robinson MK, Stotts J. An approach to allergic contact sensitization risk assessment of new chemicals and product ingredients. Am J Contact Dermatitis 1993; 4:205.
36. Gerberick GF, Robinson MK. A skin sensitization risk assessment approach for evaluation of new ingredients and products. Am J Contact Dermatitis 2000; 11:65.
37. Robinson MK, Gerberick GF, Ryan CA, et al. The importance of exposure estimation in the assessment of skin sensitization risk. Contact Dermatitis 2000; 42:251.

38. Gerberick GF, Robinson MK, Felter SP, et al. Understanding fragrance allergy using an exposure-based risk assessment approach. Contact Dermatitis 2001; 45:333.
39. Felter SP, Robinson MK, Basketter DA, et al. A review of the scientific basis for uncertainty factors for use in quantitative risk assessment for the induction of allergic contact dermatitis. Contact Dermatitis 2002; 47:257.
40. Robinson MK, Cohen C, de Fraissinette AD, et al. Non-animal testing strategies for assessment of the skin corrosion and skin irritation potential of ingredients and finished products. Food Chem Toxicol 2002; 40:573.
41. Robinson MK, Perkins MA. A strategy for skin irritation testing. Am J Contact Dermat 2002; 13:21.

10

Ethnic Itch

Daniela A. Guzman-Sanchez, Christopher Yelverton, and Gil Yosipovitch

Department of Dermatology, Wake Forest University School of Medicine, Salem, North Carolina, U.S.A.

INTRODUCTION

Itch is one of the most common dermatologic symptoms. It has a significant impact on quality of life for numerous patients suffering from skin conditions such as atopic eczema, psoriasis, urticaria and also systemic diseases such as uremia (1).

Itch shares many similarities with pain, as both are unpleasant sensory experiences and in chronic conditions lead to serious impairment in quality of life (2). Pain and itch experiences may be modified by personal, genetic and cultural factors.

In the last 10 years, a growing field of pain management has addressed perceptions of pain in ethnic populations (3–7). However, there is a lack of salient literature on itch in ethnic groups. The focus of this chapter is to discuss differences in clinical presentations of itch among ethnic groups and also to describe future directions of research in this previously unexplored field.

UNIQUE PRESENTATIONS OF ITCH IN ETHNIC POPULATIONS

Atopic Dermatitis

Recently, several reports described that the clinical picture of atopic dermatitis (AD) may differ in dark skinned individuals when compared to the classic flexural eczema seen in fair skin (8–10). Nnoruka (10) reported that in Nigerian children the most frequent presentation of AD is the extensor surface involvement of elbow, wrist, and knee joints (10).

It has been suggested that atopic children with dark skin are about six times more likely to develop severe AD (10,11). In Hispanics, the clinical picture of AD is similar to that in Caucasian. However, there are more residual pigmentary changes (12).

Dermatologists should note that erythema can be a misleading indicator of severity in these children. The difficulties of assessment due to skin pigmentation may mean that severe cases are not being detected and appropriately treated (11).

Prurigo mitis

Prurigo mitis is an itchy rash seen mostly in African Americans and is highly associated with AD. It begins early in childhood and is characterized by small, rounded, flesh-colored or erythematous, flat-topped papules, and vesicles. Severe itching leads to excoriation and scarring (13).

Lichen Amyloidosis

Cutaneous amyloidosis is classified into three major types: lichen amyloidosis, macular amyloidosis, and nodular amyloidosis. These conditions are not associated with systemic disease (14,15).

Lichen amyloidosis is the most common form of cutaneous amyloidosis and is characterized by the clinical appearance of itchy, brown papules and plaques, predominantly on the extensor areas of the extremities, back, chest, and abdomen. Pruritus is intense and may be a presenting symptom. Histopathologic findings include hyperkeratosis, hypergranulosis, and deposits of amyloid surrounded by melanophages in the papillary dermis (12,14,15).

Patients from the Middle East, Central and South America, and Asians especially, Chinese are particularly predisposed (12,14,15).

Treatments with sedating antihistamines and topical high-potency corticosteroid are partially effective. In most cases, the pigmentation disorder is not clear, although the patients report an improvement of their itch (12,14,15).

Unique Itchy Dermatosis in Japanese Skin

Prurigo Pigmentosa (Nagashima's Disease)

Nagashima first described this entity as "a peculiar pruriginous dermatosis with gross reticular pigmentation" in 1971 and named the disease "prurigo pigmentosa in 1978. It has been described mostly in Japan (16); although there are recent reports from Spain and Turkey (16–19).

While the pathogenesis is unclear, it has been speculated that CD8 lymphocyte cells and ethnic predisposition may play important roles (18).

Prurigo pigmentosa frequently affects young women and is mostly seen in the spring and summer. It is characterized by the sudden onset of reddish papules coalescing to form a reticulated pattern and accompanied by extreme pruritus (18,19).

The typical rash that is found is symmetrically distributed and tends to localize especially on the upper back, nape of the neck, clavicular region and the chest (18). These lesions last from one week to one year and some recurrences have been reported (16,18). Resolution occurs with hyperpigmentation: coexisting reticular macular hyperpigmentation with a coarse marble like appearance observed in and around the papules (16,17,19).

Histopathology findings include spongiosis, exocytosis, lichenification and, degeneration of the basal layer. Parakeratosis with elongation of the epidermal rete ridge, papillary dermal edema and dilatation of the superficial blood vessels may also be seen. A perivascular lymphocytic infiltrate is among other histopathology findings. Pigmented lesions reveal pigmentary incontinence and mild perivascular round cell infiltration (16).

Treatment includes Dapsone, Sulfametoxazole and Minocycline which have been effective at inducing a long remission (16,18,19).

Actinic Lichen Planus

Actinic lichen planus (ALP) is also known as: lichen planus tropicus, lichen planus subtropicus, lichenoid melanodermatitis, lichen planus atrophicus annularis and summertime actinic lichenoid dermatitis. These are all variants of lichen planus that affects, mainly children and teenagers and are extremely pruritic (20,21). In the series published by Bouassida, the incidence was estimated at one case per million inhabitants per year, mean age of onset was 17 years old and male to female ratio 1:2.5; and phototypes ranged from III to V (22). Most cases have been described in the Middle East (20–22).

Pathogenesis of ALP is relatively unknown. Onset typically occurs during the spring, with remission during the winter, suggesting that sunlight exposure may be the main precipitating factor (23). However, evidence for photo-induced pathogenesis is still lacking (21). Lesions are located most frequently on the face (20–22,24). Three clinical types are recognized: annular, dyschromic and pigmented. The most common form is the annular type, which consists of erythematous brownish plaques with a circular configuration (21,22). The dyschromic type presents with discrete and confluent whitish papules. The pigmented type consists of hypermelanotic patches, sometimes assuming a melasma-like appearance (24).

Histopathology is characterized by lichenoid lymphohistiocytic infiltrate, dyskeratotic kertinocytes and wedge-shaped hypergranulosis. Marked melanin incontinence and mild inflammation is usually seen (25).

Treatment with topical corticosteroids combined with sunscreen has been reported to be effective (20–24).

PAIN STUDIES IN ETHNIC SKIN: FUTURE DIRECTIONS FOR STUDIES IN ITCH

A recent large, multicenter study showed significant differences in responses to multiple painful stimuli among the ethnic groups. The authors evaluated pain thresholds using thermal, cold and pressure methods as well as through psychological questionnaires. Results suggested that African Americans had significantly lower tolerance for each of the stimuli, compared to the Caucasian group (6).

We previously studied pain perception threshold, in 49 subjects from several ethnic groups in Asia, including Chinese, Malay and Indian. We examined pain thresholds on the forehead and forearm, typical sites for cosmetic and minor surgical procedures (4). Using a quantitative sensory testing device (TSA 2001; Medoc Inc., Ramat Yishai, Israel), we measured the thermal pain thresholds using "method of limits" (the subjects were exposed to a noxious heat stimulus of changing intensity and asked to halt the stimulus increase when it first became uncomfortable). No significant differences were found in thermal pain thresholds among ethnic groups. However, this study did not address pain tolerance as an important factor in explaining the difference of pain perception among the ethnic groups (4).

The Use of Questionnaires to Study Itch in Ethnic Populations

Many studies have used validated pain questionnaires to characterize pain perception in ethnic groups (3–7). In a series published by Hastie et al. (5), questionnaires were used to evaluate pain in ethnic groups and the impact of techniques to reduce pain. The study included African Americans, Hispanic and Whites. No differences were found in pain prevalence or severity between ethnic populations. The findings showed that African Americans and Hispanics used prayer as a means for pain reduction more frequently than Whites (5). It has also been reported that ethnic minorities tend to be under treated for pain when compared to nonHispanic Whites. This is possibly related to ineffective communication between health providers and patients, adequate access to health services and differences in health beliefs between groups (6).

We have studied itch characteristics in several disease entities among different populations in Singapore (26,27). Singapore has a multiethnic society comprised. Chinese (70%), Malay (20%) and Indian (10%). We noted in several of our studies that each group has a unique itch perception. For example, in patients with chronic urticaria, Indians experimented itch associated more to pain than Chinese. This could be related to cultural or geographical issues and further studies are needed (27).

FUTURE DIRECTIONS

In conclusion, there is lack of information about patient perception of itch in ethnic groups. In addition it is important to explore the cultural behaviors and influences of cultural beliefs or preferences in racial and ethnic groups who have itch. This may enhance our understanding of racial and ethnic differences in clinical itch. Research on how economic factors, family and health support systems influence quality of life, quality of care in racial, and ethnic minorities, who are experiencing chronic itch, is of prime importance. Itch assessments that are culturally and linguistically sensitive are needed. Addressing the issues described above could help to reduce racial and ethnic disparities in itch.

REFERENCES

1. Yosipovitch G. Pruritus: an update. Curr Prob Dermatol 2003; 15(4): 135–164.
2. Yosipovitch G, W Greaves M, Schmelz M. Itch. Lancet 2003; 361:690–694.
3. Campbell C, Edwards R, Fillingim R. Ethnic differences in responses to multiple experimental pain stimuli. Pain 2005; 113:20–26.
4. Yosipovitch G, Meredith G, Huak Chan Y, Leok Goh Ch. Do ethnicity and gender have an impact on pain thresholds in minor dermatologic procedures? A study on thermal pain perception thresholds in Asian ethnic groups. Skin Res Technol 2004; 10:38–42.
5. Hastie B, Riley J, Fillingim R. Ethnic differences and responses to pain in healthy young adults. Pain Med 2005; 6(1):61–71.
6. Green C, Anderson K, Baker T, et al. The unequal burden of pain: confronting racial and ethnic disparities in pain. Pain Med 2003; 4(3):277–294.
7. Edwards R, Doleys D, Fillingim R, Lowery D. Ethnic differences in pain tolerance: clinical implications in a chronic pain population. Psychosomatic Med 2001; 63(2):316–323.
8. Halder R, Nootheti P. Ethnic skin disorders overview. J Am Acad Dermatol 2003; 48:143–148.
9. Child F, Fuller L, Higgins E, Du Vivier A. A study of the spectrum of skin disease occurring in a black population in south east London. Br J Dermatol 1999; 141:512–517.
10. Nnoruka E. Current epidemiology of atopic dermatitis in south–eastern nigeria. Int J Dermatol 2004; 43:739–744.
11. Ben–Gashir M, Seed P, Hay R. Reliance of erythema scores may mask severe atopic dermatitis in black children compared with their White counterparts. Br J Dermatol 2002; 147:920–925.
12. Arenas R. Dermatología Atlas, diagnostico y tratamiento. México: Mc Graw Hill, 2005:76–80.
13. Principles of pediatric dermatology e–book http://www.drmhijazy.com/english/chapters/chapter36.htm.
14. Al–Ratrout J, Satti M. Primary localized cutaneous amyloidosis: a clinicopathologic study from Saudi Arabia. Int J Dermatol 1997; 36:428–434.

15. Leow Yung Hian, Yosipovitch Gil. Pruritus in lichen simplex chronicus and Lichen amyloidosis. In: Yosipovitch G, Greaves M,Fleischer A, Mc Glone, ed. Itch Basic Mechanisms Therapy. New York: Marcel Dekker, 2004:255–258.
16. Boer A, Ackerman B. Prurigo pigmentosa (Nagashima's disease). Textbook and Atlas of a distinctive inflammatory disease of the skin. Chatham, Canada: Ardor Scribendi, 2004.
17. Yanguas I, Goday J, Gonzalez–Guemes M, Berridi D, Lozano M, Soloeta R. Prurigo pigmentosa in a White woman. J Am Acad Dermatol 1996; 35:473–475.
18. Gurses L, Gurbuz O, Demircay Z, Kotilog lu E. Prurigo pigmentosa. Int J Dermatol 1999; 38(12):924–925.
19. Gur–Toy G, Gungor E, Aruz F, Aksoy F, Alli N. Prurigo pigmentosa. Int J Dermatol 2002; 41(5):288–291.
20. Peretz E, Grunwald M, Halevy S. Annular plaque on the face. Arch Dermatol 1999; 135:1543–1548.
21. Handa S, Sahoo B. Childhood lichen planus: study of 87 cases. Int J Dermatol 2002; 41:423–427.
22. Bouassida S, Boudaya S, Turki H, Gueriani H, Zahaf A. Actibic lichen planus: 32 cases. Ann Dermatol Venereol 1998; 125(6–7):408–413.
23. Isaacson D, Turner ML, Elgart ML. Summertime actinic lichenoid eruption. J Am Acad Dermatol 1981; 4:404–411.
24. Salman SM, Kibbi AG, Zaynoun S. Actinic lichen planus: a clinicopathologic study of 16 patients. J Am Acad Dermatol 1989; 20:226–231.
25. Weedon D. The lichenoid reaction pattern (interface dermatitis). In: Weedon D, ed. Skin Pathology. 2nd ed. London: Churchill Livingstone, 2002:37.
26. Yosipovitch G, Goon ATJ, Wee J, Chan Y, Zucker I, Goh C. Itch characteristics in chinese patients with atopic dermatitis using a new questionnaire for the assessment of pruritus. Int J Dermatol 2002; 41:212–216.
27. Yosipovitch G, Ansari N, Goon A, Chan YH, Goh CL. Clinical characteristics of pruritus in chronic idiopathic urticaria. Br J Dermatol 2002; 147(1):32–36.

11

Age-Related Changes in Skin Microtopography: A Comparison Between Caucasian and Japanese Women

Sophie Gardinier

CE.R.I.E.S.[a], Neuilly Sur Seine Cedex, France

Hassan Zahouani

Laboratoire de Tribology et Dynamique des Systèmes, UMR CNRS 5513, Ecole Centrale de Lyon–ENI Saint–Etienne, Institut Européen de Tribologie, Ecully Cedex, France

Christiane Guinot

CE.R.I.E.S., Neuilly Sur Seine Cedex, and Computer Science Department, Ecole Polytechnique, Université de Tours, Tours, France

Erwin Tschachler

CE.R.I.E.S., Neuilly Sur Seine Cedex, France and Department of Dermatology, University of Vienna Medical School, Vienna, Austria

INTRODUCTION

Skin aging is associated with progressive changes most prominently a reduction of skin thickness and characteristic changes of the tissue architecture (1).

---

[a] The CE.R.I.E.S. is the Research Centre on Human Healthy Skin funded by CHANEL.

Morphologically, these changes manifest as wrinkles, tissue slackening and pigmentation irregularities. Type and severities of aging-associated skin changes differ among individuals and are influenced by genetic, life style and environmental factors, particularly life-time UV exposure (2,3). Besides these macroscopic changes clearly visible for the naked eye, aging is associated with changes in the skin microtopography (4–8). The skin surface is characterized by a typical relief which reflects the three-dimensional (3-D) organization of the deeper layers (9) and "may be considered as a mirror of the functional status of the skin" (10). Variations of the pattern of the skin surface microrelief during skin aging and skin diseases, as well as for the efficacy test of skin care products have been the subject of considerable interest for many years (5–7,11). Over the past decades, technological advances in the assessment of the skin surface micromorphology have led to a better understanding of the effects of intrinsic and extrinsic factors on skin microtopography. For example, it has been well established that characteristic changes in the network of skin lines occur with age, leading to digging of certain lines and vanishing of others (5–7). However, detailed and quantitative description of the evolution of skin lines with age are only rarely reported in the literature (12–14) as most of the published results are based on standard parameters which are used for the description of surface topographies in general without being specifically adjusted to the skin. For this reason, we have adapted to a 3-D white light interferometer which works with a high vertical and lateral resolution, enabling a precise characterization of the skin lines network. We used this approach to study characteristics of the skin surface topography and their association with aging by quantifying and comparing the morphological changes occurring in the microrelief of the volar forearm.

CHANGES OF THE SKIN MICRORELIEF IN JAPANESE AND FRENCH WOMEN WITH AGE

When studying changes of skin aging in two different ethnic populations, a great variety of confounding factors, in particular, deriving from a different environment and lifestyle habits (2,3), can hardly be controlled. There are valid *pro* and *contra* arguments for and against either studying a resident ethnic population and comparing it to a migrant population residing in the same area or choosing two resident populations in two different countries. When confronted with that choice, we arbitrarily chose the latter approach, with the outlook that in future studies also the former approach should be addressed. Therefore, French and Japanese volunteers who participated in this study were recruited in France and Japan respectively. Three hundred and fifty-six French-Caucasian women living in the Ile-de-France area and 120 Japanese women from Sendai, aged between 20 and 80, with an apparent healthy skin, and without systemic or topical treatment with known effects on skin, were included. Women were not allowed to apply skin care or make-up products on the investigated skin sites for at least 12 hours before skin replicas were taken with silicon rubber (Silfo®, Flexico Ltd., England) on the left volar forearm at identical sites at equal distance between wrist and elbow. In both laboratories, the room temperature was kept at (mean ± standard deviation) $21 \pm 2°C$ and the relative humidity at $50 \pm 5\%$ and all procedures were performed after a 30-minute rest period for the participating women in an air-conditioned room. Care was taken to preserve the orientation of the replica to allow for accurate interpretation.

Analysis of the skin replicas was carried out by vertical scanning interferometry (VSI), also called white-light interferometry (Interferometer Wyko NT 2000, Veeco, Germany) (15,16). In this technique, a white-light beam passes through a microscope objective to the skin replica. A beam splitter reflects half of the incident beam to the reference surface (15,16). The beams reflected from the skin replica and the reference surface combine at the beam splitter to form a pattern of interference fringes, whose intensity is recorded by a CCD Camera. Then, an algorithm processed fringe modulation data from the intensity signal to calculate the height of each point forming the topographical signal. The vertical resolution value of the VSI mode is about 3 nm with vertical range of 1000 μm. Lateral resolution is a function of the magnification objective and the chosen detector array size. The range of lateral resolution is between 0.08 μm and 3.2 μm depending on the objective size. The sampling steps and the size of the area which can be scanned depend on the choice of the objective. A major advantage of this technique is the ability to extend the area of analysis by "stitching" (15,16). The stitching method is an automatic approach to establish a composite image from several individual parts of a large sampling area (15,16). The algorithm is able to stitch together previously stored data sets or data of measurements in progress to create a larger field of view without switching to a lower magnification. This approach preserves the resolution required to depict small features within a large area, and allows viewing of the skin surface features that previously could not be imaged with a single measurement. Figure 1 shows an illustration of the stitching method.

The topographic parameters analysed included twelve standard "global parameters" traditionally used to quantify the topography of any given surface (12). Three families of global parameters were quantified: five depth parameters (SRa, SRq, SRz, SRpm, SRvm), two space parameters (Smx, Smy), and four motif parameters (SRx, SRy, SARx, SARy) (Fig. 2). In addition the total "surface developed" (SDEV) was assessed, which provides information of the proportion of relief contained in an image with respect to the whole area analysed.

Mean arithmetic depth after levelling: SRa

$$SRa = \frac{1}{NM} \sum_{i=1}^{N} \sum_{j=1}^{M} |Z_{ij}(x, y)|$$

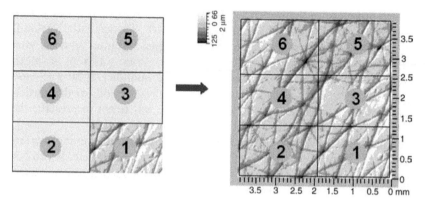

Figure 1 Stitching of elementary zones allows creating a larger sampling area by maintaining the high resolution.

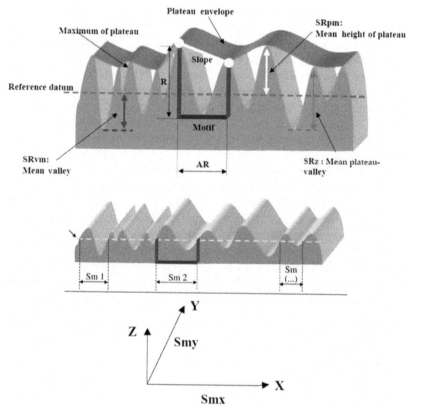

Figure 2 Global parameters of the skin microrelief.

Least mean square value of the heights distribution after levelling: SRq

$$SRq = \left[\frac{1}{NM} \sum_{j=1}^{N} \sum_{i=1}^{M} Z_{ij}^{2}(x, y) \right]^{1/2}$$

Mean value of plateau-valley height: SRz

$$SRz = \frac{1}{NM} \sum_{j=1}^{N} \sum_{i=1}^{M} (\text{Hplateau-Hvalley})\text{max}_{ij}$$

Mean height of plateau: SRpm

$$SRpm = \frac{1}{NM} \sum_{i=1}^{N} \sum_{j=1}^{M} [Z_{ij}(x) - \text{Zmoy}] \quad Z(x) > 0$$

Mean heights of valleys: SRvm

$$SRvm = \frac{1}{NM} \sum_{i=1}^{N} \sum_{j=1}^{M} [Z_{ij}(x) - \text{Zmoy}] \quad Z(x) > 0$$

In addition to these global parameters, we have defined 13 new parameters specifically computed by morphological analysis of the skin surface (12). Because they provide detailed topographical information, we will refer to them as "local parameters,"

These parameters express:

- The density of the lines according to their orientation every 20° with the body axis (9) used as the principal axis of orientation: DENS20, DENS40 ... DENS180, expressed in percentage (Fig. 3). For example, DENS20 expresses the number of primary and secondary lines between 0° and 20° as compared to the whole area analysed (0°–180°).
- The density of the lines according to their depth: DENSZ1 (lines < 30 μm of depth), DENSZ1-Z2 (lines between 30 μm and 60 μm of depth) and DENSZ2 (lines > 60 μm of depth), expressed in percentage with regard to the total number of lines detected on the whole area analysed. For example, DENSZ1 represents the number of lines smaller than 30 μm of depth as compared to the total number of lines detected in the whole area analysed.
- The anisotropy index, ANISO, which corresponds to the percentage of furrows oriented in different directions. The higher the anisotropy index the more the lines tend to be oriented in one direction, the smaller the anisotropy index the more the lines are oriented in different directions.

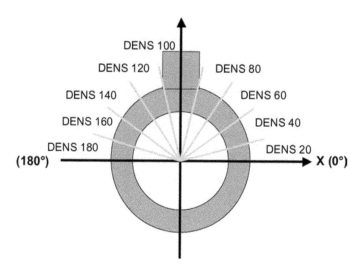

Figure 3 Parameters of density of lines according to their orientation every 20° on the replica.

The statistical analysis was performed using the SAS® software release 8.1 (17). For each population, the links between the 25 parameters were explored using principal component analysis (PCA) (18). Then, to visualize the associations between the parameters, a graphical display was produced using the two first principal components as an axes system. Finally, the individual links between each parameter and age were studied using Spearman correlation coefficients and linear regression models using R^2 (19).

To visualize the associations between the different skin surface parameters, a graphical display was produced using the two first components of the PCA as an axes system. Figure 4 represents the graphical display for Caucasian women. It showed that the global parameters (♦ diamond symbol) are grouped on the right of the figure and are opposed to almost all the local parameters (■ square symbol). These results indicated that the local parameters introduced in the present work yielded information which differed from those of the global parameters. A similar conclusion was found for Japanese women (data not shown).

Global parameters which quantify the totality of the relief were not found to be discriminatory to establish differences between Caucasian and Japanese women. In both populations, they were found to be positively correlated with age ($p < 0.0001$) except for the total "developed surface" (Table 1). As expected, standard parameters of depth (SRa, SRq, SRz, SRpm, SRvm) increased with age in both populations. Space (Smx, Smy) and motif parameters (SRx, SRy, SARx, SARy) which exhibited the highest

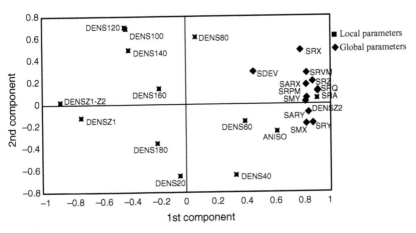

Figure 4 Graphical display of the principal component analysis results showing the relationship between the 25 parameters for Caucasian women.

Table 1 Spearman Correlation Coefficient (r) of Respective Parameters with Age

Global parameters	Caucasian r	Japanese r	Local parameters	Caucasian r	Japanese r
Depth parameters			*Density of lines according to depth*		
Sra	0.59[a]	0.53[a]	DENSZ1 (Z < 30 μm)	−0.44[a]	−0.41[a]
SRq	0.60[a]	0.56[a]	DENSZ1-Z2	−0.54[a]	−0.43[a]
			(30 μm < Z < 60 μm)		
SRz	0.47[a]	0.42[a]	DENSZ2 (> 60 μm)	0.54[a]	0.45[a]
SRpm	0.52[a]	0.40[a]	*Density of lines according to orientation*		
SRvm	0.42[a]	0.41[a]	DENS20	−0.06	−0.08
Space parameters			DENS40	0.23[a]	−0.05
Smx	0.74[a]	0.66[a]	DENS60	0.24[a]	0.04
Smy	0.76[a]	0.64[a]	DENS80	−0.01	0.06
Motif parameters			DENS100	−0.37[a]	−0.04
SRx	0.31[a]	0.32[b]	DENS120	−0.35[a]	0.01
SRy	0.44[a]	0.41[a]	DENS140	−0.29[a]	−0.00
SARx	0.55[a]	0.66[a]	DENS160	−0.12[c]	− 0.09
SARy	0.61[a]	0.68[a]	DENS180	−0.27[a]	−0.18[c]
SDEV	−0.09	0.05	ANISO	0.53[c]	0.27[b]

Note: r p-value (degree of statistical significance).
[a] p < 0.0001.
[b] p < 0.001.
[c] p < 0.05.

correlation coefficients with age were also found to increase during aging (Table 1). These results suggest changes in skin lines network organization resulting in a widening of the plateau area (the area between the lines) with age.

Deepening of the furrows with age was confirmed by analysis of local parameters of the skin microrelief. As shown in Table 1, the density of lines according to their depth was found to be correlated with age in both populations showing an increase in the density of primary lines (DENSZ2: density of lines greater than 60 μm of depth) and a rarefaction of the secondary lines (DENSZ1 and DENSZ1-Z2: density of lines less than 60 μm of depth). Interestingly, this phenomenon was found to be more pronounced in Caucasian women.

The local parameters describing the lines orientation also revealed differences between Caucasian and Japanese women. In Caucasian, DENS100, DENS120, DENS140, DENS160 and DENS180 were found to be negatively correlated with age whereas DENS40 and DENS60 significantly increased, indicating that furrows became oriented along a preferential axis (20° to 60°) with age. By contrast, no link with age was found in Japanese women (Table 1).

As a result of the increase in the density of lines deeper than 60 μm of depth and changes occurring in the orientation of lines with age, the anisotropy index showed a significant increase with age in both populations. The relationship between the anisotropy index and age followed a linear model with a slope of 0.23 for Caucasian women and a slope of 0.08 for Japanese women (Fig. 5). The R^2 values indicate that for Caucasian women, 32% of the anisotropy index variation is explained by age whereas age explains only 9% of the anisotropy index variation in Japanese women. These results indicate that changes in skin microtopography occurred in both populations but are more pronounced in Caucasian women. As illustrated in Figure 6, the characteristic polygonal pattern of the innate skin microrelief is similar in both populations early on in life, but becomes more anisotropic with aging in Caucasian than in Japanese women, leading to a reorientation of the lines in a more parallel fashion. These changes have been associated in the past with progressive loss dermal firmness, density loss and atrophy, decreased elasticity and increase in skin folding capacity (20).

Several previous studies have shown that facial features of skin aging differ between Caucasian and Asian women in their intensity and rate of occurrence, with an earlier appearance of wrinkles in Caucasian (21–24). This phenomenon has been attributed to the inherent properties of Asian skin (25,26). A higher collagen content of the dermis has been suggested to be responsible for the maintenance of a more youthful appearance in Asian individuals (27). Similarly differences of the pigmentary system between Caucasians and Asians may account for a better protection against photo-aging (28). The present study suggests that differences in the time of

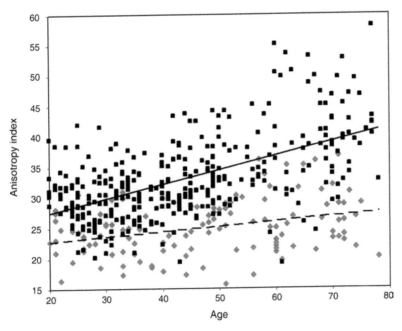

Figure 5 Evolution of the anisotropy index with age in Caucasian (■ individual values) and Japanese women (♦ individual values).

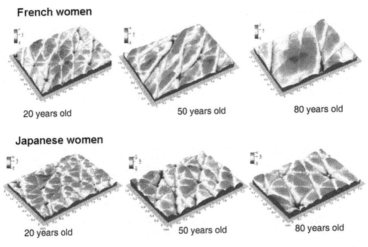

Figure 6 Images of skin replicas in women of different age, illustrating the more pronounced parallel reorganisation of the skin lines network with age more in Caucasian as compared to Japanese women.

occurrence and severity of signs of skin aging between Caucasian and Asian can also readily be verified at the level of skin microtopography.

In the present study, investigations of the skin microrelief have been carried out on the inner forearm which is an area relatively protected against UV-irradiation. Nevertheless, a certain degree of UV-exposure cannot be totally excluded on this area. We cannot exclude that the differences observed in this site were due only in part to chronological skin aging, and that different sun exposure behavior might be a contributing factor. Indeed, the increase in the density of deeper lines associated with an increase in skin anisotropy, has been described for both chronological aging and sun-damaged skin (29). To answer the question as to the contribution of involuntary sun exposure a future comparison of the skin microtopography at fully sun protected body sites will be necessary. An additional remaining question concerns the layer of the skin which contributes most to the changes in the microrelief. Most likely that the changes we observed reflect both structural alteration of the dermis as well as the epidermis (30). However, future studies involving skin biopsies and comparing the histology to the data obtained from skin surface analysis will be necessary to delineate the relative contribution of the different skin layers to the modifications of skin microrelief.

SUMMARY

Whereas differences in the appearance of signs of skin aging as well as skin sensitivity in individuals of different ethnic background have been investigated in several recent studies, studies into differences of the skin microrelief are very rare. Using the interferometry technique, we investigated the skin microtopography from negative replica performed on the left volar forearm of Caucasian and Japanese women. Results were expressed with 12 standard "global parameters" traditionally used to quantify any surface topography, and 13 "local parameters" including parameters of distribution of the lines according to their orientation every 20 degrees, their depth and an anisotropy index. We found that: (i) except for the total developed surface parameter, global parameters were positively correlated with age in both study samples, (ii) Caucasian women showed a more pronounced increase in the density of lines greater than $60\,\mu m$ of depth and a decrease of lines less than $60\,\mu m$ with age than Japanese women, and (iii) the age-related changes in the density of lines according to their orientation were far less pronounced in Japanese as compared to Caucasian women. Finally, the index of anisotropy was found to increase with age in both populations, the Japanese being less affected. Taken together, these results indicate that at the microtopographic level age-associated changes of the skin are markedly stronger in Caucasian than in Japanese women.

ACKNOWLEDGMENTS

The authors thank Isabelle Le Fur and Sabine Guéhenneux (CE.R.I.E.S., Neuilly sur seine, France) for their support, Roberto Viargolu (Ecole Centrale de Lyon, Ecully, France) and Laurence Ambroisine (CE.R.I.E.S., Neuilly sur seine, France) for their technical assistance. Particular thanks are due to Pr Hachiro Tagami (Department of Dermatology, Tohoku University School of Medicine, Sendaï, Japan) for investigations performed in his department.

REFERENCES

1. Lavker RM. Cutaneous aging: chronologic versus photoaging. In: Gilchrest BA, ed. Photodamage. BlackWell Science, Carlton, 1995:123–135.
2. Yaar M, Eller MS, Gilchrest BA. Fifty years of skin aging. J Invest Dermatol Symp Proc 2002; 7:51–58.
3. Jenkins G. Molecular mechanisms of skin ageing. Mech Ageing Dev 2002; 123:801–810.
4. Lavker RM, Kwong F, Kligman AM. Changes in skin surface patterns with age. J Gerontol 1980; 35:348–354.
5. Agache P, Mignot J, Makki S. Microtopography of the skin and aging. In: Kligman A, Takase Y, eds. Cutaneous Aging. Tokyo, Japan: University of Tokyo Press, 1988:475–499.
6. Hayashi S, Mimura K, Nishijima Y. Changes in surface configuration of the skin caused by ageing and application of cosmetics: three-dimensional analysis according to a new system based on image analysis and Fourier transformation. Int J Cosmet Sci 1989; 11:67–85.
7. Corcuff P, De Lacharrière O, Lévêque JL. Extension-induced changes in the microrelief of the human volar forearm: variations with age. J Gerontol Med Sci 1991; 46:223–227.
8. Vörös E, Robert C, Robert AM. Age-related changes of the human skin surface microrelief. Gerontology 1990; 36:276–285.
9. Corcuff P, de Rigal J, Makki S, Lévêque JL, Agache P. Skin relief and aging. J Soc Cosmet Chem 1983; 34:177–190.
10. Fisher T, Wigger-Alberti W, Elsner P. Direct and non-direct measurement techniques for analysis of skin surface topography. Skin Pharmacol Appl Skin Physiol 1999; 12:1–11.
11. Altemeyer P, Erbler H, Krömer T, Duwe HP, Hoffmann K. Interferometry: a new method for no-touch measurement of the surface and volume of ulcerous skin lesions. Acta Derm Venereol 1995; 75:193–197.
12. Zahouani H, Vargiolu R. Mesure du relief cutané et des rides. Physiologie de la peau et explorations fonctionnelles cutanées. Pr Pierre Agache, editions médicales internationales 2000:41–57.
13. Xie Y, Assoul M, Mignot J. Morphological and spectral analysis of human skin surface topography. Innov Tech Biol Med 1993; 14:575–587.
14. Lagarde JM, Rouvrais C, Black D. Topography and anisotropy of the skin surface with ageing. Skin Res Technol 2005; 11:110–119.

15. Schmit J, Creath K. Interferometric Techniques. Encyclopedia of Applied Physics, Update 2, Berlin, Germany: Wiley-VCH, 1999:67–86.
16. Harashki A, Schmit J, Wyant JC. Improved vertical scanning interferometry. Applied Optics 2000; 39:2107–2115.
17. SAS Institute Inc. SAS/STAT® User's Guide, Version 8. Cary, North Carollina: SAS Institute Inc., 1999.
18. Jobson JD. Applied multivariate data analysis. Categorical and Multivariate Methods. Vol. 2. New York: Springer-Verlag, 1992.
19. Jobson JD. Applied multivariate data analysis. Regression and Experimental Design. Vol. 1. New York, New York: Springer-Verlag, 1991.
20. Pierard GE, Uhoda I, Pierard-Franchimont C. From skin microrelief to wrinkles. An area ripe for investigation. J Cosmet Dermatol 2004; 2:21–28.
21. Hillebrand GG, Levine MJ, Miyamoto K. The age-dependant changes in skin condition in African Americans, Asian-Indians, Caucasians, East Asians and Latinos. IFSCC magazine 2001; 4:259–266.
22. Tsukahara K, Fujimura T, Yoshida Y, et al. Comparison of age-related changes in wrinkling and sagging of the skin in Caucasian females and in Japanese females. J Cosmet Sci 2004; 55:373–385.
23. Nouveau-Richard S, Yang Z, Mac-Mary S, et al. Skin ageing: a comparison between Chinese and European populations—a pilot study. J Dermatol Sci 2005; 40:187–193.
24. Tschachler E, Morizot F. Ethnic differences in skin aging. In: Gilchrest BA, Krutman J, eds. Skin Ageing. Heidelberg, Germany: Springer, 2006:24–31.
25. Lee Y, Hwang K. Skin thickness in Korean adults. Surg Radial Anat 2002; 24:183–189.
26. Fanous N. TCA peel for Asians: a new classification and a modified approach. Facial Plast Surg Clin North Am 1996; 4:195–200.
27. Mc Curdy JA. Cosmetic surgery of the Asian face. Thieme New York, New York: Medical Publishers, 1990:1–2.
28. Berardesca E, de Rigal J, Lévêque JL, Maibach HI. In vivo biophysical characterization of skin physiological differences in races. Dermatologica 1991; 182:89–93.
29. Corcuff P, Francois AM, Lévêque JL, Porte G. Microrelief changes in chronologically sun-exposed human skin. Photodermatology 1988; 5:92–95.
30. Pearse AD, Gaskell SA, Marks R. Epidermal changes in human skin following irradiation with either UVB or UVA. J Inves Dermatol 1987; 88:83–87.

12

Inter- and Intraethnic Differences in Skin Micro Relief as a Function of Age and Site

Stephane Diridollou

L'Oréal Recherche, Institute for Ethnic Hair and Skin Research, Chicago, Illinois, U.S.A.

Jean de Rigal

L'Oréal Recherche, Chevilly, France

Bernard Querleux and Therese Baldeweck

L'Oréal Recherche, Aulnay, France

Dominique Batisse and Isabelle Des Mazis

L'Oréal Recherche, Chevilly, France

Grace Yang

L'Oréal Recherche, Institute for Ethnic Hair and Skin Research, Chicago, Illinois, U.S.A.

Frédéric Leroy

L'Oréal Recherche, Aulnay, France

Victoria Holloway Barbosa

L'Oréal Recherche, Institute for Ethnic Hair and Skin Research, Chicago, Illinois, U.S.A.

INTRODUCTION

The concept of race is rooted in the idea of biological difference marked by heredity transmission of physical characteristics. According to some authors, these racial variations were selected based on natural selection to facilitate adaptations to a particular environment (1).

Nevertheless, many anthropologists agree that such strict biological classification is impossible because of the coexistence of races through extensive migrations and hybridization among human groups throughout human history, which has produced a heterogeneous world population (2).

In the face of these issues, some scientists have simply abandoned the concept of race in favor of ethnicity to refer to self-identifying groups based on belief in shared religion, language, nationality, customs, culture, geographic region, as well as criteria to such traits as skin pigmentation, color and form of hair, and physical characteristics (3).

The knowledge of ethnic differences in skin function could explain some disparities seen in dermatologic disorders (4,5) and provide adequate treatments, as well as skin care products adapted for each ethnic population (6,7).

Unfortunately, two recent overviews have pointed out that significant work remains to be performed in the area of ethnic skin to understand and quantify racial or ethnic differences in skin properties and function (7,8).

Indeed, as reported by N.O. Wesley in 2003, most of the published skin investigations using objective instrumental methods were carried out on Caucasian population did not include other ethnic groups (7). In addition, few studies on racial or ethnic differences in skin properties and physiology have been investigated (9–29), and the rare objective methods reported in the literature on physical and biochemical racial skin differences are often confusing, difficult to interpret and mainly inconclusive (7).

As regards to the literature, it seems that the three main confounding factors in studies based on skin ethnicity differences are, the small sample sizes, the incomparable climatic conditions, and geographical localizations (4,7).

The skin micro relief expresses the physical state of the integument, its mechanical properties, hydration, integrity, and its global health status.

The skin micro relief is subject to external and internal influences, such as photo aging and chronological aging. In addition, it has been suggested that there is a close relationship between the dermis architecture, the collagen and elastic networks, and the skin surface pattern (30).

Thus, a study of the skin micro relief of different ethnic groups should provide a global picture of the skin health status differences by ethnicity.

Because of this, we have carried out a set of in vivo experiments on the skin micro relief of different ethnic populations living in Chicago. The investigation was performed in the same climatic conditions, during the summer season of 2004, on 311 women from four ethnic groups. The skin micro relief was investigated using the SkinChip®, which is an in vivo and noninvasive system. Through the study of the line density and orientation, inter- and intraethnic micro relief skin differences as a function age and anatomic site are reported.

POPULATION AND METHODS

Population

Caucasian, and Mexican ethnic groups were enrolled in this study and were distributed as follows: 114 African American, 89 Chinese, 63 Caucasian, and 45 Mexican women.

The subjects' ages ranged from 18 to 87 years. The population was distributed in two age groups as follows:

1. Younger group (18–50 years): 171 women with an average age of 36 ± 9 years (mean $\pm$ SD).
2. Older group (> 51 years): 140 women with an average age of 61 ± 8 years (mean $\pm$ SD).

The distribution of the population according to these two age groups and the ethnicity is presented in Figure 1 .

There were a number of inclusion criteria for the study. It was required that the subjects had lived in Chicago for more than 2 years before the study and have parents and grand parents from the same ethnicity. They also should not have suffered from dermatological disorders or undergone dermatological therapy. Volunteers were requested not to wash or treat their skin with skin care products 1 day before measurements. The dorsal and ventral forearm skin sites, 10 cm below the elbow, were analyzed to represent sun-exposed and sun-protected areas, respectively. For convenience, the skin area that was investigated during this study was not shaved.

This study was conducted for 5 weeks, from 16th of August to 16th of September 2004. The outdoor temperature was $21.7 \pm 2°C$ (mean $\pm$ SD), and the relative humidity was $68 \pm 9\%$ (mean $\pm$ SD) during the period of the investigation.

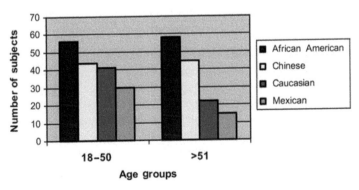

Figure 1   Distribution of the population according to two age groups versus ethnicity.

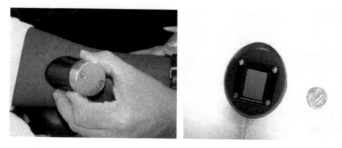

Figure 2 Pictures of the SkinChip® probe.

Methods

The skin micro relief was investigated using an in vivo, noninvasive, and real time imaging system called the SkinChip, which uses active capacitance imaging technology. The images were obtained by applying the SkinChip's probe on the skin's surface for 5 seconds (Fig. 2).

This device is based on the technology produced by ST Microelectronics for sensing fingerprints for security reasons, and was adapted for characterizing other skin sites on the body. The main advantage of this system is that it is fast and does not require any skin print as described in the literature for other systems (24, 31–34). The sensor is composed of an array of more than 92,000 micro-sensors located on a 18 mm × 12.8 mm mm surface. It has been shown to be a convenient in vivo approach to quantifying the skin micro relief, in terms of line density and line orientation (35). This apparatus can map out the micro relief of skin in real-time with a 50 μm resolution. As the micro relief modulates the capacitance between each sensor cell and the skin surface, primary and secondary lines appear accurate. Coding these images in black for high-capacitance and in white for low-capacitance, the micro relief lines appear in white on the pictures as presented in Figure 3. Using a dedicated image analysis software developed by our laboratories, the two main directions of the primary lines of the skin micro relief and the intersections of the micro relief can be detected automatically (Fig. 3).

More precisely, the detection of the main orientations was assessed through three main steps. First, preconditioning of the images (background heterogeneity was corrected) was performed, then a clustering method (k-means) was used to reduce the 256-gray level image to a 5-gray level image. Subsequently, co-occurrence matrices were calculated at different angles; the main coefficients are plotted versus the angle, and the two first peaks are representative of the two main directions. The intersections of the micro relief are calculated from the preconditioned image. After thresholding at the 170th gray level, a thinning process is carried out before the detection of "corners" at each crossing of the lines (35).

(A)   **(B)**

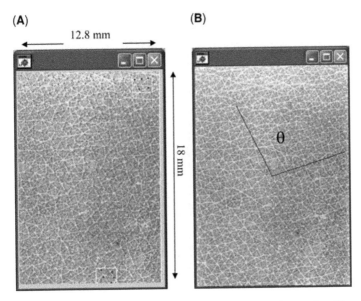

Figure 3   Images obtained on the ventral forearm from of a 35 year-old woman. (A) The white lines reflect the skin micro relief lines, the grey dots reflect the number of intersections of the micro relief lines, the white squares correspond to the areas automatically excluded to the analysis because of the uncertainty of the intersection detections, and **(B)** the two dark lines indicate the 2 main directions of the primary lines of the skin micro relief.

In this way, two parameters can be determined:

1. CD: the corner density, which reflects the number of intersections of the micro relief skin lines per cm^2.
2. $\theta = $ (Angle1-Angle2): the angle difference of the two main directions of the micro relief.

The corner density (CD) can be related to the line density of the micro relief, while the angle difference of the two main directions (θ) can be related to the level of isotropy of the skin.

The lower the CD, the lower the line density of the skin micro relief. The lesser the angle difference, the greater the two main directions of the micro relief come together, and this results in a lower level of isotropy. Two skin micro relief examples obtained on the ventral site of the forearm from of a 30 and 78 year-old women are presented in Figure 4.

Statistical Analysis

Explorative data analysis was performed using SPSS for Windows version 11.5 (SPSS Inc. Chicago, IL, USA).

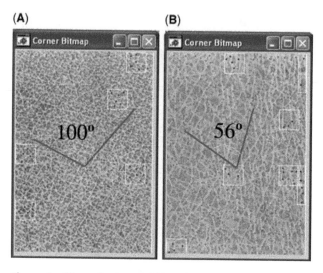

Figure 4 (*See color insert*) Skin micro relief obtained on the ventral forearm from (**A**) a 30-year-old woman (**B**) a 78-year-old woman. The density of intersections and the angle difference of the two main directions of the micro relief are 384 and $286/cm^2$, and 100 and 56°, respectively, for the 30- and 78-year-old women. In this example, a decrease in the number of intersections and a convergence of the two main directions of the micro relief are observed with increased age.

1. The inter and intraethnic micro relief characteristics have been studied as a function of age and site.
2. Statistical differences among different groups were evaluated with two-ways ANOVA test for each parameter.

A p-value < 0.05 was considered statistically significant. The results are expressed as mean $\pm 95\%$ confidence intervals on the mean for each group. All significant differences are identified on the graphs with an asterisk.

RESULTS AND DISCUSSION

Whole Sample

Properties of the skin have been studied as a function of skin site and age without considering the ethnicity from which the results came. The results are as follows:

Whole Sample/Site Difference

The results showed a significant difference between the ventral and dorsal site of the forearm (Fig. 5). The CD is significantly lower, and the angle difference of the two main directions is significantly higher on the dorsal site compared to the ventral side.

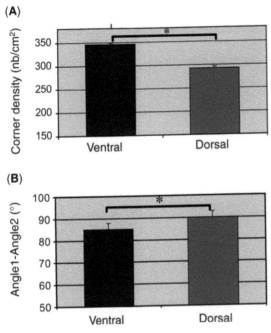

Figure 5 Whole sample: (**A**) corner density and (**B**) difference of the two chief directions of the micro relief as a function of the two forearm sites (mean $\pm$ confidence interval). Significant, $*p < 0.001$.

This revealed significant site differences between the two sides of the forearm, pointing out that the line density of the skin micro relief is lower on the dorsal than ventral site of the forearm, with a higher level of isotropy. This result suggested anatomical and/or physiological site skin differences, due to original or environmental factors including solar exposure and/or mechanical stress.

It is important to point out that the influence of the hair follicles was more predominant on the dorsal site than on the ventral site. Thus, the hair could influence how the two micro relief parameters are measured.

For further investigations, a new algorithm is being developed which improves the analysis of pictures by better distinguishing the hairs and taking them into account.

Whole Sample/Age Difference

For the whole sample, the results show that there is an inverse significant relationship between CD and age on the ventral site but not on the dorsal site (Fig. 6A). There is also an inverse significant relationship between the angle difference of the two main directions and age but on both sides of the forearm (Fig. 6B).

(A)

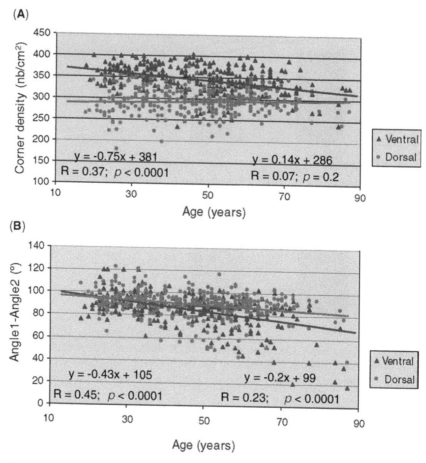

Figure 6 Whole sample: (**A**) corner density and (**B**) difference of the two chief directions of the micro relief, on the ventral (in black) and dorsal (in gray) sites as a function of age.

In conclusion, these results reveal that the line density of the skin micro relief decreases with age on the ventral site, but seems constant with age on the dorsal site. In addition, the two main directions of the micro relief come together with age on the ventral and dorsal sites, suggesting a decrease of the level of isotropy with age on both sides of the forearm.

The result regarding no apparent change of the line density of the skin micro relief on the dorsal site of the forearm with age seems surprising as this site is usually exposed to sunlight and is sensitive to the solar aging effect. Nevertheless, this result is consistent with data reported by Manuskiatti et al. in 1998 (24), who has revealed an increase of the roughness of the skin with age on the volar but not on the dorsal side of the forearm. In this case, the roughness was determined using silicon negative replica that was analyzed using a SkinVisiometer®, which is a photometric device (24).

This result can be explained by a great disparity of the data on this site (Figs. 6A and B) because of different sun exposure habits that are not directly correlated with the age factor and is strongly dependent on each subject. Nevertheless, further studies have to be done to confirm these preliminary results.

Our results obtained on the ventral side of the forearm which pointed out a decrease of the line density and level of isotropy of the skin micro relief with age are consistent with data reported in the literature that was carried out on the same area. Corcuff et al. reported a study involving 116 Caucasian subjects that used an image analysis of skin replicas. The two main directions of the micro relief became closer, and the line density of the micro relief decreased according to age (31). Lagarde et al. reported a study involving 80 Caucasian subjects (40 women and 40 men), and used silflo skin prints that were analyzed by projection of interference fringes and phase shift. That recent study had the same results in terms of an increase of the level of anisotropy and roughness with age (34).

These results are interesting and demonstrate that SkinChip's results are consistent with those obtained using other standard systems based on skin print analysis. This device takes less than 10 seconds to get a skin micro relief image and does not require any skin prints; hence, it appears to be a convenient way to investigate the skin micro relief on a large number of subjects. Our results have to be linked to skin structure change with age.

Lavker et al. suggested, in 1980, that there is a close relationship between the dermis architecture, the collagen network, and the skin surface pattern (30).

In addition, several authors have revealed that there are changes in the skin as a function of age such as: the collagen metabolism and composition become altered (36), the amounts of insoluble collagen and cross-linking increase (37), the ratio of type III to type I collagen changes (38), and there are variations in the elastic network (39). The decrease in collagen synthesis activity and the disorganization of the fibril network with age may account for the increase of the skin roughness and level of anisotropy observed particularly on the ventral side of the forearm which leads to a decrease in the number of furrows. These tend to become deeper and can change their orientation by becoming closer together with age and thus lead to the appearance of small wrinkles.

The changes of the skin structures with age have also been reported by several authors to be related to a thinner dermis (40–46), an increase of the hypo-echogenecity of the upper part of the dermis (41,43–48), a decrease of the ultrasound coefficient attenuation (49), and skin that is less elastic (17,40,44,50–54), less tense (44,55) and stiffer with age (40,44,54,56–58).

Ethnic Populations

The inter- and intraethnic micro relief skin characteristics have been studied as a function of age and site, in terms of line density and level of isotropy. The results are discussed subsequently.

Ventral Site

Ethnic Difference: *For the younger group,* the CD and the angle difference of the two main directions are significantly lower for Caucasians than for African American, Mexican, and Asian women (Figs. 7A and B).

For the older group, the CD is significantly lower for Caucasians compared to African American and Asian women. In addition, the angle difference is significantly lower for Caucasians and Asians than for African American women (Figs. 7A and B).

Thus, the line density of the skin micro relief for Caucasian women is lower and has a lower level of isotropy than the other ethnic groups. This difference is greatest when Caucasian women are compared to African American women.

For both skin micro relief measurements, the values for Mexican women seem to be between those of African American and Caucasian women (Figs. 7A and B).

In 1998, Manuskiatti et al. used a silicon negative replica to study the roughness of skin using the ventral side of the forearm of Black and White

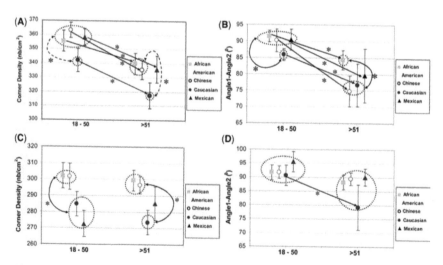

Figure 7 (A) Corner density and (B) difference of the two chief directions of the micro relief, as a function of age and ethnicity groups on the ventral forearm, and (C) and (D) on the dorsal forearm respectively (mean ± confidence interval). Significant, $^*p < 0.05$.

subjects (24). They did not see any significant difference between the different ethnicities. However, the study was conducted on only a small number of subjects, which consisted of 12 Black and 10 White females (24).

Our results obtained on 311 females from four ethnic groups are unique and reveal for the first time that the micro relief of the skin varies as a function of ethnicity and suggests that there are anatomical and/or physiological ethnic skin differences.

Age Change: For the four ethnic groups, the CD and the angle difference of the two main directions are significantly lower for the older group compared to the younger group (Figs. 7A and B). This means that the line density of the skin micro relief decreases and the two main directions of micro relief became closer as the age of the skin increased for all the ethnic groups.

Even if no statistic interaction between age and ethnicity has been observed, we have pointed out that the percentage of decrease of the CD from the younger group to elderly group is −4, −6, −7, and −8% for African American, Mexican, Caucasian, and Chinese women, respectively.

The same trend is observed for the angle difference, which is to say that the percent decrease from the younger group to older group is −8, −11, −11, and −17% for African American, Mexican, Caucasian, and Chinese women, respectively.

It seems that the age effect is less pronounced on the skin micro relief of African American women than for the three other ethnicities and suggests that the African American population is less affected with chronological aging compared to the three other ethnic groups. Further studies have to be done to confirm these results.

Dorsal Site

Ethnic Difference: *For the younger group*, the CD is significantly lower for Caucasians and Mexicans compared to African American and Asian women (Fig. 7C). The angle differences between the two main directions of the micro relief do not change as a function of ethnicity (Fig. 7D).

For the older group, the CD is significantly lower for Caucasians than for the African American and Asian women (Fig. 7C). The angle differences between the two main directions of the micro relief did not change as a function of ethnicity (Fig. 7D).

Thus, on the dorsal site of the forearm, we have revealed that the line density of the skin micro relief of Caucasian and Mexican women is lower than the other two ethnic groups. However, in comparison with the results on the ventral site, significant differences in the level of anisotropy were not observed between the four ethnic groups.

Age Change: On the dorsal site for the four ethnic groups, the CD and the micro relief angle difference of the two main directions follow the same trend with age as seen on the ventral side, which is to say that these two micro relief parameters are lower for the older group compared to the younger group. Nevertheless, in comparison with the ventral site, no significant difference has been revealed, except for the Caucasian group where there were differences seen in the angle of the micro relief (Fig. 7D). As a matter of fact, for this ethnic group, the angle difference of the two main directions of the micro relief has been revealed to be significantly lower for the older group than the younger group. This suggests that there may be a photo-aging effect that is more pronounced for Caucasians compared to the three other populations (Fig. 7D).

This is consistent with what is usually written in the literature where it states that the photo-aging effect is influenced by the photoprotective role of the melanin in skin of color. Thus, darker skin is less susceptible to the solar aging effect (5,6,17,59–63).

To specifically investigate the importance of the melanin further, future studies will consider the degree of pigmentation in the evolution of the micro relief with age.

CONCLUSION

The investigation of the skin micro relief of 311 women from four ethnic groups has revealed inter- and intraethnic differences in skin micro relief as a function of age and skin site.

We have revealed that the line density of the skin micro relief is lower and that the level of isotropy is higher on the dorsal site compared to ventral site of the forearm for the four ethnic populations.

We have also shown that the line density and level of isotropy of the skin micro relief are less pronounced in Caucasians than in the three other ethnic groups studied. The largest difference was seen between the Caucasian and the African American ethnic groups and suggests that there are anatomical or physiological property differences in ethnic skin.

Finally, it has been demonstrated that the line density and the level of isotropy of the skin micro relief decrease with age for all four ethnic groups. This leads to a decrease in the number of furrows, which become deeper and closer together with age. This age effect seems more pronounced with Caucasian skin compared to the other three ethnic populations. The African American population appears to be the ethnic group that is the least affected by age.

We have revealed that the micro relief of the skin is different according to 4 ethnic groups. We have also pointed out that the age effects may be a function of ethnicity.

This reveals, particularly, that the skin of African American women show less chronological and photo aging effects than that of the three other ethnic groups.

We have also revealed that the SkinChip is a convenient and fast way to investigate the micro relief of the skin on a large number of subjects.

A future project will be to compare these results obtained in Chicago with results obtained from other countries with different environments (Europe, Africa, South America and Asia).

This should be useful in improving our knowledge about skin of people from different ethnic populations and helping to develop specific products that are customized to all these populations.

REFERENCES

1. Coon CS. The origin of races. New York, New York: Alfred A Knopf, 1962.
2. Goldstein DB, Chikhi L. Human migrations and population structure: what we know and why it matters. Annu Rev Genomics Hum Genet 2002; 3:129–152.
3. Gordon, Milton M. Assimilation in American Life: The Role of Race, Religion, and National Origins. New York, New York: Oxford University Press, 1964.
4. Modjtahedi SP, Maibach HI. Ethnicity as a possible endogenous factor in irritant contact dermatitis: comparing irritant response among Caucasians, Blacks and Asians. Contact Dermatitis 2002; 47(5):272–278.
5. Taylor SC. Skin of color: Biology, structure, function, and implications for dermatologic disease. J Am Acad Dermatol 2002; 46:S41–S62.
6. Halder RM, Nootheti PK. Ethnic skin disorders overview. J Am Acad Dermatol 2003; 48:S143–S148.
7. Wesley NO, Maibach HI. Racial (ethnic) differences in skin properties. Am J Dermatol 2003; 4:843–860.
8. Beradesca E, Maibach H. Ethnic skin: overview of structure and function. J Am Acad Dermatol 2003; 48:S139–S142.
9. Rienertson RP, Wheatley VR. Studies on the chemical composition of human epidermal lipids. J Invest Dermatol 1959; 32:49–69.
10. Johnson LC, Corah NL. Racial differences in skin resistance. Science 1963; 139:766–769.
11. Freeman RG, Cockerell EG, Armstrong J, Knox JM. Sunlight as a factor influencing the thickness of epidermis. J Invest Dermatol 1962; 39:295–297.
12. Thomson ML. Relative efficiency of pigment and horny layer thickness in protecting the skin of European and Africans against solar ultraviolet radiation. J Physiol (London) 1955; 127:236–246.
13. Weigand DA, Haygood C, Gaylor JR. Cell layers and density of Negro and Caucasian stratum corneum. J Invest Dermatol 1974; 62:563–568.
14. Wilson D, Berardesca E, Maibach HI. In vitro transepidermal water loss: differences between black and white human skin. Br J Dermatol 1988; 119:647–652.
15. Rebora A, Guarrera M. Racial differences in experimental skin infection with *Candida albicans*. Acta Derm Venereol (Stockholm) 1988; 68:165–168.
16. Corcuff P, Lotte PC, Rougier A, Maibach HI. Racial differences in corneocytes: a comparison between black, white and oriental skin. Acta Derm Venereol 1991; 71:146–148.
17. Beradesca E, De Rigal J, Leveque JL, Maibach HI. In vivo biophysical characterization of skin physiological differences in races. Dermatologica 1991; 182:89–93.

18. La Ruche G, Cesarini JP. Histology and physiology of black skin. Ann Dermatovenereol 1992; 119:567–574.
19. Sugino K, Imokawa G. Maibach HI. Ethnic difference of stratum corneum lipid in relation to stratum corneum function. J Invest Dermatol 1993; 100:597.
20. Kompaore F, Marty JP, Dupont C. In vivo evaluation of the stratum corneum barrier function in Blacks, Caucasians and Asians with two noninvasive methods. Skin Pharmacol 1993; 63:200–207.
21. Reed JT, Ghadially R, Elias PM. Skin type, but neither race nor gender, influence epidermal permeability barrier function. Arch Dermatol 1995; 131:1134–1138.
22. Warrier AG, Kligman AM, Harper RA, Bowman J, Wickett RR. A comparison of black and white skin using noninvasive methods. J Soc Cosmet Chem 1996; 47:229–240.
23. Reilly DM, Ferdinando D, Johnston C. The epidermal nerve fibre network: characterization of nerve fibres in human skin by confocal microscopy and assessment of racial variations. Br J Dermatol 1997; 137:163–170.
24. Manuskiatti W, Schwindt DA, Maibach HI. Influence of age, anatomic site and race on skin roughness and scaliness. Dermatology 1998; 196:401–407.
25. Beradesca E, Pirot F, Singh M. Differences in stratum corneum pH gradient when comparing White Caucasian and Black African American skin. Br J Dermatol 1998; 139:855–857.
26. Sueki H, Whitaker-Menezes D, Kligman AM. Structural diversity of mast cell granules in Black and White skin. Br J Dermatol 2001; 144:85–93.
27. Harding CR, Moore AE, Rogers JS, et al. Dandruff: a condition characterized by decreased levels of intercellular lipids in scalp stratum corneum and impaired barrier function. Arch Dermatol Res 2002; 294:221–230.
28. Jsourdain R, De Lacharriere O, Bastien P, Maibach HI. Ethnic variations in self-perceived sensitive skin: epidemiological survey. Contact Dermatitis 2002; 46:162–169.
29. Hicks SP, Swindells KJ, Middelkamp-Hup MA, Sifakis MA, Gonzalez E, Gonzalez S. Confocal histopathology of irritant contact dermatitis in vivo and the impact of skin color (black and white). J Am Acad Dermatol 2003; 48:727–734.
30. Lavker RM, Kwong F, Kligman AM. Changes in skin surface patterns with age. J Gerontology 1980; 35:348.
31. Corcuff P, de Rigal J, Makki S, Agache P, Leveque JL. Skin relief and ageing. J Soc Cosmet Chem 1983; 34:177–190.
32. Leveque JL. EEMCO guidance for the assessment of skin topography. J Eur Acad Dermatol Venereol 1999; 12:103–114.
33. Zahouani H, Vargiolu R. Skin line morphology: tree and branches. In: Agache P, Humbert P, eds. Measuring the skin. Berlin, Germany: Springer, 2004; 5:41–59.
34. Lagarde JM, Rouvrais C, Black D. Topography and anisotropy of the skin surface with ageing. Skin Res Technol 2005; 11:110–119.
35. Leveque JL, Querleux B. SkinChip, a new tool for investigating the skin surface in vivo. Skin Res Technol 2003; 9:343–347.
36. Uitto J. Connective tissue biochemistry of the aging dermis: age-related alterations in collagen and elastin. Dermatol Clin 1986; 4:443–446.
37. Quaglino D, Bergamini G, Boraldi F, Pasquali Ronchetti I. Ultrastructural and morphometrical evaluations on normal human dermal connective tissue, the influence of age, sex and body region. Br J Dermatol 1996; 134:1013–1032.

38. Epstein EH. 1 (III), 3 human skin collagen: release by pepsin digestion and preponderance in fetal life. J Biol Chem 1974; 249:3225–3231.
39. Lavker RM, Zheng P, Dong G. Aged skin: a study by light, transmission electron, and scanning electron microscopy. J Invest Dermatol 1987; 88:S44–S51.
40. Escoffier C, De Rigal J, Rochefort A, Vasselet R, Lévêque JL, Agache P. Age related mechanical properties of human skin: an in vivo study. J Invest Dermatol 1989; 93:353–357.
41. De Rigal J, Escoffier C, Querleux B, Faivre B, Agache P, Lévêque JL. Assessment of aging of the human skin on vivo ultrasonic imaging. J Invest Dermatol 1989; 5:621–625.
42. Hoffmann K, Dirsckka TP, Stucker M, El Gammal S, Altmeyer P. Assessment of actinic skin damage by 20 MHz sonography. Photodermatol Photoimmunol Photomed 1994; 10:97–101.
43. Seidenari S, Pagnoni A, Di Nardo A, Giannetti A. Echographic evaluation with: image analysis of normal skin: variations according to age and sex. Skin Pharmacol 1994; 7:201–209.
44. Diridollou S, Vabre V, Berson M, et al. Skin ageing: changes of physical properties of human skin in vivo. Int J Cosmetic Sci 2001; 23:353–362.
45. Diridollou S, Black D, Lagarde JM, et al. Sex- and site-dependent variations in the thickness and mechanical properties of human skin in vivo. Int J Cosmetic Sci 2000; 22:421–435.
46. Diridollou S, Patat F, Gens F, et al. In vivo model of the mechanical properties of the human skin under suction. Skin Res Technol 2000; 6:214–221.
47. Gniadecka M, Gniadecki R, Serup J, Sondergaard J. Ultrasound structure and digital image analysis of the subepidermal low echogenic band in aged human skin: diurnal changes and interindividual variability. J Invest Dermatol 1994; 102:362–365.
48. Richard S, De Rigal J, De Lacharriere O, Berardesca E, Leveque JL. Noninvasive measurement of the effect of lifetime exposure to the sun on the aged skin. Photodermatol Photoimmunol Photomed 1994; 10:164–169.
49. Guittet C, Ossant F, Remenieras JP, Pourcelot L, Berson M. High-frequency estimation of the ultrasonic attenuation coefficient slope obtained in human skin: simulation and in vivo results. Ultrasound Med Biol 1999; 25:421–429.
50. Couturaud V, Coutable J, Khaiat A. Skin biomechanical properties: in vivo evaluation of influence of age and body site by non invasive method. Skin Res Technol 1995; 1:68–73.
51. Ishikawa T, Ishikawa OM. Measurement of skin elastic properties with a new suction device (I): Relationship to age, sex and the degree of obesity in normal individuals. J Dermatol 1995; 22:713–717.
52. Iida I, Noro K. An analysis of the reduction of elasticity on the ageing of human skin and the recovering effect of a facial massage. Ergonomics 1995; 9:1921–1931.
53. Quan MB, Edwards C, Marks R. Non invasive in vivo techniques to differentiate photodamage and ageing in human skin. Acta Derm Venereol (Stockholm) 1997; 77:416–419.
54. Barrel AO. Mechanical function of the skin: state of the art. Inc: Skin Bioengineering Techniques and Applications in Dermatology and Cosmetology. Current Problems in Dermatology 26. Basel, Switzerland: Karger, 1998:69–83.

55. Alexander H, Cook TH. Variations with age in the mechanical properties of human skin in vivo. In: Kennedi RM, ed. Bedsore. Biomechanics. Bath, England: Mc Millan Press, 1976:109–118.
56. Agache P, Monneur C, Leveque JL, De Rigal J. Mechanical properties and Young's modulus of human skin in vivo. Arch Dermatol Res 1980; 269:221–232.
57. Leveque JL, De Rigal J, Agache P, Monneur C. Influence of ageing on the in vivo extensibility of human skin at a low stress. Arch Dermatol Res 1980; 269:127–135.
58. Grahame R, Holt PJL. The influence of ageing on the in vivo elasticity of human skin. Gerontologia 1969; 15:121–139.
59. Pathak MA, Fitzpatrick TB. The role of natural photoprotective agents in human skin. In: Pathak MA, Fitzpatrick TB, Harber LC, Seiji M, Kukita A, eds. Sunlight and Man. Tokyo, Japan: University of Tokyo Press, 1974:725–750.
60. Kligman AM. Solar elastosis in relation to pigmentation. In: Pathak MA, Fitzpatrick TB, Harber LC, Seiji M, Kukita A, eds. Sunlight and Man. Tokyo, Japan: University of Tokyo Press, 1974:157–163.
61. Montagna W, Prota G, Kenney JA. Black skin: structure and function. San Diego: Academic Press, 1993:1–12.
62. Fitzpatrick TB, Szabo G, Wick MM. Biochemistry and physiology of melanin pigmentation. In: Lowell AG, ed. Biochemistry and physiology of the skin. New York, New York: Oxford University Press, 1983:687–712.
63. Kaidbey KH, Poh AP, Sayre M. Photoprotection by melanin: a comparison of Black and Caucasian skin. J Am Acad Dermatol 1979; 1:249–260.

13

Stratum Corneum Lipids and Water Holding Capacity: Comparison Between Caucasians, Blacks, Hispanics and Asians

Alessandra Pelosi and Enzo Berardesca

*Department of Dermatology, San Gallicano Dermatological Institute (IRCCS),
Rome, Italy*

Joachim W. Fluhr

*Department of Dermatology, San Gallicano Dermatological Institute (IRCCS),
Rome, Italy, and Friedrich Schiller University,
Jena, Germany*

Philip Wertz

Dows Institute, University of Iowa, Iowa City, Iowa, U.S.A.

**Jocélia Lago Jansen, Angela Anigbogu, Tsen-Fang Tsai, and
Howard I. Maibach**

*Department of Dermatology, University of California at San Francisco
School of Medicine, San Francisco, California, U.S.A.*

INTRODUCTION

In dermatology, topical therapies need to be adapted to different environmental human behaviours. Pharmacological response depends upon the percutaneous absorption and the activity of the chemical once absorbed into the biological system. For this reason it is extremely important to take into account the racial variations, if existing, in skin physiology in terms of percutaneous penetration and skin reactivity (1). The mechanism might involve stratum corneum structural variations.

Structural data (obtained comparing Caucasian *versus* Black skin) suggest that cell cohesion and desquamation of corneocytes are increased in Blacks (2). This observation contrasts with functional data reporting increased transepidermal water loss (TEWL), both in vivo and in vitro, associated with reduced transcutaneous penetration in Blacks. In the literature, conflicting findings have been reported in terms of sensitivity to cutaneous irritants. Marshall, Lynch and Smith (3) reported a decreased skin irritability in Blacks while Weigand (4) found Blacks to be more resistant to irritant reactions. More recently Blacks and Hispanics were found developing stronger irritant reactions to 2% sodium lauryl sulphate (SLS) proportional to the individual TEWL basal values (5); in particular Blacks showed an increased TEWL compared to Caucasians when SLS (0.5% and 2%) was applied on a preoccluded site (6).

Scant attention has been paid to Asian skin reactivity and barrier function. Robinson (7) investigated acute and cumulative skin irritation in Asians and Caucasians and found a wide variation of skin responsiveness in both races without any clear difference.

Despite the lack of definitive data it is widely stated that no differences in TEWL baseline values exist between races (6,8). Furthermore, it seems that differences in physiological responses become evident when removal of corneocytes and damage to the barrier are involved (9). In the current investigation the water holding capacity (WHC) of four racial groups was compared, using the plastic occlusion stress test (POST). This assay is confirmed to be a sensitive technique to investigate in vivo the efficacy of the skin barrier (10,11). The aim of this investigation was to assess whether stratum corneum could be a relevant structure modulated in different races by related cutaneous reactions, focusing on the relationship between barrier function and changes in lipid composition of the stratum corneum.

MATERIALS AND METHODS

POST and TEWL Measurements

Four groups, Caucasian, Black, Hispanic and Asian were investigated. The study was performed on 12 healthy volunteers from each race (6 males/6 females), age ranging from 20 years to 65 years (mean age 41.0 ± 10.3) Institutional Review Board approval and informed consent were obtained. Caucasians were American of Anglo-Saxon origin, Blacks were African Americans with dark skin, Hispanics were Mexicans and Asians were South-eastern Asians. All subjects had four grandparents with the same ethnic self-identity. Room temperature ranged between 19°C and 21°C with relative humidity between 58% and 60% (12). The subjects rested 30 minutes before measurements. Three sites were randomised on the volar forearms, two on one forearm and one on the contra lateral forearm. Prior to the procedures, basal values of TEWL were measured on each site with an evaporimeter (Tewameter, TM 210, Courage-Khazaka, Cologne, Germany). The measurement was performed according to the published guidelines (13,14). Two percent SLS (99% pure, Sigma, St. Louis, MO) in aqueous solution was applied by mean of a filter paper disc on the first site. Chloroform/methanol (2:1) was used to remove lipids from the stratum corneum on the second site: the solution (1 ml) was applied inside a glass cylinder, 2 cm in diameter, for 1 minute and then removed, and the skin site was wiped with a gauze (15). Empty aluminium chambers of 12 mm diameter (Epitest Ltd, Helsinki, Finland) were applied on the two sites tested and on an additional one that served as a control. An occlusive film (Transpore, 3M, St. Paul, MN) was placed for 24 hours to secure each chamber in place. All the chambers were removed after 24 hours, excess water was dried for two seconds with tissue paper and TEWL measured on each site immediately (0 min) and then every five minutes for 30 minutes. This procedure is known as the post occlusive stress test (POST).

Lipids Extraction

Skin surface lipids were collected from additional six subjects for each race (Caucasian, Black, Asian and Hispanic) of both genders, age ranging from 24 years to 36 years (mean age 31.3 ± 3.5). Volunteers were requested not to use any moisturizing product during the two weeks before the test. Three sites were selected on the volar forearms (between the wrist and the cubital fossa), two on one forearm and one on the contra lateral forearm. A glass cylinder, 3 cm in diameter, open at both ends, was pressed against the skin of the first preselected site and filled with 5 ml of ethanol. After five minutes the solvent was removed and discarded. Then 5 ml of cycloexane/ethanol solution (1:4) was pipetted into the cylinder and, after 1 minute of contact, removed and saved. This extraction was repeated twice for a total of 15 ml of cycloexane/ethanol. The entire procedure was then repeated on the two additional sites. The ethanol prewashes were discarded and the combined cycloexane/ethanol washes from the three sites were combined and dried under nitrogen (Evaporating unit, Pierce Chemical company, Rockford, Illinois). The extracted lipids were stored in glass tubes (12 ml) with Teflon-lined screw caps at $-20°C$ until analysis.

Thin Layer Chromatography

Glass plates (20 × 20 cm) coated with 0.25 mm thick silica gel G (Adsorbosil-plus-1; Alltech Associates; Deerfield IL, U.S.A.) were washed with chloroform: methanol (2:1), activated in a 110°C oven, and the adsorbent was poured into 6 mm wide lanes. Samples were dissolved in 100 μl of chloroform:methanol (2:1), and 10 μl were applied 2–3 cm from the bottom edge of the plate using calibrated glass capillaries. The chromatograms were with chloroform:methanol:water (40:10:1) to 10 cm, followed by chloroform:-methanol:acetic acid (190:9:1) to 20 cm, followed by hexane:ethyl ether:acetic acid (70:30:1) to 20 cm. This multiple development regimen resolves cholesterol sulphate, six series of ceramides and cholesterol. The less polar lipids, which are predominantly of sebaceous origin, are near the top edge of the plate. After development, chromatograms were air dried, sprayed with 50% sulphuric acid, and slowly heated to 220°C on an aluminium slab on a hot plate. After two hours, charring was complete, and the chromatogram was quantitated by photodensitometry.

Statistics

Statistical analysis was performed using ANOVA for repeated measures and Fisher LSD test for post hoc comparison; a level of $p < 0.05$ was considered significant.

RESULTS

Evaporimetry Measurements

No significant differences were found in the mean basal TEWL values between the four groups; however, obvious differences were detected between the 3 test sites (delipidized, control and SLS): At 0 minutes, TEWL values were higher in Hispanics on the delipidized site compared to the control site ($p \leq 0.03$) and to the SLS site ($p \leq 0.005$) while in Blacks, the values were higher on both, delipidized and control, compared to the SLS site ($p \leq 0.04$). From 5 minutes to 30 minutes, in all races, TEWL values were higher on the SLS site compared to the control $p \leq 0.004$) and to the delipidized site ($p \leq 0.0007$) with no statistically significant differences observed between the control and the delipidized site. On the delipidized site Hispanics showed higher TEWL values compared to Asians ($p \leq 0.02$) within the first 10 minutes and compared to Caucasians ($p \leq 0.02$, Table 1) within the first 5 minutes (Fig. 1). Blacks showed higher TEWL values compared to Asians ($p \leq 0.02$) within the first 20 minutes and compared to Caucasians ($p \leq 0.02$, Table 1) at 5 minutes and 15 minutes time points (Fig. 1). At 25 minutes and 30 minutes no statistically significant differences were detected at this site. On the control site Blacks showed higher values at 5 minutes and 10 minutes compared to Asians ($p \leq 0.05$) while Hispanics showed higher values compared to Asian ($p \leq 0.05$) only at 10 minutes (Fig. 2). From 15 minutes to 30 minutes no statistically significant differences were detected at this site among races.

Table 1   Delipidized Site

	Hispanics	Blacks	Caucasians	Asians
Hispanics		NS	0, 5 min p ≤ 0.02	0, 5, 10 min p ≤ 0.02
Blacks	NS		5, 15 min p ≤ 0.02	0, 5, 10, 15, 20 min p ≤ 0.02

Note: Hispanics show higher transepidermal water loss (TEWL) values compared to Asians (p ≤ 0.02) within the first 10 minutes and compared to Caucasians (p ≤ 0.02) within the first 5 minutes. Blacks show higher TEWL values compared to Asians (p = 0.02) within the first 20 minutes and compared to Caucasians (p ≤ 0.02) at the 5 and 15 minutes time points.

On the SLS site the highest values of TEWL were obtained in Caucasians at 5 minutes (59.71 ± 0.8 mg/m^2/h) the lowest in Blacks (33.1 ± 0.2 mg/m^2/h) and Hispanics (33.3 ± 0.3 mg/m^2/h) at 30 minutes but no significant differences were detected among races at this site.

Lipid Data Analysis

The following classes of lipids were extracted (Table 2): cholesterol sulphate, ceramide 6, ceramide 4/5, ceramide 3, ceramide 2, ceramide 1, and free

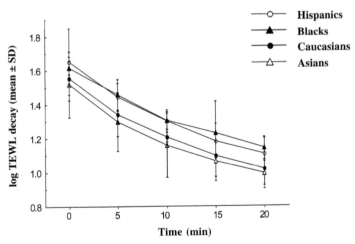

Figure 1   TEWL (log g/m^2/h) on the delipidized site. Hispanics show higher values compared to Asians within the first 10 min and compared to Caucasians within the first 5 min (p ≤ 0.02). Blacks show higher TEWL values compared to Asians within the first 20 minutes and compared to Caucasians at the 5 and 15 min time points (p ≤ 0.02).

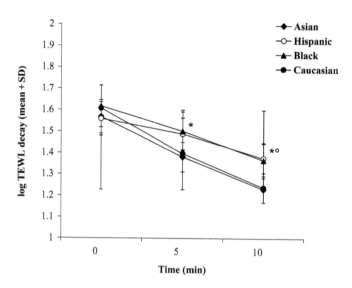

Figure 2 TEWL on the control site. Blacks (∗) show higher values compared to Asians at 5 and 10 minutes while Hispanics (°) show higher values compared to Asians at the 10 min time point (p ≤ 0.05).

cholesterol. Results are shown in Table 2. Blacks showed higher absolute values composition of cholesterol sulphate compared to Asians and Caucasians (p ≤ 0.03). Blacks and Caucasians showed higher levels of ceramide 3 compared to Asians (p ≤ 0.034) Caucasians showed higher levels of ceramide 2 compared to Asians and Hispanics (p ≤ 0.02) while Blacks had higher levels compared only to Asians (p ≤ 0.03). Hispanics showed higher levels of free cholesterol compared to Caucasians, Blacks and Asians (p ≤ 0.014). No significant differences in ceramides 4/5 and 6 were found among the different races.

Table 2 Absolute Composition Values (mean ± SD) of Different Classes of Lipids in Different Races

	CS (µg)	CER 3 (µg)	CER 2 (µg)	CH (µg)
Hispanics	7.2 ± 3.6	11.4 ± 2.1	5 ± 1.9	23.9 ± 7
Asians	♦ 2.7 ± 3.5	♦• 7.5 ± 3.8	♦• 3.5 ± 2	■ 9.6 ± 9
Blacks	13.2 ± 11.2	12.7 ± 5.7	6.5 ± 2.8	■ 15.3 ± 5.3
Caucasians	♦ 5.1 ± 0.9	12.2 ± 3.2	8.4 ± 2.6	■ 13.5 ± 4.9

Note: (♦) lower values compared to Blacks (p ≤ 0.021); (•) lower values compared to Caucasians (p ≤ 0.035); (■) lower values compared to Hispanics (p ≤ 0.014).
Abbreviations: CS, cholesterol sulphate; CER 3, ceramide 3; CER 2, ceramide 2; CH, free cholesterol.

DISCUSSION

The present study assessed the stratum corneum water holding capacity (WHC) using transepidermal water loss (TEWL) measurements for 30 minutes following 24 hours of occlusion. Skin occlusion results in an increased hydration because of inhibition of water evaporation. This method, POST (post occlusion stress test), was first used by Orsmark, Wilson and Maibach (16), who measured the WHC of the skin of the diapered area of infants using a paraffin film. In our study the method has been modified using aluminium chambers attached to skin with plastic tape. Hydration achieved by occlusion results in an increased TEWL after removal of the chamber and TEWL decay curves are related to the capacity for binding water (17). Racial differences on skin barrier function and holding capacity have been investigated previously. No differences in TEWL baseline values between Blacks, Caucasians, and Hispanics have been reported (6); similar results have been observed in a study performed on Chinese, Indians and Malays (8). Our data support these observations. Since no statistically significant differences on TEWL baseline values exist among races, the skin was stressed by irritation and delipidization to detect WHC differences (17). Dark skin has been reported to be less susceptible than light skin to cutaneous irritants (3), although this difference is not detectable when the stratum corneum is removed. Blacks and Caucasians are known to have a broader range of TEWL response to SLS. Since this range is wider in normal than in stripped skin, presumably the stratum corneum partially modulates the racial responses. In our study we found no statistically significant differences among races after SLS exposure. However, we could detect differences between races when the skin was delipidized. Chloroform/methanol, an efficient solvent that extracts lipids from the skin after a short application time, removes mainly ceramides and other polar lipids that regulate skin water retention function. When we delipidized the skin, Hispanics and Blacks showed higher TEWL values compared to Caucasians and Asians within the first 15 minutes. Furthermore they showed higher values on the delipidized site compared to the SLS site at 0 minutes.

To explore possible racial differences in stratum corneum lipid composition, an in-vivo extraction of stratum corneum lipids from the different racial groups was performed. Direct solvent extraction is a superficial non-invasive technique, which allows one to collect a representative sample of stratum corneum lipids suitable for analysis. Stratum corneum lipids, located within the intercellular space between corneocytes, include cholesterol esters, fatty acids, free cholesterol, and more polar lipids such as ceramides and cholesterol sulphate. These lipids play important roles in cell differentiation, cohesion, and desquamation and in the permeability barrier of the skin and water holding properties of the stratum corneum (18). Ceramides are important in the skin hydration state (19,20). Many studies have contributed to the understanding of lipids in the stratum corneum. For example, epidermal differentiation is associated with changes in lipid content and, although the total amount of collected stratum corneum lipids does not vary with age, in the elderly there is an increase in the percentage of polar stratum corneum lipids (21). Moreover, in atopic dry skin, a reduced proportion of certain ceramide fractions has been reported, confirming that these polar lipids may have a protective effect on skin barrier impairment (22). Other findings indicate that alteration in barrier function regulates rates of epidermal lipid synthesis and that TEWL is a likely regulatory factor of the process (23,24). Grubauer, Feingold, Harris and Elias (25), studying the skin permeability barrier in mice, found a linear correlation between TEWL and amount of polar lipids removed. Recently Coderch, De Pera, Fonulllosa, De La Maza and Parra (26) could show that liposomal stratum corneum lipids were able to increase the water holding capacity in two differently aged groups. Little is known about racial differences in stratum corneum lipids. Reinertson and Wheately (27) found higher total lipid contents in Blacks compared to Caucasians. Our findings demonstrate that there are racial differences in total extracted lipid content, with the lowest levels in Asians, the next lowest in Caucasians, compared to Blacks and Hispanics. Moreover racial differences in absolute values of different classes of epidermal lipids seem to exist: Asians have a tendency to have less ceramide 3 compared to Blacks and Caucasians, decreased ceramide 2 compared to Caucasians, less cholesterol sulphate compared to Blacks and decreased values of free cholesterol compared to Hispanics. These findings correlate well with TEWL recordings performed after delipidization under stressed condition (POST): less polar lipids result in decreased bound water and a lower TEWL. The reason these differences in TEWL are evident only under stress is unclear. We are aware of the complexities of defining race and attempting to generalize on the basis of small population samples. Yet, we are impressed by the discriminating power of the "stress tests" (POST and delipidization) and the lipid analysis; together with racial skin differences may be far greater than colour.

REFERENCES

1. Berardesca E, Maibach HI. Racial differences in skin pathophysiology. J Am Acad Dermatol 1996; 34:667–672.
2. Corcuff P, Lotte C, Rouger A. Racial differences in corneocytes. A comparison between black, white and oriental skin. Acta Derm Venereol 1991; 71:146–148.
3. Marshall EK, Lynch V, Smith HV. Variation in susceptibility of the skin to dichloroethylsulphide. J Pharmacol Exp Ther 1919; 12:291–301.
4. Weigand DA, Gaylor JR. Irritant reaction in Negro and Caucasian skin. South Med J 1974; 67:548–551.
5. Berardesca E, J de Rigal, Lévêque JL, Maibach HI. In vivo biophysical characterization of skin physiological differences in races. Dermatologica 1991; 182:89–93.

6. Berardesca E, Maibach H. Sodium lauryl sulphate induced cutaneous irritation. Comparison of White and Hispanic subjects. Contact Dermatitis 1988; 19: 136–140.
7. Robinson MK. Racial differences in acute and cumulative skin irritation responses between Caucasian and Asian population. Contact Dermatitis 2000; 42:134–143.
8. Goh CL, Chia SE. Skin irritability to sodium lauryl sulphate as measured by skin water vapour loss by sex and race. Clin Exp Dermatol 1988; 13:16–19.
9. Berardesca E, Pirot F, Singh M, Maibach HI. Differences in stratum corneum pH gradient when comparing white Caucasian and black African American skin. Br J Dermatol 1998; 139:855–857.
10. Berardesca E, Maibach HI. Monitoring the water-holding capacity in visually non irritated skin by plastic occlusion stress test (POST). Clin Exp Dermatol 1990; 15:107–110.
11. Berardesca E, Vignoli GP, Fideli D, Maibach HI. Effect of occlusive dressings on the stratum corneum water holding capacity. Am J Med Sci 1992; 304:25–28.
12. Mathias T, Wilson DM, Maibach HI. Transepidermal water loss as a function of skin surface temperature. J Invest Dermatol 1981; 77:219–222.
13. Pinnagoda J, Tupker RA, Agner T, Serup J. Guidelines for transepidermal water loss (TEWL) measurement. Contact Dermatitis 1990; 22:164–178.
14. Rogiers V. EEMCO guidance for the assessment of transepidermal water loss in cosmetic science. Skin Pharmacol Appl Skin Physiol 2001; 14:117–128.
15. Berardesca E, Herbst R, Maibach HI. Plastic occlusion stress test as a model to investigate the effects of skin delipidization on the stratum corneum water holding capacity in vivo. Dermatology 1993; 187:91–94.
16. Orsmark D, Wilson D, Maibach H. In vivo transepidermal water loss and epidermal occlusive hydration in new-born infants: anatomical region variation. Acta Derm Venereol 1980; 60:403–407.
17. Middleton JD. The mechanism of water binding in stratum corneum. Br J Dermatol 1968; 80:437–450.
18. Wertz PW. Epidermal lipids. Semin Dermatol 1992; 2:106–113.
19. Imokawa G, Akasaki S, Minematsu Y, Kawai M. Importance of intercellular lipids in water-retention properties of the stratum corneum: induction and recovery study of surfactant dry skin. Arch Dermatol Res 1989; 281:45–51.
20. Lintner K, Mondon P, Girard F, Gibaud C. The effect of a synthetic cermide 2 on transepidermal water loss after stripping or sodium lauryl sulphate treatment: an in vivo study. Int J Cosmet Sci 1997; 19:15–25.
21. Saint-Léger D, Agache PG. Variations in skin surface lipids during life. In: Léveque JL, Agache PG, eds. Ageing skin. Properties and functional changes. New York, Basel, Hong Kong, 1993:251–261.
22. Di Nardo A, Wertz P, Giannetti A, Seidenari S. Ceramide and cholesterol composition of the skin of patients with atopic dermatitis. Acta Derm Venereol 1998; 78:27–30.
23. Elias PM, Feingold KR. Lipids and the epidermal water barrier: metabolism, regulation and pathophysiology. Semin Dermatol 1992; 1:176–182.
24. Meguro S, Arai Y, Masukawa Y. Relationship between covalently bound ceramides and transepidermal water loss (TEWL). Arch Dermatol Res 2000; 292:463–468.

25. Grubauer G, Feingold KR, Harris RM, Elias PM. Lipid content and lipid type as determinant of the epidermis permeability barrier. J Lipid Res 1989; 30:89–96.
26. Coderch L, De Pera M, Fonulllosa J, De La Maza A, Parra J. Efficacy of stratum corneum lipid supplementation on human skin. Contact Dermatitis 2002; 47:139–146.
27. Reinertson RP, Wheatley VR. Studies on the chemical composition of human epidermal lipids. J Invest Dermatol 1959; 32:49–51.

14

The Impact of Skin Disease in "Ethnic" Skin

Gary J. Brauner

Mount Sinai School of Medicine, New York, New York, U.S.A.

INTRODUCTION

The pursuit of Science requires focus and refinement, and must always be kept separate from sociopolitical desires and agendas, which serve only to confuse the issues of such pursuit. This author, therefore, takes umbrage from the intellectual dishonesty in the present day use of such a nomenclature for "ethnic" and "skin of color."

Merriam-Webster's definition of "ethnic" is clear. Its etymology is "from Greek *ethnikos* national, gentile, from *ethnos* nation, people; akin to Greek *Ethos* custom ... of or relating to large groups of people classed according to common racial, national, tribal, religious, linguistic, or cultural origin or background." This definition has no consideration for the amount of pigment visible in the epidermis as a unifying feature but relates to the social bonding and associations of groups. Our definition should be as clear too, though it is now entirely not (1–3).

In her landmark supplement to the Journal of the American Academy of Dermatology in 2002 (4), Taylor attempted to classify what she meant as "people of skin of color" in the following confusing array (author's italics) of a huge genetically and phenotypically diverse population.

"Defining pigmented skin or skin of color obviously entails a discussion of the various races and ethnic groups of our species... Based on this system of classification, most of these racial groups would consist of people with skin of color. *Even certain Caucasoids (e.g., Indians, Pakistanis, and Arabs) have pigmented skin*... In the United States, the racial and ethnic classification of those individuals with pigmented skin or skin of color would include *African-American black* persons (including Caribbean American black persons), *Asian and Pacific Islanders (including those of Filipino, Chinese, Japanese, Korean, Vietnamese, Thai, Malaysian, Laotian, or Hmong descent), Native Americans, Alaskans, and Aleuts,* and those who report Latino or Hispanic ethnicity (including people of *Mexican, Cuban, Puerto Rican, Central American, or Spanish descent).* Also included are certain people traditionally categorized as *Caucasoids, such as the majority of Indians, Pakistanis, and those of Middle Eastern origin"* (4).

As apolitical dermatologist-scientists we all know that except for totally vitiliginous persons or tyrosinase-negative albinos the entire human race is one of "people of color" (5). For the sake of defining our chapter subject, therefore, this author will consider scientific categorization by the traditional Coons' (6,7) anthropologic definitions of race which contain elements of separation and genetic phenotypism, definitions which do continue to be accepted, citing the Capoid, Negroid, Australoid, and Mongoloid races and will consider their cutaneous biology as well as cultural adaptations by members of these racial groups, both of which features subsequently influence cutaneous disease.

A brief review of the "impact of skin disease in ethnic skin" must be a tripolar reflection. First, it is the impact of "ethnicity" or a more narrowed and scientifically appropriate terminology (i.e., "race") on the clinical presentation of cutaneous diseases. Second, it is the social or environmental impact of certain skin diseases as viewed by different cultural groups or races. Certain cutaneous conditions have much more social significance and burden in different groups. Conversely, cultural practices frequently give rise to differing prevalence of disease in different groups (8–11). The third consideration is economic impact, wherein the socioeconomic position of members of those groups (i.e., the effects of geography or poverty) may influence the prevalence of cutaneous disease in those different groups (11–13).

THE IMPACT OF RACE ON THE FREQUENCY AND CLINICAL APPEARANCES OF CUTANEOUS DISEASE

Cutaneous processes are clearly different in their frequencies in racial groups by virtue of phenotypic clustering (Tables 1 and 2). In the black

Table 1 Cutaneous Processes Exaggerated in black Races

Pigment lability-dyschromias
Follicular responses and follicular diseases
Mesenchymal responses—fibroplastic and granulomatous
Bullous disease

Table 2 Cutaneous Processes Exaggerated in Mongoloid Race-Weighted Prevalence

Congenital and acquired dyschromias (not postinflammatory)
Eczemas
Cutaneous amyloids

and Mongoloid races, solely on the basis of their increased production of melanin, one would expect and does see a disproportionate incidence of disfiguring dyschromias, both hyper- and hypopigmentation (or even both in the same lesion) as compared to Caucasians of light coloration. The more active melanocytes of darker races are more likely to disgorge visibly increased numbers of melanosomes into the epidermis or the dermis, and members' of those darker races keratinocytes (with the least inflammatory provocation) dump pigment into the dermis. Conversely, even a small temporary interference with pigment transfer from melanocyte to keratinocyte leaves a visible lighter blotch in a darkly pigmented person as seen in pityriasis alba. Sensitivity to azelaic acid elaborated by *Malassezia furfur* in tinea versicolor is more obvious, more disfiguring, and seemingly more common in the dark-skinned.

The Mongoloid race (Table 3) has a weighted prevalence for a variety of congenital and acquired (not postinflammatory) dyschromias as compared to Caucasians and the black races. Transient congenital Mongolian spots appear in up to 96% of East Asian newborns, and Nevus of Hori, Ota, or Ito as well as melasma are not uncommon.

Certain diseases such as spontaneous hair knotting (14) or woolling of scalp hair secondary to pruritus, either of which leads to trichorrhexis nodosa, or the appearance of papules, pustules, and hyperpigmentation from transfollicular or reentry transepidermal penetration by sharpened

Table 3 Congenital and Acquired Dyschromias in Mongoloid Race (not Postinflammatory)

Congenital Mongolian spot	96%
Nevus of Ota	0.8% Japanese outpatients
Nevus of Ito	
Reticulated and patterned acquired dyschromias	
Riehls melanosis postinflammatory	
Melasma more freq in Asian than white women	
	40% in women in Thailand
	0.25–4% of derm visits
Acquired bilateral nevus of Ota-like macules (Japanese)	

Source: From Ref. 10.

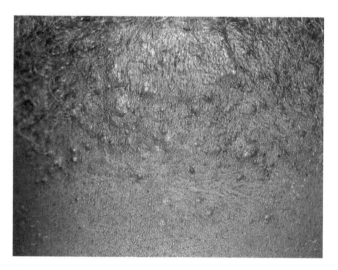

Figure 1 (*See color insert*) Acne keloid.

hairs in pseudofolliculitis barbae in the three woolly-haired or ulotrichous (and coincidentally darker complected black) races are directly related to the inherited curvature of the follicle and the inherited flattened, ovoid, curly, spiral, or helical hairs produced as well (15–19).

Scarring follicular diseases (which appear almost only or exclusively in Africans and African Americans) such as "acne keloidalis" or folliculitis papillaris capillitii of Kaposi (Fig. 1), central centrifugal scarring alopecia of the scalp (Fig. 2), and dermatitis cruris pustulosa et atrophicans of Harman almost all involve benign pharmacologically sensitive *Staphylococcus aureus*. A possible genetic abnormality in desmoglein 1 which may allow for more disruption of the hair follicle by staphylococci in these races is suggested by the phage types and epidermolysin production of the staph involved which seem to attack desmoglein 1 and also suggested by the rare, recently described, genetic associations of inherited woolly hair and desmoplakin or desmoglein mutations, the former associated with arrhythmogenic right ventricular dysplasia and cutaneous disease (6,19–29).

In former eras of higher prevalence of syphilis follicular patterns of papules and even pustules were seen in as many as 5% of African American patients (30) and never in Caucasians. Eczemas in African American and African Caribbean patients are more frequently follicular and nummular-follicular (31,32). What the possible genetic predisposition is for such patterning is not at all even surmised.

The incidence of eczemas in East Asians seems higher than in Caucasians in several studies of Japanese patients though the results are

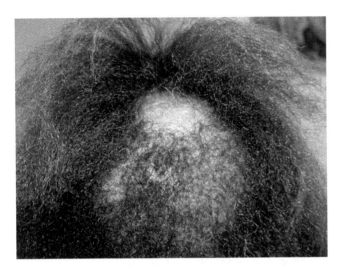

Figure 2   (*See color insert*) Centrifugal central scarring alopecia.

controversial because it is not uniformly confirmed in Asian populations in various continents (10). Follicular accentuation and eczemas are reported as more common in Japanese children also.

Black races have an increased prevalence of a variety of exaggerated mesenchymal responses ranging from relative peripheral lymphocytosis to increased prevalence of luetic juxta-articular nodes, endocardial fibroelastosis, uterine fibroids, endemic Kaposi's sarcoma, leiomyosarcoma, dermatofibrosarcoma protuberans, ainhum, and keloids (33–35). Relative prevalence of keloids in surveys has ranged from 2:1 to 19:1 in blacks versus Caucasians (36). Genetic information is in its infancy, but preliminary results from a Japanese family and an African American family with familial keloids recently showed the first genetic evidence of keloidal linkage to chromosome 2q23 for the Japanese family whereas the African American family showed evidence for a keloid susceptibility locus on chromosome 7p11 (25).

With respect to granulomatous disease, sarcoidosis in black inductees in World War II was 18 times that of whites (37). A similar disparity still exists 50 years later regardless of place of birth in the United States (38). South-American blacks (39) and South-African Bantus (40,41) also seem to have a higher prevalence than whites. Iannuzzi et al. recently studied 229 African American families with two or more sibs, with a history of sarcoidosis, and found multiple suggestive regions for genetic linkage; the multiplicity suggested that more than one gene influences susceptibility to sarcoidosis in African Americans (42,43). Sarcoidosis is the 21st century great mimic as lues once was. Because there can be literally dozens of varied clinical presentations (even multiple in the same patient) of sarcoidosis in

African Americans ranging from subtle hypopigmented or ichthyosiform patches through lichenoid, pityriasiform, psoriasiform, papular, gelatinous nodular, verrucoid, ulcerative, etc., one must consider this diagnosis in almost any eruption in an African American.

Predisposition or resistance to infections may be on a genetic or racial basis in certain instances. Although an increased prevalence of cutaneous diseases in Africans and African Americans associated with staphylococci may be explainable on a cultural rather than genetic basis (vide infra) the reasons for the total absence of pediculosis capitis (44) infestations in young African Americans and conversely the presently exclusively African American affliction with tinea capitis, (*Trichophyton tonsurans* in the United States but *Trichophyton violaceum* in Africa) remain enigmas (45,46). Four typical clinical patterns may appear in *T. tonsurans* infections of the scalp: (i) seborrheic dermatitis- or atopic dermatitis-like, (ii) alopecia areata-like, (iii) oil folliculitis-like, (iv) furuncle-like and (v) even tinea incognita with minimal hair loss and no scale or erythema may occur.

There is suggestive evidence that blacks do not handle coccidioidomycosis well immunologically (47,48). Allergic manifestations, of which erythema nodosum is the most common, are seen in only 2% of deeply pigmented males with this disease compared with up to 30% in white females. Wide dissemination and a higher fatality rate after dissemination are notable in blacks (47).

Kawasaki's disease is seen predominantly in Asians even when occurring in mixed populations—in San Diego Asian or Pacific islanders are twice as likely as white infants to be affected (49). Mollusca contagiosa are more common in East Asian children in this author's heavily Asian practice.

The prevalence of mesenchymal disease also differs for the Mongoloid race. Depositional cutaneous diseases such as frictional amyloidosis, macular amyloid, lichen amyloid, and ano-sacral amyloid are more common in East Asians (Table 4) as are wasting diseases such as lipodystrophia centrifugalis abdominalis infantilis (10).

Table 4 Cutaneous Inflammatory Processes Exaggerated in Mongoloid Race

Cutaneous Amyloid
   Friction amyloid (Japan)
   Macular amyloid
   Lichen amyloid (Chinese)
   Ano-sacral (Japanese and Chinese)
Lipodystrophia centrifugalis abdominalis infantilis (esp Japanese)
Kikuchi-Fujimoto necrotizing lymphadenitis
Actinic prurigo (native Americans)

Source: From Ref. 10.

Table 5 Patterns of Bullous Disease in blacks

Disease	Frequency
Miliaria	Rare in blacks?
Staphylococcal scalded skin	Rare in blacks
Neonatal pustular melanosis	Unique to blacks
Acropustulosis of infancy	Predominantly blacks
Bullous lupus erythematosus	Predominantly blacks
Porphyria cutanea tarda	Predominantly blacks
Dermatitis herpetiformis	Very rare in blacks
Lues, follicular pustular	Unique in blacks
Reiter's syndrome	Different HLA in blacks?

Abbreviation: HLA, human leukocyte antigen.

The prevalence of bullous disease shows a distinct pattern in the black races presumably on an as yet unknown genetic basis (Table 5). Almost no black has ever been reported with dermatitis herpetiformis. Staphyloccoccal scalded skin syndrome and even miliaria are rare. Bullous systemic lupus (but only those categories including coexistent EBA or pemphigoid and lupus) (50–55) is evident more commonly in blacks as are porphyria cutanea tarda and acropustulosis of infancy (56,57). Neonatal pustular melanosis (58) is today and follicular pustular lues in the past was nearly unique to blacks.

THE IMPACT OF CULTURE

In the more heavily pigmented non-Caucasian races dyschromias are a more obvious and discomforting clinical sequel to a variety of cutaneous inflammatory diseases. In East Asian populations, even neoplastic (facial nevi, seborrheic keratoses, and lentigines) or acquired noninflammatory progressive dyschromias bear an unhappy significance not evident in lighter Caucasians. The only equivalent cultural obsession with dyschromia in Caucasians is perhaps the pursuit of a tanned "healthy" look with resultant abuse of epidermis and dermis by natural and artificial ultraviolet sources and its resultant carcinogenesis and elastosis.

Such desire for evenness of pigmentation in darker-skinned Africans has led to abusive applications of hydroquinone and other bleaches to lighten normal skin to lighter shades. When inflammatory responses to hydroquinones appear, the dark-skinned victim may become a mutilated hyper-and hypopigmented marbled and spotted persona with leukomelanoderma (59); if hydroquinone abuse is combined with intense unprotected sunlight exposure, ochronosis may develop (60).

Even xerosis becomes linguistically elevated to "ashy skin" for African Americans. The liberal use of greasy emollients by dark-skinned. Africans and African Americans to maintain a smoothly brown and not two-toned

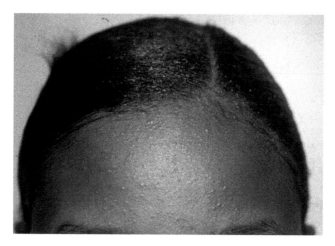

Figure 3 (*See color insert*) Pomade acne.

pattern has led to a variety of folliculitides, both sterile and staphylococcal, not seen in Caucasians or Asians.

Use of greasy pomades or silicone-based nongreasy "shine" products to manage style-ability of hair and produce a sheen on the hair, and to diminish scalp scaling is almost universal in African American communities. The pomades leach out onto the forehead resulting in pomade acne (Fig. 3).

The application of a variety of emollients such as petrolatum, mineral oil, cocoa butter, Shea butter etc., in other areas to minimize the so-called "ashy" appearance of xerotic skin may induce, particularly when following frictional or abrasive rubbing, oil folliculitis and an increased prevalence of acne keloid, scarring folliculitis decalvans-like scalp oil folliculitis, vaselinoderma of the face, or segmental folliculitis (22,61). Chronic scalp folliculitis, folliculitis decalvans, traction alopecia, dermatitis cruris pustulosa et atropicans, folliculitis papillaris capillitii (acne keloid), vaselinoderma, and pomade acne all result from customary cutaneous hygiene and maintenance practices.

Such desire for evenness of pigmentation in East Asians brings patients often to the derma-surgeon for removal of even the tiniest 1 or 2 mm brown facial macule. Most Asians avoid the sun and do not actively seek a tan. Chinese consider dark spots below the eye and on the shoulders unlucky and particularly undesirable (62,63). Brown lesions are thought related to diet especially excess protein; some may attempt dietary alteration hoping that lentigines or nevi will fade. Dark brown–black spots are considered marks of prior illness and of fever in certain organs (Fig. 4). The increased prevalence of more disfiguring and expansive dyschromias such as Nevus of Ota, Mongolian spots, and melasma in East Asians may also contribute to a heightened social anxiety over even small pigmented lesions.

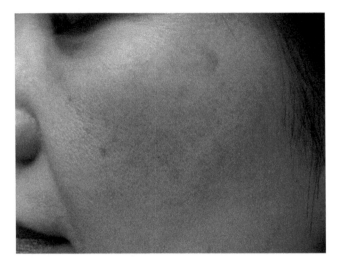

Figure 4 (*See color insert*) Facial lentigo on Asian skin.

Increased exposure to higher concentrations of para-phenylenediamine in darker hair dye shades may be reflected as an increased incidence of contact dermatitis in African Americans to such products (64).

Keloids appear with at least 10-fold increased risk in black populations versus Caucasian (36). What may seem a biologic disadvantage has been taken as an advantage socially to reflect ritualistic life passage episodes. Because of the community's understanding of this likely result of trauma,

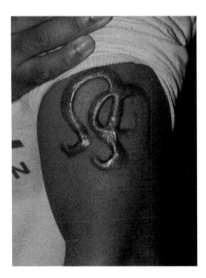

Figure 5 (*See color insert*) Fraternity keloid.

many different African tribal groups use scarification (knowing keloids will develop in the programmed cutting sites) to mark children's passage to adolescence or marriageability. Leni Reifenstahls' landmark photos of East African Kau tribal ritual support some of the most graphic documentation of this body art (65). African American college students similarly may scarify Greek letters in their fraternity initiation rites (Fig. 5).

Asian populations are more likely to employ alternative homeopathic medical remedies such as cupping or moxibustion, both of which produce traumatic injury, purpura and cutaneous burns, respectively (10,62). They also are more likely to use nontraditional medications some of which in Chinese and Korean medicine contain arsenic and can produce clinical arsenicalism. Chinese herbal balls, a Chinese "Sin-Luk" pill for asthma and Korean herbal preparations used to treat hemorrhoids include arsenic (62).

MELANIN AND DERMATOSES IN "ETHNIC" SKIN

Because the defining feature (4) of the misnomer "ethnic" seems to be the darkness of a person's untanned skin, thus including those persons of Asian, sub-Saharan African, and Hispanic-American ancestry but excluding only all light-skinned non-Hispanic Caucasians, melanin's ability to obscure or accentuate the classic textbook descriptions of cutaneous diseases must be our starting point.

One must learn to mentally add to or subtract from (Fig. 6) (15) the patient's usual skin color these classic textbook descriptions which are primarily based on appearance in Caucasians. Dark skin color can easily impair the physician's ability on initial impression of the patient to suspect anemia, cyanosis, or jaundice. Urticaria is easily missed when the edematous wheal is not a pink papule but a slightly lighter than normal raised area.

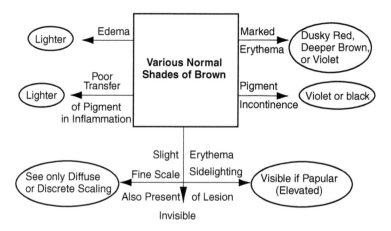

Figure 6 Adding and subtracting background color. *Source*: From Ref. 15.

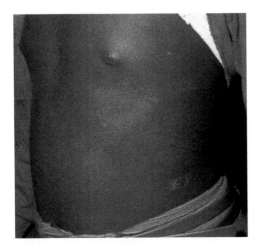

Figure 7 (*See color insert*) Scale highlights lesions of pityriasis rosea.

Erythema may be occult and found only if accompanied by some tell-tale white scale whose presence conversely is made more obvious by a darker skin tone background (Fig. 7). Erythema commonly has a violaceous tinge. Excoriation may produce a gray color. Fixed drug eruptions, because of the

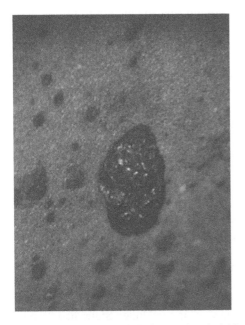

Figure 8 Black seborrheic keratosis mimicking modular melanoma.

intensity of the dermal accumulation of incontinent pigment, may be jet-black. Histologically normal nevi can appear ominously black (Fig. 8).

THE IMPACT OF GEOGRAPHY AND POVERTY

Third world populations are overwhelmingly those of the non-Caucasian. When one considers that upward mobility of these populations by migrating to predominantly Caucasian-populated first world nations still has left most of them in urban poverty, it is no wonder that population surveys seem to show a different prevalence of cutaneous diseases and their severity than one sees in a better-heeled Caucasian populace. Moy et al. (13) note that in the United States in 1996 "the incomes of 28% of Latinos, 28% of African Americans, and 14% of Asians versus 11% of American-Whites were at or below the poverty level." Minimal income (66) dictates lack of health insurance, lack of paid healthcare providers in the community, lack of transportation to visit a physician, and no childcare to allow mobility for physician visits. Fear of deportation for those residing as illegal immigrants and a sense of cultural or racial insensitivity of caregivers make visiting those caregivers a last resort. All these elements of poverty and more, thus, delay care and allow for more serious presentations of cutaneous and other diseases. African Bantus may traditionally first visit the witch doctor for herbal or caustic remedies before making a long journey to the white physician; therefore, by the time the white physician sees them, any disease that may be present has become extraordinarily severe. It is thought that the high mortality of acral lentiginous melanomas in blacks, wherein 30% of patients with pedal lesions may already have nodal metastases at the time of the first visit, may be due to both poor public education and delayed financial access. For the first third of the 20th century, American dermatologists considered lupus erythematosus to be extremely rare in blacks, probably because almost none saw a black patient (67). Taylor (68) cites Fox in 1908 (69) who even then claimed that blacks "were only apt to seek treatment for affections of the skin which cause positive annoyance or pain."

These third- and first-world underclass populations are subject to all the medical degradations of such poverty, that is overcrowding, lack of adequate sanitation, and lack of balanced and adequate diet, all increasing susceptibility to diseases in general. Poverty, not race, is the major contributing factor to the apparently high prevalence of pyodermas in blacks of the southern United States and the high prevalence of pyodermas, pyodermic eczemas, tropical ulcers, pellagra, scabies, parasitoses, leprosy, tuberculosis, and so on and the low prevalence of rosacea and xanthomas in the Bantu (40,41).

In her review of the epidemiology of skin disease in different ethnic groups, Taylor (68) suggests that studies early in the 20th century performed as retrospective surveys of public clinic visits in the United States had "top 6" or "top 12" lists of incidences of diseases in essence similar to other series including only whites. In reality, the outpatient incidence of infectious diseases, even in a U.S. black population, such as syphilis, tineas, tinea versicolor, etc., was significantly higher in both early and late century than that of Whites (70–72).

Many African studies of dermatologic disease are heavily weighted, with a reported 22% to 79% prevalence of black patients seen for nonluetic infectious diseases versus 10% to 40% in African whites, about 9% in American whites, and about 3% in English whites (32,73–77). The corresponding prevalence of primary dermatoses (e.g., psoriasis) in blacks is, therefore, frequently much lower, and most authors still neglect to report on the basis of true incidence or prevalence by considering disease occurrence versus population at risk and not versus overall outpatient visits, as they mistakenly do.

Despite attempts to consider the spectra of cutaneous diseases afflicting blacks, Asians, and Caucasians the same, the spectra may overlap but are not the same at all. The strength of perspicacious dermatologists such as Hazen, Kenny, and few others has been to discern and to abstract from surveys so heavily weighted by infections and infestations as to otherwise obscure the truly unique patterns of cutaneous disease and responses of different races.

REFERENCES

1. Halder R, ed. Ethnic skin disease. Dermatol Clin 2003; 21:596–768.
2. Holloway V, Halder R, eds. Ethnic hair and skin: what is the state of the science? J Amer Acad Dermatol 2003; 48(suppl):S105–S148.
3. Johnson B, Moy R, White G, eds. Ethnic Skin. St Louis, Missouri: Mosby, 1998.
4. Taylor S. Skin of color: biology, structure, function, and implications for dermatologic disease. J Amer Acad Dermatol 2002; 46:S41–S62.
5. Montagna W, Prota, G, Kenney J, eds. Black Skin: Structure and Function. San Diego: Academic Press, 1993.
6. Coon, Carlton, The Origin of Races. New York, New York: Alfred Knopf, 1962.
7. Sarich V, Miele F. Race: the reality of human differences. Cambridge, Massachusetts: Westview Press, Perseus books, 2004.
8. Halder R, Roberts C, Nootheti PR. Cutaneous diseases in the black races. Dermatol Clinics 2003; 21:679–687.
9. Jackson B. Cosmetic considerations and nonlaser cosmetic procedures in ethnic skin. Dermatol Clinics 2003; 21:703–712.
10. Lee C, Lim H. Cutaneous diseases in Asians. Dermatol Clinics 2003; 21: 669–677.
11. Sanchez M. Cutaneous disease in Latinos. Dermatol Clinics 2003; 21:689–697.
12. Bravo F. Sanchez, M, New and re-emerging cutaneous infectious diseases in Latin America and other geographic areas. Dermatol Clinics 2003; 21:655–668.
13. Moy J, McKinley-Grant L, Sanchez M. Cultural aspects in the treatment of patients with skin diseases. Dermatol Clinics 2003; 21:733–742.
14. Dawber R. Knotting of scalp hair. Br J Dermatol 1974; 91:169.
15. Brauner G. Cutaneous disease in black children. Am J Dis Child 1983; 137:488.
16. Khumalo N, Doe P, Dawber R, et al. What is normal black African hair? A light and scanning electron-microscopic study. J Am Acad Dermatol 2000; 430:814–820.

17. Steggerda M. Cross sections of human hair from four racial groups. J Hered 1940; 31:475.
18. Steggerda M, Seibert H. Size and shape of head hair from six racial groups. J Hered 1941; 32:315.
19. Sugathan P, Zacariah J, Joy M. Folliculitis cruris pustulosa et atrophicans. Int J Dermatol Venerol 1973; 39:35.
20. Alcalai R, Metzger S, Rosenheck S, et al. A recessive mutation in desmoplakin causes arrhythmogenic right ventricular dysplasia, skin disorder, and woolly hair. Am Coll Cardiol 2003; 42:319–327.
21. Brauner G. Oil folliculitis: a paradigm in African Americans? AAD Annual meeting Washington DC, February 2004.
22. Harman R. Dermatitis cruris pustulosa et atrophicans. In: Marshall J, ed. Essays on Tropical Dermatology. Amsterdam, Netherlands: Excerpta Medica, 1972.
23. Kanzaki H, Ueda M, Morishita Y, Akiyama H, Arata J, Kanzaki S. Producibility of exfoliative toxin and staphylococcal coagulase types of Staphylococcus aureus strains isolated from skin infections and atopic dermatitis. Dermatology 1997; 195:6–9.
24. LoPresti P, Papa C, Kligman A. Hot comb alopecia. Arch Dermatol 1968; 98:234.
25. Marneros A, Norris J, Watanabe S, et al. Genome scans provide evidence for keloid susceptibility loci on chromosomes 2q23 and 7p11. J Invest Dermatol 2004; 122:1126–1132.
26. Prevost G, Couppie P, Monteil H. Staphylococcal epidermolysins. Curr Opin Infect Dis 2003; 16:71–76.
27. Sperling L, Skelton H, Smith K, et al. Follicular degeneration syndrome in men. Arch Dermatol 1994; 130:763–769.
28. Sperling L, Homoky C, Pratt L, et al. Acne keloidalis is a form of primary scarring alopecia. Arch Dermatol 2000; 136:479–484.
29. Sperling L, Sau P. The follicular degeneration syndrome in black patients: 'hot comb alopecia' revisited and revised. Arch Dermatol 1992; 128:68–74.
30. Hazen H. Syphilis and skin diseases in the American Negro. Arch Dermatol 1935; 31:316.
31. Vollum D. Skin markings in Negro children from the West Indies. Br J Dermatol 1972; 86:260.
32. Walshe M. Dermatology in Jamaica. Trans St. Johns Hosp Dermatol Soc 1968; 54:46.
33. Marshall J. Skin diseases in Africa Capetown, South Africa: Maskew Miller Ltd., 1964.
34. Polednak A. Connective tissue responses in Negroes in relation to disease. Am J Phys Anthropol 1974; 41:49.
35. Scott F. Skin diseases in the South African Bantu. In: Marshall J, ed. Essays on Tropical Dermatology. Amsterdam, Netherlands: Excerpta Medica, 1972.
36. Koomin A. The etiology of keloids: a review of the literature and a new hypothesis. S Afr Med J 1964; 38:913.
37. Michael M. Cole R, Beeson P, et al. Sarcoidosis Am Rev Tub 1950; 62:403.
38. Israel H. Influence of race and geographic origin on sarcoidosis. Arch Environ Health 1970; 20:608.

39. Canizares O. Epidemiology of Dermatoses of Latin America. In: Marshall J, ed. Essays on Tropical Dermatology. Amsterdam, Netherlands: Excerpta Medica, 1972.
40. Morrison J. Sarcoidosis in the Bantu. Necrotizing and mutilating forms of the disease. Br J Dermatol 1974; 90:649.
41. Schulz E, Findlay G, Scott T. Skin disease in the Bantu. S Afr Med J 1962; 36:199.
42. Iannuzzi M, Iyengar S, Gray-McGuire C, et al. Genome-wide search for sarcoidosis susceptibility genes in African Americans. Genes Immun 2005; 6:509–518.
43. Schurmann M. Genetics of sarcoidosis. Semin Respir Crit Care Med 2003; 24:213–222.
44. Kanof N. Of lice and man. J Am Acad Dermatol 1980; 3:91.
45. Honig P, Smith L. Tinea capitis masquerading as atopic orseborrheic dermatitis. J Pediatr 1979; 94:604.
46. Prevost E. Nonfluorescent tinea capitis in Charleston S.C. Jnl Amer Med Ass 1979; 244:1765.
47. Emmons C, Binford C, Utz J. Medical Mycology. Philadelphia: Lea and Febiger, 1970.
48. Wilson J. Coccidiodomycosis. In: Marshall J, ed. Essays on Tropical Dermatology. Amsterdam, Netherlands: Excerpta Medica, 1972.
49. Bronstein D, Dille A, Austin J, et al. Relationship of climate, ethnicity and socioeconomic status to Kawasaki disease in San Diego County, 1994 through 1998. Pediatr Infect Dis J 2000; 19:1087–1091.
50. Gammon W. The relationship between epidermolysis bullosa acquisita, systemic lupus erythematosus and bullous SLE, AAD Annual Meeting Washington DC, December 7, 1988.
51. Gammon W, Briggaman R. Bullous SLE: a phenotypically distinctive but immunologically heterogeneous bullous disorder. J Invest Dermatol 1993; 100:28S–34S.
52. Jacoby R, Abraham A. Bullous dermatosis and systemic lupus erythematosus in a 15-year-old boy. Arch Dermatol 1979; 115:1094–1097.
53. Sontheimer R. The lexicon of cutaneous lupus erythematosus—a review and personal perspective on the nomenclature and classification of the cutaneous manifestations of lupus erythematosus. Lupus 1997; 6:84–95.
54. Sontheimer R. The vesiculobullous manifestations of lupus erythematosus AAD annual meeting Washington DC, December 7, 1988.
55. Ting W, Stone MS, Racila D, et al. Toxic epidermal necrolysis-like acute cutaneous lupus erythematosus and the spectrum of the acute syndrome of apoptotic pan-epidermolysis (ASAP): a case report, concept review and proposal for new classification of lupus erythematosus vesiculobullous skin lesions. Lupus 2004; 13(12):941–950.
56. Jarratt M, Ramsdell W. Infantile acropustulosis. Arch Dermatol 1979; 115: 834–836.
57. Kahn G, Rywlin A. Acropustulosis of infancy. Arch Dermatol 1979; 115: 831–833.
58. Barr R, Globerman L, Werber F, Transient neonatal pustular melanosis, Int J Dermatol 1979;18:636–638.
59. Dogliotti M, Caro I, Hartlegen R, et al. Leucomelanoderma in blacks. S Afr Med J 1974; 48:1555.

60. Hardwick N, Van Gelder L, Vandermerwe C, et al. Exogenous ochronosis: an epidemiologic study. Br J Dermatol 1989; 120:229.
61. Harman R. Dermatitis cruris pustulosa et atrophicans, the Nigerian shin disease. Br J Dermatol 1968; 80:97.
62. Goh C, Chua S, NG S, (eds). The Asian skin: a reference color atlas of dermatology. Singapore: McGraw-Hill, 2005.
63. Kushi M. Your face never lies. Wayne, New Jersey: Avery Publishing, 1983.
64. Deleo V, Taylor S, Belsito D, et al. The effect of race and ethnicity on patch test results. J Amer Acad Dermatol 2002; 46:S107–S112.
65. Reifenstahl L. People of Kau. New York, New York: Harper and Row, 1976.
66. Pierce H. Dermatologic involvement with black youth. J Nat Med Assoc 1971; 63:58.
67. Cummer C. Etiology of lupus erythematosus: occurrence in the Negro. Arch Dermatol 1936; 33:434.
68. Taylor S, Epidemiology of skin diseases in ethnic populations. Dermatol Clinics 2003; 21:601–607.
69. Fox H. Observations on skin diseases in the Negro. J Cutan Dis 1908; 26:67.
70. Halder R, Grimes P, McLaurin C, et al. Incidence of common dermatoses in a predominantly black dermatologic practice. Cutis 1983; 32:388–390.
71. Hazen H. Personal observations upon skin diseases in the American Negro. J Cutan Dis 1914; 32:704.
72. Schachner L, Ling N, Press S, Statistical analysis of a pediatric dermatology clinic. Pediatr Dermatol 1983; 1:157–164.
73. Harman, R. Letter from Ibadan. Br J Dermatol 1962; 74:416.
74. Kenney J. Management of Dermatoses peculiar to Negroes. Arch Dermatol 1965; 91:126.
75. Okoro A. Skin disease in Nigeria. Trans St. Johns Hosp Dermatol Soc 1973; 59(1):68–72.
76. Somorin A. The secular changes of skin and venereal diseases in Nigeria. Int J Dermatol 1979; 18:59–62.
77. Vollum D. An impression of dermatology in Uganda. Trans St. Johns Hosp Dermatol Soc 1973; 59:120–128.
78. Dinehart S, Herzberg A, Kerns B, et al. Acne keloidalis: a review. J Dermatol Surg Oncol 1989; 15:642–647.
79. Vernall D. A study of the size and shape of cross sections of hair from four races of men. Am J Phys Anthropol 1961; 19:345.
80. Taylor S, ed. Understanding Skin of Color. J Amer Acad Dermatol 2002; 46:S41–S124.
81. Murono K, Fujita K, Yoshioka H. Microbiologic characteristics of exfoliative toxin-producing Staphylococcus aureus. Pediatr Infect Dis J 1988; 7:313–315.
82. Amagai M, Matsuyoshi N, Wang Z, et al. Toxin in bullous impetigo and staphylococcal scalded-skin syndrome targets desmoglein 1. Nat Med 2000; 6: 1275–1277.
83. Verhagen A. Pomade acne in Black skin (Letter). Arch Dermatol 1974; 110:465.
84. Sperling L, Solomon A, Whiting D. A new look at scarring alopecia. Arch Dermatol 2000; 136:235–242.

85. Brauner G, Flandermeyer K. Pseudofolliculitis barbae II, treatment. Int J Dermatol 1977; 16:520.
86. Jacyk W. Clinical and pathologic observations in dermatitis cruris pustulosa et atrophicans. Int J Dermatol 1978; 10:802.
87. Brauner G. Acne keloid: neither acne nor keloidal [abstr]. 16th Int Congress Dermatol Tokyo 1982.
88. Brauner G. Cutaneous disease in the Black races. In: Moschella S, ed. Dermatology. Philadelphia, Pennsylvania: Saunders, 1990.

15

Acne and Scarring

Andrew F. Alexis and Susan C. Taylor

Skin of Color Center, St. Luke's-Roosevelt Hospital and Columbia University College of Physicians and Surgeons, New York, New York, U.S.A.

INTRODUCTION

Acne vulgaris is a frequently encountered dermatologic condition in people of color who live in the Americas, Europe, Africa, and Asia. Although there are many similarities in acne between people of color and Caucasians, differences in the presenting complaint, clinical presentation, cultural skin and hair care practices, treatment selection and adverse events have been described. Acne vulgaris is an inflammatory disorder with sequelae that may have profound consequences in individuals with skin of color. These sequelae may include postinflammatory hyperpigmentation (PIH) and keloidal scarring. PIH is often the primary presenting complaint for acne patients with darker skin types. This is because a typical acne lesion resolves within two weeks, but the hyperpigmentation that results from acne may remain for months or even years in these individuals. Hence, lesions of PIH are often of greater concern to this patient population than the acne. Education of skin of color patients about the necessity of treatment of acne is a distinguishing feature in these patients.

 Whereas, the primary treatment options for acne vulgaris arc similar across skin phototypes, races, and ethnicities, the selection of specific modalities may differ. All approved therapies are ultimately utilized to one degree or another in this patient population, but modifications are often instituted to avoid adverse events such as irritation-induced hyperpigmentation.

Furthermore, certain topical and oral medications may be preferred in this population for their ability to treat concomitant disorders such as PIH.

Finally, a knowledge of culturally specific skin and hair care practices, particularly the use of hair pomades in the African American population, impacts treatment recommendations and therapy.

Acne vulgaris, a seemingly routine cutaneous disorder, has several unique features in individuals with skin of color. This chapter will highlight the important differences in this leading disorder in individuals with skin of color.

EPIDEMIOLOGY

Data regarding the epidemiology of cutaneous diseases in individuals with skin of color is limited. Insight into skin diseases, including acne, in these populations is often based upon health-care service utilization data such as retrospective private and clinic practice surveys as well as dermatologists' published reports of their personal experience (1–5). The data indicates that acne vulgaris is indeed a disorder for which many individuals of color seek health-care services. Acne vulgaris has been reported as the most common diagnosis seen in black patients in published surveys in the United States (1) and the United Kingdom (2). A survey of Latino patients in the United States, indicated that acne vulgaris was the most common dermatologic disease in this ethnic group (3). In Asians, data from a practice survey in Singapore found acne to be the second most frequent diagnosis observed in adult patients (4). Similarly, in the Middle East, a study from Kuwait reported acne vulgaris to be the third most common dermatosis observed in preadolescent children (5). Because acne vulgaris is clearly a disorder which occurs with frequency in the skin of color population, it is imperative that dermatologists are well versed in the diagnosis and treatment of this disorder.

PATHOGENESIS

There is no data that conclusively supports the notion that the pathogenesis of acne vulgaris in individuals with skin of color is different from that in Caucasian skin. A review of the literature reveals that there is no data to suggest that there are differences in desquamation of the pilosebaceous epithelium with abnormal follicular keratinization and plugging, in the proliferation of *Propionibacterium acnes,* or in sebum production (1). Studies evaluating ethnic differences in *P. acnes* colonization as well as sebum production have been performed but report conflicting results and have generally been hampered by small sample sizes and/or suboptimal designs. Therefore, there is insufficient evidence to suggest racial or ethnic differences in these factors. However, the evolution of the acne lesion and the degree of inflammation at clinical presentation may vary in darker skin types.

Histologic differences in acne vulgaris in black skin have been reported. A study by Halder et al. (2) examining biopsies of 30 African American women with acne found marked histologic inflammation. Most notably, significant polymorphonuclear cell infiltration was observed even in clinically noninflammatory lesions (e.g., comedones). Furthermore, in inflammatory papules and pustules, the inflammatory infiltrate was extensive and located at a substantial distance from the actual papule or pustule. This finding may explain the propensity toward PIH commonly observed in dark-skinned individuals with acne.

Although the pathogenesis of PIH is unclear, the release of inflammatory mediators such as interleukin-1 alpha and prostaglandin E2 have been identified in a porcine model of PIH from oleic acid–induced acne (3).

CLINICAL FEATURES

The characteristic lesions of acne vulgaris in individuals with skin of color include inflammatory lesions—papules, pustules, nodules, and cysts—and noninflammatory lesions—open and closed comedones. However, given the histologic data regarding comedones, perhaps these lesions should be classified as inflammatory in the skin of color patient (7). The relative frequency of comedonal and noncomedonal lesions may differ between various racial and ethnic groups.

A 1970 study of 1646 inmates in Michigan (893 whites, 753 blacks) found a significantly higher prevalence of nodulocystic acne in whites (5%) compared to blacks (0.5%) (4). By contrast, no racial differences in the anatomic distribution (face, back, chest, and neck) of acne lesions were found.

A more recent survey of 313 patients (239 black, 55 Hispanic, and 19 Asian and other) conducted at the Skin of Color Center in New York City reported cystic acne in 18.0%, 25.5%, and 10.5% of blacks, Hispanics, and Asians/other ethnicities-respectively (1). In the same study, papules and comedones were the predominant lesion types in all three ethnic groups, affecting approximately three-quarters and one-half of patients, respectively.

The most notable clinical difference observed in acne in ethnic skin is the frequent presence of PIH or acne hyperpigmented macules (AHMs). AHMs are often the chief complaint of dark-skinned patients with acne and, in extensive cases, can cause significant disfigurement and adversely affect self-esteem (1). AHMs were reported in 65% of blacks, 52% of Hispanics, and 47% of Asians studied in the above survey of 313 patients (1). The average duration of the AHM was reported to be four months or longer. In the authors' experience, AHMs are frequently of equal or greater concern to the dark-skinned patient than the acne itself, and therefore warrant prompt treatment. Patient's terminology regarding AHMs is not limited to hyperpigmentation but terms such as scarring, blemishes, spots, and dark marks are frequently used. Furthermore, at the time of presentation to the dermatologist, there may be a paucity of acneiform lesions present which may be in contrast to many prominent AHMs. In this situation, patients of color may be reticent to use acne medications and instead are only motivated to seek and use skin-lightening medications. It is imperative that dermatologists discuss the importance of treating even mild acne to prevent the further occurrence of PIH.

Acne scarring appears to be less prevalent in blacks compared to other racial groups, and this may be related to the lower prevalence of nodulocystic acne (1). Ice pick scarring has been observed in cases of moderate-to-severe acne in this patient population. However, the risk of keloid scarring secondary to inflammatory acne is a major consideration in patients with skin of color. This is most commonly seen as a sequela of truncal acne with the chest and back as common sites but can also appear on the face, especially in the area of the jawline (unpublished clinical observation). The possible formation of keloidal scarring is a compelling reason for the institution of immediate treatment of acne in the skin of color population. Prevention of keloidal scars is preferable to treating this form of scarring, which is often a therapeutic challenge.

Pomade acne is a unique clinical variant of acne vulgaris which occurs primarily in African Americans, in whom it was first described (5). Pomade acne is diagnosed clinically by the presence of multiple closed comedones and occasionally scattered papulopustules in the distribution of the forehead and temples. Pomade acne occurs secondary to the use of occlusive oil-based products to groom and improve the manageability of the hair. Furthermore, women with skin of color, in an attempt to camouflage PIH, may select oil-based cosmetic products that may likewise lead to comedonal acne.

THERAPY

The treatment of acne vulgaris in patients with skin of color does not differ dramatically from that of other patients. Standard therapeutic modalities including benzoyl peroxide preparations, topical and oral antibiotics, topical and oral retinoids, as well as hormonal therapies may be appropriate in certain skin of color patients. Additionally, a unique treatment consideration in skin of color is the prevention as well as the treatment of PIH. To that end, therapies that treat both active acne and PIH are preferable. Furthermore, therapeutic agents that are well tolerated and have the least propensity for irritation and resulting PIH are also of benefit in this population.

Topical retinoids are particularly important in the treatment of acne in skin of color patients. The three retinoids commonly used in the United States are adapalene, tazarotene, and tretinoin. Each of the retinoids has been studied in darkly pigmented skin and has been demonstrated to be effective in treating both acne lesions and associated PIH (10–16). It is theorized that topical retinoids are able to improve hyperpigmentation by several mechanisms including the following:

- Inhibition of tyrosinase induction in melanocytes
- Enhancement of desquamation that speeds up sloughing of melanin in keratinocytes
- inhibition of melanosome transfer from melanocytes to keratinocytes
- Redistribution or dispersion of epidermal melanin

Effectiveness in treating acne-induced PIH in dark skin has been demonstrated with 0.1 % (6) and 0.025% (7) retinoic acid (tretinoin) cream, adapalene 0.1% gel (8–11), and tazarotene 0.1% cream (12). Adapalene appears to be well tolerated in numerous ethnic groups studied, including black South Africans (8), US and European blacks (9), and Chinese (10,11).

Although topical retinoids have been demonstrated to be effective in the treatment of acne-induced PIH, minimizing irritation from these agents is especially important in darker skin in order to prevent irritation-induced PIH. As such, the selection of an appropriate vehicle for a given patient's skin type is paramount. In general, cream vehicles are better tolerated and are preferred in patients with sensitive or dry skin. Gels can be reserved for patients with oily skin and/or patients who have developed a tolerance to topical retinoid creams after extended use. Several therapeutic maneuvers serve to improve tolerability of retinoids such as every other day dosing for the first two to four weeks of therapy, applying a small amount of the medication to completely dry skin and moisturizing liberally after application. Equally important is advising patients to eliminate potentially drying topical agents including toners, astringents, masks, and scrubs which may reduce the tolerability to topical retinoids. Initiating therapy with a low concentration topical retinoid preparation (e.g., tretinoin 0.025% cream or tazarotene 0.05%) and gradually increasing the strength as tolerated is also a helpful strategy in maximizing tolerability and efficacy in patients with skin of color.

It is theorized that oral retinoids may be underutilized in the treatment of severe acne in the African-American–skin of color population (6). The perception among clinicians that acne is less severe in African Americans may be the reason why African Americans appear to be prescribed isotretinoin less often than Caucasians. The oral retinoid, isotretinoin, was reported to not only improve acne but also moderate PIH in a case report of an Asian patient (13).

Benzoyl peroxide preparations are also important therapeutic modalities in the treatment of acne in skin of color patients. Combination products containing 5% benzoyl peroxide and a topical antibiotic (clindamycin or erythromycin) are particularly useful in mild-to-moderate acne, given their antimicrobial and anti-inflammatory effects. A special consideration for these preparations in ethnic skin is the need to prevent irritation-induced PIH. As such, higher concentrations of benzoyl peroxide (i.e., greater than 5%) should be avoided unless the skin is deemed oily. In addition, the selection of a nondrying vehicle that is well tolerated is important. Aqueous gels are, in general, better tolerated in this skin type than alcohol-based gels.

Azelaic acid is another potentially useful topical agent in the treatment of acne in darker skin types. In particular, 20% azelaic acid cream has been shown to be effective in treating inflammatory and noninflammatory acne lesions as well as associated hyperpigmentation (14). Its effect on hyperpigmentation—via reversible inhibition of tyrosinase—makes azelaic acid especially suitable for the treatment of acne in ethnic skin. However, the clinical experience of these authors' is that azelaic acid is less effective in the treatment of acne and AHMs than topical retinoids (unpublished clinical observation).

As PIH is one of the greatest concerns in dark-skinned acne patients, the use of adjunctive bleaching agents to address this issue is particularly helpful. Formulations containing 4% hydroquinone are the most widely used for the treatment of AHMs. Clinical experience suggests that 4% hydroquinone is effective in hastening the resolution of AHMs in skin of color (1), and can be employed concurrently as part of a combination regimen in the treatment of acne. However, the potential for a halo of hypopigmentation surrounding an AHM is a potential complication of this therapy; this effect is reversible and resolves over several weeks after discontinuation of hydroquinone. A novel use of a combination treatment of mequinol 2%/ tretinoin 0.01% solution with a unique applicator tip has been reportedly effective in the treatment of PIH (15).

Other adjunctive therapies for acne in ethnic skin include superficial chemical peels and microdermabrasion. The safety and efficacy of salicylic acid (20% and 30%) (16) and glycolic acid (30–50%) (17) peels in darkly pigmented skin has been reported by several authors. Salicylic acid peels are particularly advantageous in the treatment of acne as they are effective comedolytic agents and can help reduce hyperpigmentation (likely via increased epidermal turnover and enhanced penetration of concomitantly used bleaching agents). The safety of chemical peels in the treatment of acne in skin of color hinges on minimizing the risk of PIH. This can be achieved by initiating therapy at the lowest concentration (e.g., 20% salicylic acid) and titrating upward as tolerated, discontinuing topical retinoids one week prior to a peel, and ensuring sunscreen use after peels. When used as a concomitant adjunctive therapy in the treatment of acne, chemical peels are conveniently performed at four-week intervals (however many authors advocate two-week intervals). The safety of microdermabrasion in darker skin complexions has also been reported and can be used to treat AHMs and mild acne scarring (18). However, there is no evidence to suggest that microdermabrasion is more effective than chemical peeling (19). As with peels, PIH is a potential complication when the procedure is performed in dark skin.

Light-based therapies for acne are the newest addition to our therapeutic armamentarium for acne and acne scarring. However, the safety of these procedures in darker skin has not been studied extensively. A pilot study involving 19 patients with Fitzpatrick skin types I to VI reported safety and efficacy of long-pulsed dye laser-mediated photodynamic therapy combined with topical therapy for mild-to-severe comedonal, inflammatory, or cystic acne (20). Another study evaluated nonablative 1450-nm diode laser in the treatment of facial atrophic acne scars in Asians with Fitzpatrick skin types IV to V. Nonablative resurfacing for atrophic acne scars with the pulsed 1320-nm Neodymium: yttrium aluminum garnet (Nd:YAG) laser has also been studied in skin types I to V (21,22). Although reportedly safe, hyperpigmentation remains a potential adverse event of nonablative lasers in darker skin types. Further research into the use of light-based therpies for acne in skin of color is warranted.

SUMMARY

Acne vulgaris is one of the most common reasons individuals of all races and ethnicities seek consultation by a dermatologist. In skin of color, differences in the prevalence, histology, clinical presentation, and approach to treatment have been described. Understanding these differences is important in the diagnosis and treatment of this leading disorder in ethnic skin.

REFERENCES

1. Taylor SC, Cook-Bolden F, Rahman Z, Strachan D. Acne vulgaris in skin of color. J Am Acad Dermatol 2002; 46(suppl 2):S98–S106.
2. Halder RM HY, Bridgeman-Shah S, Kligman AM. A clinical pathological study of acne vulgaris in black females. J Invest Dermatol Clin 1996; 106:888.
3. Kitawaki A TY, Takada K. New Findings on the mechanism of post-inflammatory hyperpigmentation [abstr]. Pigment Cell Res 2003; 16(5):603.
4. Wilkins JW Jr., Voorhees JJ. Prevalence of nodulocystic acne in white and Negro males. Arch Dermatol 1970; 102(6):631–634.
5. Plewig G, Fulton JE, Kligman AM. Pomade acne. Arch Dermatol 1970; 101(5):580–584.
6. Haider RM. The role of retinoids in the management of cutaneous conditions in blacks. J Am Acad Dermatol 1998; 39(2 Pt 3):S98–S103.
7. Tu P, Li GQ, Zhu XJ, Zheng J, Wong WZ. A comparison of adapalene gel 0.1 % vs tretinoin gel 0.025% in the treatment of acne vulgaris in China. J Eur Acad Dermatol Venereol 2001; 15(Suppl 3):31–36.
8. Zhu XJ, Tu P, Zhen J, Duan YQ. Adapalene gel 0.1 %: effective and well tolerated in the topical treatment of acne vulgaris in Chinese patients. Cutis 2001; 68(suppl 4):55–59.

9. Grimes P, Callender V. Tazarotene cream for postinflammatory hyperpigmentation and acne vulgaris in darker skin: a double-blind, randomized, vehicle-controlled study. Cutis 2006; 77(l):45–50.

10. Winhoven SM, Ahmed I, Owen CM, Lear JT. Postinflammatory hyperpigmentation in an Asian patient: a dramatic response to oral isotretinoin (13-cis-retinoic acid). Br J Dermatol 2005; 152(2):368–369.

11. Fitton A, Goa KL. Azelaic acid A review of its pharmacological properties and therapeutic efficacy in acne and hyperpigmentary skin disorders. Drugs 1991; 41(5):780–798.

12. Taylor SC, Young M. A multicenter, 12-week, nonrandomized phase 3b trial: combination solution of mequinol 2%/ tretinoin 0.01% vs hydroquinone 4% cream in the treatment of mild-to-moderate postinflammatory hyperpigmentation. Poster presentation at the 64th Annual Meeting of the American Academy of Dermatology, San Francisco, CA, March 3–7, 2006.

13. Grimes PE. The safety and efficacy of salicylic acid chemical peels in darker racial-ethnic groups. Dermatol Surg 1999; 25(1):18–22.

14. Jacyk WK. Adapalene in the treatment of African patients. J Eur Acad Dermatol Venereol 2001; 15(Suppl 3):37–42.

15. Czernielewski J, Poncet M, Mizzi F. Efficacy and cutaneous safety of adapalene in black patients versus white patients with acne vulgaris. Cutis 2002; 70(4): 243–248.

16. Bulengo-Ransby SM, Griffiths CE, Kimbrough-Green CK, et al. Topical tretinoin (retinoic acid) therapy for hyperpigmented lesions caused by inflammation of the skin in black patients. N Engl J Med 1993; 328(20):1438–1443.

17. Roberts WE. Chemical peeling in ethnic/dark skin. Dermatol Ther 2004; 17(2):196–205.

18. Grimes PE. Microdermabrasion. Dermatol Surg 2005; 31(9 Pt 2):1160–1165 discussion 5.

19. Alam M, Omura NE, Dover JS, Arndt KA. Glycolic acid peels compared to microdermabrasion: a right-left controlled trial of efficacy and patient satisfaction. Dermatol Surg 2002; 28(6):475–479.

20. Alexiadcs-Aimenakas M. Long-pulsed dye laser-mediated photodynamic therapy combined with topical therapy for mild to severe comedonal, inflammatory, or cystic acne. J Drugs Dermatol 2006; 5(1):45–55.

21. Jeong JT, Kye YC. Resurfacing of pitted facial acne scars with a long-pulsed Er:YAG laser. Dermatol Surg 2001; 27(2):107–110.

22. Tanzi EL, Alster TS. Comparison of a 1450-nm diode laser and a 1320-nm Nd;YAG laser in the treatment of atrophic facial scars: a prospective clinical and histologic study. Dermatol Surg 2004; 30(2 Pt 1):152–157.

16

Black Skin Cosmetics: Specific Skin and Hair Problems of African Americans and Cosmetic Approaches for Their Treatment

Christian Oresajo and Sreekumar Pillai

Engelhard Corporation, Stony Brook, New York, U.S.A.

INTRODUCTION

According to U.S. Census Bureau, the population of the three main ethnic groups in the United States, blacks, Hispanics, and Asians, are expected to reach 87 million and comprise more than 30% of the population by 2005. Industry tracking shows that members of these groups tend to spend a greater portion of their income on personal care products. This has prompted skin-care product developers and cosmetic companies to pay more attention to the ethnic consumer (1). Hispanic and African American women use four times more personal care products than Caucasian women (2). One of the factors influencing this success is African Americans' purchasing power, which has been steadily rising in recent years, according to the Selig Center for Economic Growth at the University of Georgia. black purchasing power reached $533 billion in 1999, up 73% from $308 billion in 1990. Industry executives said this trend is expected to continue (2). Up until recently, there were only few ethnic personal care product makers. They were mostly small, family owned and managed mostly by African Americans. However, in recent years many major cosmetic companies have begun to give attention to black skin and hair problems as evidenced by the start of new programs and institutions devoting to research in African American skin and hair problems. An example is the L'Oreal Institute for Ethnic Hair and Skin Research started in 2001 in Chicago.

In many respects, people with black skin are faced with greater challenges than fair-skinned people. Black skin, for instance, is more prone to hyperpigmentation and scarring following injury or other inflammations. To prevent these, they need to always guard against acne and to continually protect their skin from the sun. In fact, any conditions that irritate skin, such as picking blemishes, shaving or plucking hair, can result in black skin producing more melanin and creating dark spots. During pregnancy too, many dark-skinned women experience the "mask of pregnancy," or a darkening of skin around the neck due to hormonal changes. Generally black women also tend to have oily facial skin, which can be compounded by more than just the skin's natural oils. Ironically, although black women are prone to excessive facial oils, they also have dry, ashy body skin. Thus, the cosmetic industry is challenged by special needs of black skin to design and formulate special cosmetic formulations to address these special needs. In this chapter, we summarize some of the racial differences in black skin, identify some specific skin, hair, and nail problems faced by black skin, and then address some of the specific cosmetic products in the market that addresses these problems.

RACIAL DIFFERENCES IN THE SKIN AND HAIR

Stratum Corneum and the Permeability Barrier

There is evidence that black skin is more prone to dryness, suggesting racial differences in lipid content of skin. Studies by Reed et al. (3) suggested that there may be lipid differences in the dark vs. lighter skin. The darkly pigmented skin showed a more resistant barrier and recovered more quickly after perturbation by tape strippings than skin of individuals with lighter pigmentation. This would suggest higher rate of lipid synthesis in darker skin. Other studies have also suggested that the lipid content of black skin may be higher than that of Caucasian skin (4). Investigators have observed higher lipid content in black epidermis, greater cellular cohesion, less permeability to certain chemicals, and more difficulty in stripping off the black skin stratum corneum (SC). A greater number of strippings were required for removal of stratum corneum in blacks than was required in Caucasians; black subjects were also found to have a greater variance in the thickness of stratum corneum layers as well as with stratum corneum stripping (4). A difference in the pH gradient is also reported between black and white skin (5). The initial three to six tape strippings showed significantly increased water loss and decrease in pH in black skin as compared to white skin. An increase in spontaneous desquamation in blacks, compared to other races has also been reported. This was attributed to a difference in the composition of the intercellular cement of the stratum corneum. In a study by Sugino et al. (6), blacks were found to have the lowest levels of ceramides in the stratum corneum compared to Caucasians, Hispanics, and Asians. Other studies could not find differences in the stratum corneum properties between black and white skin. Despite differences in age, anatomic areas of skin for skin roughness, scaliness, and stratum corneum hydration, there were no significant differences between black and white skin (7). Skin hydration, roughness, or scaliness was similar between different races (7). In summary, although several studies tend to suggest differences in structure of stratum corneum, barrier properties, and lipid composition between black and white skin, conclusive evidence for these differences have not been established.

Epidermal Structure

Differences in the thickness of the epidermis between black (6.5 μm) and Caucasian groups (7.2 μm) have been reported, although individual variations were also evident (8). The stratum lucidum consists of one to two layers in the non-sun-exposed skins in both black and Caucasian groups. In blacks, the stratum lucidum is compact and unaltered in sun-exposed skin, while in White individuals, stratum lucidum appeared thicker. In both groups the stratum granulosum consists of up to three layers (8). Major differences in the hair follicle, an important component of the epidermal structure, exist between blacks and Whites. Differences in the hair follicle structure determine the shape and quality of hair. This is discussed in the later section on hair.

Dermal Structure

Some differences have been reported in literature between the dermal structures of black and white skin. Black dermis is generally thick and compact, when compared to white dermis, which is thinner and less compact (9). The papillary and reticular layers are more distinct in white skin. They also contain larger collagen fiber bundles and the fiber fragments are sparse. Smaller collagen fiber bundles are present in blacks with close stacking, and a surrounding ground substance. Fiber fragments are more prominent and numerous in black skin. Both black and white skin have numerous melanophages; however, they are larger in blacks. Fibroblasts and lymphatic vessels are more numerous in black skin; they are dilated empty lymph channels usually surrounded by masses of elastic fibers (9). In general, because of the high melanin content of black skin, the intensity of photodamage is usually less apparent in black skin. However, despite the common perception that black skin shows less chronologic aging than white skin, a detailed study suggests that black skin shows similar chronologic changes as white skin with age (10). Biomechanical properties related to elasticity of the skin, such as skin extensibility, skin elastic recovery, and skin elastic modulus also showed some variability between races. Differences were observed between blacks and whites in dorsal (sun exposed) and volar (unexposed) sites on the forearm skin extensibility differed significantly between both sites in whites but not in blacks. These may be due to the different degrees of damage due to solar exposure between the volar and dorsal sides of the forearm in whites versus blacks.

Melanocytes

The major color determinant in the skin is the pigment melanin, a product of a specialized cell known as melanocytes. Human melanin is composed of two distinct polymers, dark brown/black eumelanin, and yellow/red pheomelanin (11). Eumelanin is made and deposited in ellipsoidal melanosomes which contain fibrillar internal structure, whereas pheomelanin is synthesized in spherical melanosomes and is associated with microvesicles (12). Black-skinned people have higher content and synthesis of eumelanin versus pheomelanin.

There are no differences in the number of melanocytes between the skin of a black person versus white person. However, the melanocytes of the dark-pigmented person are much more active in producing the dark-pigmented melanin, eumelanin. The morphology, content, and distribution of melanosomes also differ between races. Black skin contains more of eumelanin. The melanosomes are uniformly distributed, and do not appear to have a limiting membrane and they are stuck together closely. Caucasian skin melanin contain higher ratio of pheomelanin (the ratio of eu to pheo melanin depends on the particular skin color), the melanosomes are smaller, round and contain limiting membrane, and distributed in clusters with spaces between them, giving a lighter color. In lighter skin individuals the melanin content is much less in the upper layers of stratum corneum due to increased breakdown of the melanosomes. In summary, in black skin, melanocytes are more active in making melanins, melanosomes are packed and distributed and broken down differently than in white skin. In addition, the keratinocytes in the black skin also play a role in melanin distribution. Melanosomes are distributed individually by keratinocytes in dark skin whereas they are distributed in membrane-bound clusters by keratinocytes in white individuals (13). These results suggest that regulatory factors within the keratinocytes determine recipient melanosome distribution patterns.

Sebaceous and Sweat Glands

The pilosebaceous unit which comprises of the sebaceous glands, eccrine sweat glands, and apocrine sweat glands (sweat glands are also referred to as sudoriferous glands). The ratio of sebaceous gland to sweat glands is believed to be higher in blacks and the sweat glands in darker skin are believed to be larger providing better tolerance to hot climates (14). However, carefully controlled clinical studies suggest no significant differences between black and white skin with regard to the amount of sweat and sebaceous glands (4). Some studies have suggested racial differences in sebaceous glands' size and activity (14); however, no significant difference has been shown in sebum production between black and white skin. A comparison of 649 male and female subjects of different races found no consistent differences in sebaceous gland activity between black and white skin. These findings are consistent with the clinical impression and epidemiological data that the incidence of acne is similar between blacks and whites (15).

Hair Follicles and Hair Structure

The hair fiber is produced by the mitotic activity of the hair follicle, which is one of the most proliferative cell types in the human body. Structurally, hair consists of an outer cortex and a central medulla. Enclosing the hair shaft is a layer of overlapping keratinized scales, the hair cuticle, that serves as protective layers. The hair follicle is a unique composite organ, composed of epithelial and dermal compartments interacting with each other in a surprisingly autonomous way. Of the four hair types, the majority of blacks have spiral hair. The hair of blacks is naturally more brittle and more susceptible to breakage and spontaneous knotting than that of Whites. The difference in the shape of the hair shaft is intrinsically programmed from the bulb, indicating a genetic difference in hair follicle structure (16). Some characteristics observed on cross-sectional evaluation of black hair include a longer major axis, flattened elliptical shape; they also have curved follicles. In a comparative study of different racial and ethnic groups, there were no significant differences in the thickness of the cuticle, scale size and shape, and cortical cells of whites compared to blacks. black hair has an elliptical shape, while Asians have round shaped, straight hair; Caucasian hair is intermediate. The length and degree of curliness is determined genetically. The curly nature of black hair is believed to result from the shape of the hair follicle (17). In studies of the hair follicles, blacks were found to have fewer elastic fibers anchoring the hair follicles to the dermis, when compared to White subjects. Melanosomes were found to be in both the outer root sheath and in the bulb of vellus hairs in blacks but not in white. Black hair also has more pigment and on microscopy has larger melanin granules. There is no difference in keratin types between hair from different races, and no difference has been found in the amino-acid composition of hair from different races (18), although one study found variation in the levels of some amino acids between black and white hair (19). Black subjects had significantly greater levels of tyrosine, phenylalanine, and ammonia in the hair, but were deficient in serine and threonine (19).

PROBLEMS SPECIFIC TO BLACK SKIN

Pigmentary Disorders

People with darker skin often experience hyperpigmentation (discoloration or dark spots). This discoloration results from a variety of causes that lead to inflammation and activation of melanocytes. The causes include: acne, insect bites, scratches, abrasions, or overexposure to sun. Typical areas of discoloration are joints (e.g., knees, elbows, etc.) and eye area. Uneven skin pigmentation resulting from this hyperpigmentation often results in uneven light reflectance and differences in the skin optical properties of black skin. This results in certain areas of skin, especially areas that are prone to be dry with flaky skin as looking "ashy."

Ashy Skin

Dry skin is a problem for individuals of all skin colors, but may be very distressing to persons with black skin. Dry skin, especially in areas such as elbows and knees can be flaky and gives a gray, ash-like appearance. It is easily noticed in persons with black skin. Using moisturizers regularly can help reduce this condition. Ashiness can also affect the scalp. Use of moisturizers, hair oils, and hair-dressing agents (pomades) that make the hair more manageable can decrease scalp dryness.

Folliculitis

Pomade can spread to the forehead and block pores, causing pimples called pomade acne. Pomade can also contribute to a bacterial infection of the scalp called folliculitis. Folliculitis produces pus, bumps, and redness around the hair. It can also cause hair loss or can spread infection. Some black men, especially those who use razors for cutting hair on the back of their necks, develop keloid-like scars on the back of their necks, this condition is referred to as "Pseudofolliculitis Barbae". The area may itch and sometimes becomes infected. Treatment consists of oral antibiotics, topical acne products, and topical or injected cortisone. In severe cases it can cause scarring and keloid-like lesions on the chin and face.

Scarring and Keloids

A keloid is an overgrowth of fibrous tissue on the skin, following trauma (e.g., acne, vaccination, shaving wounds, ear piercing, insect bite, or surgical incision). It can be due to the overproduction of collagen, or due to deficiency of metalloproteases. The tissue response is abnormal to the normal process of wound healing or repair. The result is a raised, firm, thickened red/brown scar that may grow for a prolonged period and develop claw-like projections. Genetics and age play a role in keloid development. Although seen in black skin, it is less prevalent than in East Indian and Polynesian skin.

Irritation and Contact Dermatitis

In general, it is believed that black skin is prone to less irritation than Caucasian or Asian skin. Cutaneous reactions to 1% dichloroethylsulfide showed erythema in 58% of White subjects but in only 15% of black subjects (20). Blacks were found to be less susceptible to cutaneous irritants before the stratum corneum was removed by tape stripping (21). Darkly pigmented South African blacks were found to have lower incidence of industrial contact dermatitis (22). On the other hand, after testing many topical materials on both black and White subjects, there was no significant difference in the two races (23).

Altered Immune Responses

A difference in the cutaneous cell-mediated immunity between fair- and dark-skin people has been described (24). Fair-skinned people (skin type 1/II who are sun sensitive and tan poorly) are more sensitive to UVR (typically 1 hour noonday exposure to sun) in protection from erythema and suppression of contact hypersensitivity than skin type III/IV individuals. A race-specific immune response to UVB appears to be mediated by skin and may partly explain the resistance of blacks to photodependent skin cancer (25). An ultrastructural difference in the mast cell morphology has been reported (26). Mast cells in black skin contain larger granules than those in white skin due to increased fusion of smaller granules. Black skin mast cell granules appear to contain higher amount of cathepsin G reactivity than white skin.

Vitiligo

Vitiligo is a common condition where pigment cells are destroyed and irregular white patches on the skin appear. The cause of this is still under intense investigation. The extent of color loss differs with each person and there is no way to predict how much pigment a person will lose. Some people lose pigment over their entire bodies. Most patients with vitiligo do not regain skin color without treatment. Several methods are used to treat vitiligo, but none is perfect. The most common method is Psolaren Ultraviolet A rays therapy, combining light treatments and medication. In cases where vitiligo affects most of the body it is sometimes best to destroy the remaining normal pigment.

PROBLEMS SPECIFIC TO BLACK HAIR AND NAIL

Oily Skin and Hair

Generally speaking, due to the curly nature of the black hair, it looks more oily. In addition, it is also likely that the scalp of black skin contains larger and/more numbers of sebaceous glands that produce more oil. The amount of oil in a person's hair and skin varies, depending on race and time of year (e.g., sun and wind, temperature, and humidity). Skin looks the oiliest in hot, humid weather. Androgens, or male hormones, control the production of oil by the sebaceous glands in the skin. Higher relative levels of androgens can make the skin more oily. For example, this can occur during puberty and when taking performance-enhancing steroids.

Brittle Hair, Hair Breakage, and Hair Loss

Certain techniques and preparations used to style black hair can lead to a variety of problems. Hair loss or broken hairs at the scalp margins in women may be a problem. It may be caused by repeated or frequent tight braiding (traction alopecia), hair straightening agents (i.e., perms, relaxers), or tight rollers, and as a result of hair styled in a ponytail or single braid style. Hair straighteners use strong chemicals to change the structure of the hair. While straightened hair is easier to style, it may also become brittle and break easily. Excessive brushing, backcombing, or other stresses also cause breakage. Most hair loss from breakage is temporary because it does not affect normal hair growth. Hair will usually grow back just as it does after it has been cut. Changing hairstyles can solve these problems. In most cases, if discovered early the hair loss from these causes can be reversed.

Ingrown Hairs of the Beards (Razor Bumps)

The hair shafts of African Americans are curved. This is true of beard hair as well as other body hair. After shaving, especially close shaving, the beard's sharp pointed hair may turn back into the skin. It may pierce the wall of the hair follicle, causing a reaction resulting in bumps. Dermatologists call this condition "Pseudofolliculitis Barbae." Men with ingrown hairs (hair bumps) should try different methods of hair removal. Shaving with special types of safety razor, softening the beard using special shaving soaps before shaving, shaving only in the direction of the hair growth, not stretching the skin during shaving and restricting the number of shavings can all help treat this condition. Electrolysis, the permanent removal of hair performed by an experienced operator, may be an effective solution for this problem.

Hyperpigmentation of Nails

Dark streaks or bands on multiple fingernails and toenails in African Americans are usually normal. They tend to increase in number as a person ages. However, the development of a new single dark band on a nail could be a sign of a dangerous type of skin cancer called malignant melanoma and should be checked by a dermatologist.

   The skin, hair, and nail conditions common among African Americans are generally not serious. They can easily be recognized and usually are successfully treated. Some of the less severe problems can be masked or treated using cosmetic products that are specially designed for treatment of such conditions.

POTENTIAL COSMETIC INGREDIENTS TO ADDRESS SPECIFIC PROBLEMS FOR BLACK SKIN AND HAIR

Treatment of "Ashy" Skin and Dry Brittle Hair

Most used strategy is to use increased level of moisturizers to treat ashy skin and dry brittle hair. Dryness caused by extreme cold weather can also cause ashy skin and brittle hair in blacks. Dark skin may be less tolerant to cold weather and therefore more susceptible to damage. Heavy oily materials such as lanolin and mineral oils are generally avoided because they can cause allergy and can aggravate dark skin. Moisturizers containing ingredients such as avocado oil, wheat proteins, cationic conditioners, amino acids, silicones, and trehalose in addition to high amounts of glycerin, pyrrolidon carboxylic acid (PCA) and sodium lactate can be used. Barrier protecting and moisture-retaining creams containing petrolatum, shea, and cocoa or mango butter can also be used to prevent loss of moisture from skin and hair. The use of natural butters and vitamins and natural extracts are preferred to synthetic materials such as petrolatum. In addition to moisturization, ashy skin is also treated with exfoliating agents such as alpha or beta hydroxy acids that will remove the flaky lose scales of stratum corneum from the affected area providing skin with a soft smooth feel. The use of natural exfoliating agents (e.g., fruit extracts) are preferred to more irritating alpha hydroxy acids.

Treatment of Hyper- and Hypopigmentation and Other Skin Color Problems

Skin color problems relating to melanocyte functions such as hyper- and hypopigmentation, dark spots from pregnancy, sun sensitivity, and inflammation-induced pigmentation changes are common in people with skin of color. Several strategies can be used to treat these conditions. Skin-lightening products containing concentrated natural extracts, hydroquinone up to 2% levels, vitamin complexes or other ingredients can be used. Some of the potential skin-lightening materials that are available for a cosmetic chemist and their classes based on their mode of action is shown below:

- Copper chelators that inactivate the enzyme tyrosinase. This group includes compounds such as kojic acid, cysteine, thiols, hydroxamates, and salicylic acid.
- Substrate analogues of tyrosinase such as hydroquinone, arbutin, azelaic acid, phenols, and plant polyphenols.
- Melanin composition modulators (change the melanin content from the more darker eumelanin to the lighter pheomelanin) such as procysteine (L-2-oxothiazolidine-4-carboxylic acid), *N*-acetyl cysteine.
- Antioxidants that reduce the polymerization (and thus dark color) of melanin such as: ascorbic acid, tocopherol, and plant-derived antioxidants.

- Sunscreens to prevent further activation of melanocytes by UVB: oxybenzone and titanium dioxide.
- Melanocyte cytotoxic agents such as hydroquinone derivatives and azalaic acid.
- Melanosome transfer inhibitors (that blocks transfer of melanosomes from melanocytes to keratinocytes) such as serine protease inhibitors.
- Endothelin receptor inhibitors (endothelin stimulates melanocytes to make more melanin): chamomile extract and synthetic inhibitors.
- Plant-derived skin lighteners used in cosmetic products also include: mushroom extracts, wheat, grass, and chamomile extracts.

Sebum Suppression and Antiacne Treatments

Black skin is believed to have higher numbers and/or larger size of sebaceous glands, that secrete sebum. Increased sebum secretion is one of the factors (not the only factor) contributing to increased acne formation.

Acne is one of the most common skin diseases of teenagers and young adults. It is more common in males because of androgen secretions. A square inch of facial skin can contain as many as 5000 sebaceous glands. Hormonal changes that occur at puberty and in adolescence cause these sebaceous glands to grow larger and secrete excess sebum. Acne begins when the ducts or openings of these glands become plugged with dead skin cells, debris, bacteria, and sebum. As the plug grows, it may become visible on the surface of the skin as a small white bump or "white-head." If the plug stretches the duct open, air reaches the materials in the plug and causes darkening or "black-heads." The distended ducts can open into the surrounding tissue, releasing sebum and skin cells resulting in inflammation. Inflammation is also caused by a bacterium called *Propionobacterium acnes*, that lives normally on the skin, but can thrive within the blocked pore. This infection causes inflammation, which is responsible for the redness and swelling of a spot. Sometimes as in severe acne, the pocket of inflammation within a pore can rupture, causing damage to the skin that can result in scarring.

General strategy for the treatment of excessive oil/acne skin is to control the oil secretion in skin and use of agents such as astringents that dry out pimples. The most common over-the-counter remedy for acne is an antibacterial benzoyl peroxide, which can also dry out the skin and encourage it to shed the surface layer of dead skin. Other topical treatments are:

- Azelaic acid, which is an alternative to benzoyl peroxide, which may cause less skin soreness.
- Salicylic acid is an alternative that exfoliates the skin and helps keep acne pores open. Salicylic acid is also an antibacterial that prevents colonization of *P. acne* into acne pores.

- Topical retinoids, which are drugs based on vitamin A, and are rubbed into the skin once or twice a day. They work by encouraging the outer layer of skin to flake off, and may cause irritation and skin peeling at the start of treatment. Disadvantages of this treatment include making the skin hypersensitive to sunlight.
- Isotretinoin is a powerful oral retinoid drug, which also exists in topical form. It tends to be used in severe forms of acne that have proved resistant to other treatments. It works by drying up oily secretions.
- Hormone treatment: For women, a standard combined oral contraceptive pill (containing an estrogen and a progestogen) can improve acne symptoms. Several cosmetically acceptable hormone mimetics are available such as soy isoflavones, red clover extracts, black cohosh, and wild yam extracts containing dehydroepiadrostenedione mimetics.

Ingrown Hairs and Razor Bumps

Ingrown hair is a hair that curls and penetrates the skin with its tip, causing inflammation. Ingrown hairs are more common among people with very curly hair and African Americans. Most ingrown hairs occur in the beard area. The most common symptom of an ingrown hair is inflammation of the skin, followed by pus formation. In the case of chronic ingrown hairs, treatment may include: allowing the hair to grow longer; or remove the hair using a depilatory agent or electrolysis (to remove the hair).

A general strategy for cosmetic control of ingrown hair is the use of anti-inflammatory, antioxidant, moisturizer, or skin-soothing ingredients. Anti-inflammatory topical creams or lotions provide temporary relief. A variety of products in the market containing different plant extracts (such as Billberry, Sugar Cane, Sugar Maple, Orange, Lemon, Matricaria, Willow Bark, and Comfrey) or skin-soothing and moisturizing agents such as allantoin, panthenol, sodium lactate, sodium PCA, fructose, urea, niacinamide, inositol, etc.; or antiseptics and antioxidants such as sodium benzoate, menthol, ascorbic acid, and vitamin E are used. Agents that soften hair and reduce the growth of hair from hair follicles are becoming more popular in recent years.

CURRENTLY MARKETED PRODUCTS FOR SKIN AND HAIR CARE

Several companies such as BioCosmetics (Black Opal) and Johnson Publishing Co. (Fashion Fair) are ranked among the top 100 black-owned industrial/service businesses by black Enterprise magazine (27). Several smaller ethnic hair and skin-care manufacturing companies have been acquired by large multinationals. For example, L'Oreal bought Soft Sheen and Carson, Alberto-Culver purchased Pro-Line, Colomer bought African Pride, and recently Wella Personal Care North America Acquired Johnson Products (28). Most products directed at the African American skin care are aimed for the treatment of the frequent complaints namely, hyperpigmentation, dryness and ashy skin, blemishes, oilyness, acne breakouts, dark spots, and razor bumps. Major needs addressed in the hair category are treatment of hair damage caused by chemicals and heat such as breakage, loss of elasticity, split ends, and dryness.

Products That Correct Pigmentation Problems

black Opal, a subsidiary of BioCosmetics Research Laboratory sell products to correct skin tone and prevent hypopigmentation, primarily attributed to healing acne. Interface Cosmetics have introduced "Disappearing Acts" a cream that fades dark spots with botanicals.

Advanced complex fade cream containing 2% hydroquinone to fade dark spots is a product sold by Clear Essence Cosmetics U.S. Inc. Another product from this company, Skin-Lightening Serum® contains a concentrated natural extract mixture to achieve same results.

Sonya Dakar, a Los Angeles-based ethnic skin-care company introduced a product "Complexion corrector," a skin lightener that can be worn both at day and night. The product contains vegetable base with natural extracts such as mushroom, wheat, grass, chamomile, and lactic extracts.

Products for Oily Skin, Blemishes, and Acne

Generally speaking, black skin gets oilier and more acne prone as they get older. Black Opal's Blemish line of adult acne products includes astringent, wash, soap, and a gel that dries out pimples. The products contain salicylic acid, resorcinol, camphor, witch hazel, menthol and rosemary extracts to minimize breakouts, inhibit oil production and freshen, and soothe skin.

Interface Cosmetics, Long Island City, New York, U.S.A. makers of Prestige® brand cosmetics for black skin, sell products addressing the excessive oilyness and large pores. These products such as toners and cleansers refine pores, cleanse deeply and inhibit oil production within sebaceous glands.

Color Me beautiful, distributes the Iman Undercover Agent Oil Control Lotion®, containing silicate-based lotion that helps to control sebum, minimize pores and eliminate shine, and create a matte finish on skin without creating a masked look. Other cleansing products available from the company include: papaya enzyme cleanser, surface exfoliating serum® with microbeads and Interface Pore Management Pore Clarifying Sea Clay mask with algae, eucalyptus oil, and sea clay.

Dermablend Corrective Cosmetics, a division of L'Oreal launched Acne Treatment® cleansing gel with 2% salicylic acid, Acne Treatment foundation with 0.5% salicylic acid, and Acne Treatment Spotgel with 2% salicylic acid. These products are sold in kits that range in color from ivory to brown to match different skin color tones.

Products for "Ashy" Skin

BeautiControl (a subsidiary of Tupperware corporation) has introduced Skin Equations®, a sensitive skin line for all skin tones that is hypoallergenic, preservative, oil lanolin fragrance dye, and colorant-free product to control ashy skin. It is a skin hydrator, that reduces ashy appearance. Another product, Demarkable is a product designed to reduce scarring caused by acne

Black Opal offers a line of extramoisturizing cocoa butter products, "cocoa butter Extreme Team," which includes cream, spray lotion, soap concentrated wax with natural butters, emollients, and vitamins to moisturize dry ashy skin.

Sacha Cosmetics, a Trinidad-based cosmetic company introduced oil-free moisturizer products that control sebum secretion. They moisturize skin without making it oily and reduce ashyness. This product is to be used along with a nighttime Overnight Renewal Lotion® containing alpha hydroxy acid that gently exfoliates the dead cells to reduce ashy appearance.

Andrew Jergens, a subsidiary of Kao Corporation, Japan introduced Jergens Ash Relief™, a moisturizer containing a mixture of shea and cocoa butters and beta hydroxy acids for exfoliation and long-lasting moisturization.

Black & Beautiful, a division of ET BROWNE DRUG & CO, introduced a multipurpose skin and hair moisturizer. The product contains shea butter spray for skin and hair as natural emollients.

Clear Essence Cosmetics, a division of Bluefield Associates, Ontario, California, U.S.A. sells a series of light-weight body oils to keep skin soft and moisturized containing ingredients such as tea tree oil, vitamin E, and aloe vera extract.

Products for Razor Bumps

Carson Products Inc. (a subsidiary of L'Oreal) sells a product for African American men to treat razor bumps. Clear Essence® toner and astringent removes dirt and oil that clog skin pore and the alpha hydroxy acid revitalizes razor bump skin with new layer of cells. This product also contains a sunscreen agent for sun protection. Carson also makes Magic Shave® line, a line of shaving and depilatory products designed to treat razor bumps. These include products for after shave application, Magic Conditioning aftershave cleanser, and Magic Moisturizing aftershave lotion.

Black Opal makes Shaving Survival System® that contains advanced treatment to prevent razor bumps.

Halsik Ltd, Wilmette, Illinois, U.S.A. offers Formula 103®, a depilatory cream that helps remove coarse and sensitive facial hair for African American men who suffer from ingrown hairs. These products contain Herbazine, a proprietary herbal blend of skin-softening agents such as chamomile, matricaria, calendula, linden, and hypericum. The product dissolves hair without damaging the roots and use calcium hydroxide, calcium thioglycolate, and lithium hydroxide to eliminate razor bumps.

Hair Treatment Products

Hair-relaxing chemicals are very damaging to hair, causing breakage, loss of elasticity, and dryness. John Frieda introduced a product Frizz-Ease Relax® for relaxed hair. The product remoisturizes the hair and make it look sleek. The product contains a shampoo, conditioner, and texture-correcting serum that make hair more manageable.

Carson/Soft Sheen (a division of L'Oreal) launched Breathru®, a moisturizing and fortifying hair care line for relaxed hair using patented ceramide technology. The basis of using ceramide was that ceramides bind to hair cuticle and strengthen and resist hair breakage. A breakthrough heat-activated product contains glucosamine, sugars, ceramides, natural softening emollients, hydrolyzed wheat, oats, and sucrose.

Colomer U.S.A.'s "creame of nature + style" products are designed to deal with issues of hair breakage, fizzing, and heat damage of African American hair. This line's hair-fortifying serum smoothes strands with an antibreakage formula and Shine and control elixir eliminates frizz and puffy edges.

Palmer's Hair Food Formula contains conditioning ingredients to help shaping wax styles and adds definition and shine to hair. Black & Beautiful skin-care line also features hair care products with ingredients such as shea butter and cocoa butter. Palmer's coconut oil formula conditioner is another shine-enhancing product.

African Pride products offer shampoo, Braid & Weave Ease Out® spray, and Braid Sheen spray to help consumers maintain health and form of their hairdo. It softens hair and reduces frizzles.

A holistic hair product line from Barry Fletcher Products, "Afrodisiac" is a holistic approach to treat hair in a natural relaxed manner. It contains fragrances, essential oils and natural humectants, and emollients.

Johnson Products Ultra Sheen® brand introduced a children's hair care line that contains natural ingredients to preserve the natural state of hair, as an alternative to using chemicals to alter the structure of the hair.

FUTURE OPPORTUNITIES IN BLACK SKIN AND HAIR COSMETICS

Despite the increase in the population and the buying power of African Americans, personal care product market is not catching up with new innovations or new technologies that cater to this segment of population. Specific research targeting the needs of black skin is lagging. Clinical trials conducted on black subjects to study the skin response to various agents and conditions are sparse. Major cosmetic companies have carried out studies on Asian skin and demonstrated Asian skin is more sensitive than Caucasian skin. Similar types of studies on African American skin are few and inconclusive. Establishment of new research centers such as the L'Oreal center for Ethnic skin and hair research is a step in the right direction. Such centers and research programs from other large skin-care companies that cater to the growing population of African Americans, and black skin population in general would be helpful. It is especially important considering the fact that the black purchasing power is expected to show an annual growth rate of 6.1%, according to Selig Center's study as reported in Happi magazine of October 2003 (2).

Some specific areas of need where new research could improve African American skin and hair care would be acne and sebum suppression, pigmentation disorders, folliculitis, razor bumps, scars and keloids, and specific hair problems. Although, there are several products addressing the acne and sebum/sebaceous gland activity in skin, no products address the issues specific for black skin. For example, does the composition of sebum differ between races? Are sebaceous glands in black skin regulated by hormones in a different manner than that of other skin types? Does the hormonal levels in black skin vary from other skin types? Does the sebaceous gland morphology in the black hair follicle differ from other skin types? Does the effect of climate on sebum and acne differ between races? New research into natural hormone modulators such as phytoestrogens and androgen modulators can be evaluated specifically in black skin for their unique benefits. Novel sebum suppression and sweat-suppressing agents and their combination need to be studied for their benefits. Antiacne agents with sebum suppression strategy need to be evaluated in black skin.

Although there are several products in the market to address skin pigmentation disorders for black skin, none of them use novel technologies. Skin lightening is an area that has received maximum attention from skin-care product companies. This is mainly due to the skin-lightening needs of Asian and Japanese population. Same technologies can be applied to black skin cosmetics. New technologies described in a previous section in this review (potential cosmetic ingredients) should be useful for cosmetic application in black skin cosmetics.

Folliculitis and associated hair and shaving conditions is an area that can benefit from more research. What are the causes and how can they be prevented? Can it be controlled by agents that slow down hair growth, hair-softening agents, antimicrobial agents, or other novel actives? A relationship between hair shape and folliculitis is well established; however, does it vary between different subtypes of hair in African Americans? No unique products are in the market place specifically addressing these issues. Specific products including agents that reduce hair growth, make hair and hair roots softer and more flexible need to be evaluated for treatment of folliculitis.

Benefits of anti-inflammatory, antioxidant, anti-infective, and antimicrobial agents either alone or in combination with hair-softening agents need to be evaluated.

Scar prevention is an area that is receiving attention in recent years. Several products in the market claim reduction of scars by suppressing collagen synthesis or by activating their degradation. This strategy can be specifically applied to scars and keloids in black skin. No studies have been carried out using this strategy. Keloids and scars are major issues with black skin.

In the hair category, several unmet needs exist, among them, hair breakage, excessive oiliness, ingrown hairs, and management of chemically treated and heat treated hair. Some of these issues can be addressed by effective delivery of already existing actives. Agents for strengthening hair physically is an area that needs more investigation. Products that are substantive to hair that also strengthens hair is a possibility. Substances that can be bound to hair, that provide hair strength either by physical or biological means can be explored. For dry and ashy skin and hair, better moisturizers including better substantivity in better delivery vehicle is an opportunity.

In recent years, significant advances have been achieved in specialized delivery systems for skin- and hair-care products. Among them liposomes, cationic liposomes, micellar delivery systems, etc. offer excellent opportunities. Utilization of new and emerging encapsulation technologies for specific and targeted delivery of actives to black skin would be useful. Several companies offer patented technologies for cosmetic delivery systems. These may offer special opportunities to deliver actives to African American skin and hair.

In summary, although there are various products in the market place targeted to black skin, there are still opportunities for improvement. Discovery of new actives along with the use of special delivery systems would be an area worth exploring.

REFERENCES

1. Ethnic Skin Care Market: Feature Story. Happi Magazine, October 1992.
2. MacDonald. Ethnic Skin Care: Facing the Future: Happi, October 2003.
3. Reed JT, Ghadially R, Elias PM. Skin type, but neither race nor gender, influence epidermal permeability barrier function. Arch Dermatol 1995; 131: 1134–1138.
4. La Ruche G, Cesarini JP. Histology and physiology of Black skin. Ann Dermatol Venerol 1992; 119:567–574.

5. Beradesca E, Pirot F, Singh M, Maibach H. Differences in stratum corneum pH gradient when comparing White Caucasian and Black African American skin. Br J Dermatol 1998; 139:855–857.
6. Sugino K, Imokawa G, Maibach FF. Ethnic difference of stratum corneum lipid in relation to stratum corneum function [Abstr]. J Invest Dermatol 1993; 100:597.
7. Manuskiatti W, Schwindt DA, Maibach HI. Influence of age, anatomic site and race on skin roughness and scaliness. Dermatology 1998; 196:401–407.
8. Montagna W, Carlisle K. The architecture of Black and White facial skin. J Am Acad Dermatol 1991; 24:929–937.
9. Montagna W, Giusseppe P, Kenney JA (eds). The structure of Black skin. In: Black Skin Structure and Function. Barlington, Massachasetts, Academic Press, 1993:37–49.
10. Herzberg AJ, Dinehart SM. Chronologic aging in Black skin. Am J Dermato- pahtol 1989; 11:319–328.
11. Jimbow K, Fitzpatrick TB, Wick MM. Biochemistry and physiology of melanin pigmentation. In: Goldsmith LA, ed. Physiology, Biochemistry and Molecular Biology of the Skin. New York, New York: Oxford University Press, 1991:893.
12. Jimbow K, Oikawa O, Sugiyama S, Takeuchi T. Comparison of eumelanogenesis and pheomelanogenesis in retinal and follicular melanocytes: role of vesiculo- globular bodies in melanosome differentiation. J Invest Dermatol 73:278–284.
13. Minwalla L, Zhao Y, Le Poole IC, Wickett RR, Boissy RE. Keratinocytes play a role in regulating distribution patterns of recipient melanosomes in vitro. J Invest Dermatol 2001; 117:341–347.
14. Nicolaides N, Rothman S. Studies on the chemical composition of human hair fat: the overall composition with regard to age, sex and race. J Invest Dermatol 1952; 21:90.
15. Pochi PE, Strauss JS. Sebaceous gland activity in Black skin. Dermatol Clin 1988; 6:349–351.
16. Bernard BA. Hair shape of curly hair. J Am Acad Dermatol 2003; 48(suppl 6):S120–S126.
17. Brooks O, Lewis A. Treatment regimens for "styled" Black hair. Cosmet Toilet- ries 1983; 98:59–68.
18. Gold RJM, Schriver CH. The amino acid composition of hair from different racial origins. Clin Chem Acta 1971; 33:465–466.
19. Menkart J, Wolfram L, Mao I. Caucasian hair, Negro hair and wool: similarities and differences. J soc Cosmet Chem 1966; 17:769–787.
20. Foy V, Weinkauf R, Whittle E, Basketter DA. Ethnic variation in the skin irri- tation response. Contact Dermatitits 2001; 45:346–349.
21. Weigand DA, Haygood C, Gaylor JR. Cell layers and density of Negro and Cau- casian stratum corneum. J Invest Dermatol 1974; 62:563–556.
22. Mushall I, Heyl T. Skin diseases in the Western Cape Province. S Afr Mod J 1963; 37:1308.
23. Epstein W, Kligman AM. The interference phenomenon on allergic contact der- matitis. J Invest Dermatol 1958; 31:175.
24. Kelly DA, Young AR, McGregor JM, Seed PT, Potten CS, Walker SL. Senstivity to sunburn is associated with susceptibility to UV radiation-induced suppression of cutaneous cell-mediated immunity. J Exp Med 2000; 191:561–566.

25. Matsuoka LY, McConnachie P, Wortsman J, Holick MF. Immunological responses to UVB radiation in Black individuals. Life Sci. 1999; 64:1563–1569.
26. Sueki H, Whitaker-Menezes D, Kligman AM. Structural diversity of mast cell granules in Black and White skin. Br J Dermatol 2001; 144:85–93.
27. MacDonald V. Ethnic Skin Care, Happy October 2000.
28. MacDonald V. Ethnic Hair, Happi April 2002.

17

Ethnical Aspects of Skin Pigmentation

Olivier de Lacharrière and Rainer Schmidt
Life Sciences, L'Oréal Recherche, Clichy, France

MELANIN AND SKIN PIGMENTATION

The major source of skin color in humans is melanin. The pigment melanin is produced in highly specialized cells, the melanocytes, which are located in the basal layer of the epidermis. These dendritic cells are in close contact with the neighboring keratinocytes, forming the so-called epidermal melanin unit (1). One epidermal melanin unit is composed of one melanocyte in contact with approximately 36 keratinocytes. Within this unit, keratinocytes are not only in close contact with melanocytes but also have a profound influence on their physiology, controlling melanocytes proliferation as well as the quantity and quality of melanin synthesis (2,3).

Melanin is a complex group of heterogeneous biopolymers. The rate-limiting enzyme for the synthesis of melanin is tyrosinase (monophenol L-DOPA: oxygen oxydoreductase, E.C. 1.14.18.1). Melanin is synthesized in specific cell organelles, the melanosomes, whose phenotype usually relates to the type of melanin they produce (4). In human skin, we distinguish two types of melanin, the black, brown eumelanin and the red, yellow pheomelanin, both of which exhibit distinct physical and biological properties. Synthesized from a common precursor tyrosine, eumelanin is a polymer of 5,6-dihydroxyindole and 5,6-dihydroxyindole-2-carboxylic acid whereas pheomelanin is made of benzothiazine units derived from cysteinyldopa.

Melanin is implicated in the protection of the skin against ultraviolet (UV) radiation–induced damages. Eumelanin is generally recognized as a photostable and photoprotective polymer, based on its ability to absorb, scatter, and reflect light of different wavelengths, sequester redox-active metal ions, and scavenge oxidizing free radicals (5). Pheomelanin, on the contrary, is photolabile and considered as being a photosensitizer (6–9). Recent findings point into the direction that it is the ratio between the two types of melanin that determines the protective properties and the color of skin (10,11).

A locally increased or reduced rate of melanin synthesis is often the cause of hyper- or hypopigmented skin lesions (12). Many cellular targets are known, or have recently been identified, as being able to modulate melanogenesis.

Among these are the following:

1. Mediators of inflammation (cytokines), known to stimulate pigmentation.
2. Endothelins.
3. Proopiomelanocortein peptides, able to stimulate melanogenesis via the MC1 receptor.
4. Modulators of cAMP level and other compounds that modulate PK-c and PK-a activity.
5. Agonists and antagonists of the protein-activated receptor 2, which affect the transfer of melanin into the keratinocytes.
6. The microphtalamia transcription factor, a ubiquitous transcription factor implicated amongst others in the regulation of the expression of the melanogenic enzymes tyrosinase and TRP-1.

ETHNICAL MELANOCYTE SPECIFICITIES AND SKIN COLOR

To better understand the cellular and molecular mechanisms involved in skin pigmentation and related disorders, in vitro models can be used (Figs. 1 and 2). The possibility of culturing normal human melanocytes and introducing them into reconstructed skin models, which results in pigmented epidermis, has considerably contributed to better understand their physiology (13).

The type of pigmentation depends exclusively on the ethnic origin of the melanocytes. Caucasian melanocytes will reproduce a light pigmentation of the reconstructed epidermis, whereas melanocytes of African origin will generate a dark pigmentation (Fig. 3). The observed differences in pigmentation are mainly based on a different rate of melanin synthesis, because the number of melanocytes in the different ethnic models is identical.

Only little is known about the melanosomes distribution and their degradation within the keratinocytes after their transfer. Whereas in Caucasian skin, melanosomes are degraded during the differentiation process of keratinocytes, they persist in African skin throughout the whole epidermis

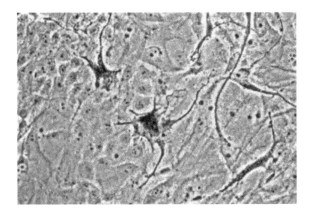

Figure 1 (*See color insert*) Cell coculture of melanocytes and keratinocytes.

and are eliminated by desquamation. The persistence of the melanosomes in African epidermis accounts mainly for the dark color. Using the pigmented reconstructed epidermis, generated with cells of different ethnic origin, we are presently trying to identify the characteristics of the different ethnic melanin units and the particular role of the keratinocytes in the processing of the melanosomes.

Boissy and coworkers (14) have investigated in more detail the complexion coloration in different ethnic groups in vivo, which varies dramatically from dark to light, as exemplified by the skin of central African and northern Scandinavian individuals, respectively, despite the fact that the density of melanocytes in the skin of these two extreme skin types is identical (15,16). An important determinant of skin coloration is the variation in the quantity, packaging, and distribution of epidermal melanosomes within keratinocytes of different ethnic groups (17). It is well documented that the

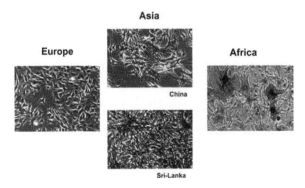

Figure 2 (*See color insert*) Morphology of melanocytes in monoculture according to their ethnical origin.

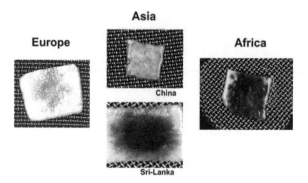

Figure 3 (*See color insert*) Pigmented reconstructed skin according to melanocyte ethnical origin.

melanosomes within keratinocytes of dark skin are distributed individually in the cytosol, predominantly over the nucleus of the keratinocytes, whereas the melanosomes within keratinocytes of light skin are clustered together in membrane-limited groups of two to eight melanosomes. Another important factor is the progressive variation in melanosome size with ethnicity— African skin having the largest melanosomes, European skin the smallest melanosomes, and the melanosomes in Indian, Mexican, and Chinese skin being intermediate in size (18–21).

Using the reconstructed pigmented human skin model, Hearing an coworkers (22) have analyzed the distribution pattern of melanosomes in keratinocytes of Asian skin using electron microscopy. They determined the melanosome size within keratinocytes of Asian skin and compared the data with other skin types. They revealed the correlation between melanosomes size and skin color. They confirmed that the size and the distribution (packing) of melanosomes have a profound effect on skin color.

SKIN PIGMENTED LESIONS, UV RADIATIONS, AND ETHNICAL FACTORS

The best-known inducer of melanin production is UV light. Sun exposure increases the melanin content of the skin, which in turn increases skin pigmentation, generally described as tanning. Tanning is considered as a defense mechanism to protect the skin against UV radiation–induced damages. The UV-induced pigmentation does not always generate a homogeneous tanning; in some individuals and certain populations, it produces hyperpigmented lesions.

In vitro studies have mainly focused on UVB (290–320 nm)-induced pigmentation in normal human melanocytes (23–30). Cellular and molecular mechanisms involved in UVA (320–400 nm)-induced pigmentation are poorly understood (31–35), even though it is now generally accepted that this part of the UV spectrum contributes largely to the tanning process (36,37), being the major stimulus for increased melanogenesis in phototypes III and IV skin (38).

Knowing that within the epidermis melanocytes and keratinocytes are in close contact, forming the epidermal melanin unit, we have developed keratinocyte–melanocyte cocultures (Fig. 1) and pigmented reconstructed skin models, which perfectly reproduce the epidermal melanin unit in vitro (13).

Using a specific assay to determine the rate of melanin synthesis (39), we observed striking differences in the melanogenic response of normal human melanocytes to UVA and UVB, depending on the presence of keratinocytes. Exposure of cocultures to UVB irradiation triggered, already at low doses ($5\,mJ/cm^2$), an increase in melanin synthesis; whereas in melanocyte monocultures, UVB doses up to $50\,mJ/cm^2$ had no melanogenic effect, indicating that keratinocytes mediate UVB-induced pigmentation. On the contrary, UVA-stimulating pigmentation was identical in mono- and cocultures, indicating that UVA affects directly the melanocytes. Another interesting observation was that melanocytes in monocultures synthesize almost exclusively phaeomelanin, whereas in contact with keratinocytes the eumelanin synthesis is strongly increased, reflecting levels observed in normal human skin (40). However, these observations are limited to Caucasian melanocytes.

Pigmented Lesions and Skin Aging—Actinic Lentigos

Skin aging is clinically characterized by flaccidity, changes in skin texture, wrinkles, and actinic lentigos. Those are hyperpigmented macules or pigmented spots, localized on skin photoexposed area (Fig. 4). It is admitted that actinic lentigos do not tan. The link between actinic lentigos and chronic sun exposure is established (41).

Recently, we demonstrated by comparison of matched groups of women living in France and China that appearance of wrinkles and pigmented spots during aging are distinct (42). Wrinkles in Caucasians appear before pigmented spots, whereas in Chinese population we observe the contrary; i.e., Chinese women develop pigmented lesions much earlier and at a higher rate compared to their French counterparts.

Furthermore, this study suggests that a more frequent sun exposure during childhood increases the risk of developing pigmented lesions, later during adult life. Those observations are in agreement with the hypothesis of Ortonne who postulated that repeated UV exposure increases definitively the number of melanocytes (43).

In a previous study, done in China in the Suzhou area (44), we compared the number, color, and size of facial pigmented spots of women living in the country (155 farmers) versus women living in the city (155 urban

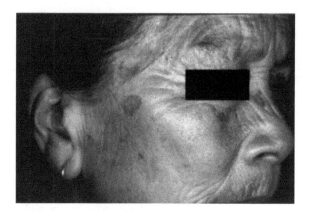

Figure 4 Actinic lentigos.

women). The two groups of women were age balanced (18–80 years). The results show that the number of facial pigmented spots (all types) was significantly higher, in equivalent age classes, for the group of women living in the country (Fig. 5). In addition, the spot-size was bigger and the color of the pigmented lesions darker for of the women living in the country than for urban women (Fig. 6).

We have also investigated the impact of the latitude on pigmented spots, on 2000 Chinese women (18–75 years) divided into age-matched groups in four cities: Beijing and Harbin (northern cities) and Chengdu and Suzhou (southern cities) (45). Over the age 26, more than 60% of the women exhibited facial pigmented lesions; this percentage remained stable until the age of 60. On the other hand, over the age of 41, there was a linear increase in the number of women affected (20% at 40 years and 80% at 70 years). According to the latitude, facial or hand pigmented

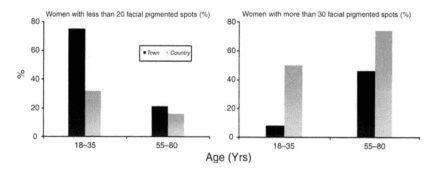

Figure 5 Number of facial pigmented spots on two groups of 155 women living in the Suzhou area (Jiangsu, China).

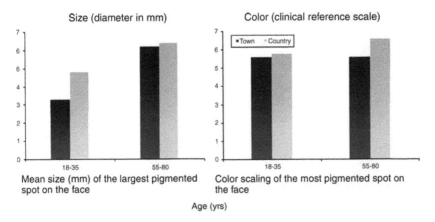

Figure 6 Size and color of facial pigmented spots on two groups of 155 women living in the Suzhou area (Jiangsu, China).

lesions were more pronounced in women from southern cities than in those from northern cities.

In Chinese women, we have observed that the clinical aspect of facial pigmented lesions differs with age. From the age of 18 to 40, the number of small pigmented lesions, defined as less than 6 mm, increases and decreases after the age of 40. The number of pigmented spots larger than 6 mm in diameter, i.e., actinic lentigos, increased constantly after the age of 30. Irrespective of the age classes, pigmented lesions were always more pronounced on the face than on the hands.

Furthermore, it is generally believed that with age, the skin becomes lighter in European populations and turns yellow in Asiatic population. However, no controlled study has quantified or scientifically explained this assertion.

MELASMA

Melasma, also called chloasma, is a pigmented lesion usually localized on face (Fig. 7). Rarely, it could be also observed on the neck or forearms. Its clinical presentation is usually in the form of symmetric large pigmented plaques, with irregular border. Its localization on the face could be classified in three types: (i) mediofacial form involving the forehead, cheeks, upper lip, nose, and chin, (ii) malar form involving the cheeks and nose, and (iii) mandibular form, specifically localized on the ramus part of he mandibula (46). According to the histological localization of the melanin, it is classical to distinguish epidermal forms, dermal forms, and mixed forms. This distinction is important for therapy, the epidermal form responding better than the dermal one to therapy. It is currently admitted that the examination of melasma with Wood lamp (UVA light) gives indication on the position of melanin in

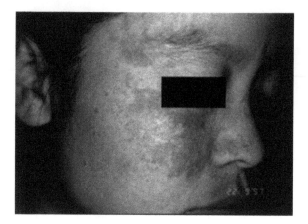

Figure 7   Melasma.

the skin for phototype I, II, and III. For darker skin, the examination with UVA does not enable us to get similar results (47).

It appears usually in women, in the third decade (48–50). The color of the melasma is usually inhomogeneous. It could be light brown or dark brown. Sun tanning increases the visibility of the melasma. Women are much more concerned than men; however men could also be concerned.

Although it is very common, the prevalence in the general population is not precisely known. Several studies indicate that melasma is more frequently observed on darker skin phototypes, i.e., IV, V, and VI. Sanchez et al. (46) have reported that Latin-American and Asiatic people are more concerned with melasma than European population. In Southeast Asia, melasma accounts for 0.25% to 4% of cases seen in dermatology institutes. In a study of 679 patients, Sivayathorn have reported a prevalence of 39.9% for women, although the condition was severe in only 16.7%. In men, the prevalence was 20.6%, with 18% having a severe involvement (51). Recently, in a study of 2000 women in China, we have reported a prevalence of melasma of 20%, with a peak of 28% in the fourth decade (52).

REFERENCES

1. Fitzpatrick TB, Breathnach AS. Das epidermale Melanin-Einheit System. Dermatol Wochenschr 1963; 147:481–489.
2. Gordon PR, Mansur CP, Gilchrest BA. Regulation of human melanocyte growth, dendricity, and melanization by keratinocyte derived factors. J Invest Dermatol 1989; 92:565–572.
3. Quevedo WC Jr., Fitzpatrick TB, Pathak MA, Jimbow K. Light and skin color. In: Fitzpatrick TB, Pathak MA, Harber LC, Seiji M, Kukita A, eds. Sunlight and Man. Tokyo, Japan: University of Tokyo Press, 1974:165–194.

4. Hearing VJ, Phillips P, Lutzner MA. The fine structure of melanogenesis in coat color mutants of the mouse. J Ultrastruct Res 1973; 43:88–106.
5. Sarna T, Swartz HM. The physical properties of melanins. In: Nordlund JJ, Boissy RE, Hearing VJ, King RA, Ortonne J-P, eds. The Pigmentary System, Physiology and Pathophysiology. New York, New York: Oxford University Press, 1998:333–357.
6. Agin P, Sayre RM, Chedekel MR. Photodegradation of pheomelanin: an in vitro model. Photochem Photobiol 1980; 31:359–362.
7. Chedekel MR. Photochemistry and photobiology of epidermal melanins. Photochem Photobiol 1982; 35:881–885.
8. Sarna T, Menon IA, Sealy RC. Photosensitization of melanins: a comparative study. Photochem Photobiol 1985; 5:529–532.
9. Cesarini J-P. Photo-induced events in the human melanocytic system: photoaggression and photoprotection. Pigment Cell Res 1988; 1:223–233.
10. Vincensi MR, D'Ischia M, Napolitano A, et al. Phaeomelanin versus eumelanin as a chemical indicator of ultraviolet sensitivity in fair-skinned subjects at high risk for melanoma: a pilot study. Melanoma Res 1998; 8:53–58.
11. Wenczl E, Van der Schans G, Roza L, et al. (Pheo)melanin photosensitizes UVA-induced DNA damage in cultured human melanocytes. J Invest Dermatol 1998; 111:678–682.
12. Ortonne J-P, Nordlund JJ. Mechanisms that cause abnormal skin color. In: Nordlund JJ, Boissy RE, Hearing VJ, King RA, Ortonne J-P, eds. The Pigmentary System, Physiology and Pathophysiology. New York, New York: Oxford University Press, 1998:489–502.
13. Régnier M, Duval C, Galey J-B, et al. Keratinocytes-melanocyte co-cultures and pigmented reconstructed human epidermis: models to study modulation of melanogenesis. Cell Mol Biol 1999; 45:969–980.
14. Thong HY, Jee SH, Sun CC, Boissy RE. The patterns of melanosome distribution in keratinocytes of human skin as one determining factor of skin color. Br J Dermatol 2003; 149:498–505.
15. Szabo G. The number of melanocytes in human epidermis. Br Med J 1954; 4869:1016–1017.
16. Staricco RJ, Pinkus H. Quantitative and qualitative data on the pigment cells of adult human epidermis. J Invest Dermatol 1957; 28:33–45.
17. Szabo G, Gerald AB, Pathak MA, Fitzpatrick TB. Racial differences in the fate of melanosomes in human epidermis. Nature 1969; 222:1081–1082.
18. Konrad K, Wolff K. Hyperpigmentation, melanosome size, and distribution patterns of melanosomes. Arch Dermatol 1973; 107:853–860.
19. Jimbow K, Fitzpatrick TB, Wick MM. Biochemistry and physiology of melanin pigmentation. In: Goldsmith SA, ed. Physiology, Biochemistry, and Molecular Biology of the Skin. Vol. 2. 2nd ed. New York, New York: Oxford University Press, 1991: 873–909.
20. Minwalla L, Zhao Y, Le Poole C, et al. Keratinocytes play a role in regulating distribution patterns of recipient melanosomes in vitro. J Invest Dermatol 2001; 117:341.
21. Alaluf S, Atkins D, Barrett K, et al. Ethnic variation in melanin content and composition in photoexposed and photoprotected human skin. Pigment Cell Res 2002; 15:112–118.

22. Yoon TJ, Lei TC, Yamaguchi Y, Batzer J, Wolber R, Hearing VJ. Reconstituted 3-dimensional human skin of various ethnic origins as an in vitro model for studies of pigmentation. Anal Biochem 2003; 318:260–269.

23. Friedmann PS, Gilchrest BA. Ultraviolet radiation directly induces pigment production by cultured human melanocytes. J Cell Physiol 1987; 133:88–94.

24. Libow LF, Sheide S, Deleo VA. Ultraviolet radiation acts as independant mitogen for normal human melanocytes in culture. Pigment Cell Res 1998; 1:397–401.

25. Ramirez-Bosca A, Bernd A, Werner R, Dold K, Holzmann H. Effect of the dose of ultraviolet radiation on the pigment formation by human melanocytes in vitro. Dermatol Res 1992; 284:359–362.

26. Aberdam E, Romero C, Ortonne J-P. Repeated UVB irradiations do not have the same potential to promote stimulation of melanogenesis in cultured normal human melanocytes. J Cell Sci 1993; 106:1015–1022.

27. Abdel-Malek Z, Swope V, Smalara D, Babcock G, Dawes S, Nordlund JJ. Analysis of the UV-induced melanogenesis and growth arrest of human melanocytes. Pigment Cell Res 1994; 7:326–332.

28. Casberg CJ, Warenius HM, Friedmann PS. Ultraviolet radiation-induced melanogenesis in human melanocytes. Effects of modulating protein kinase C. J Cell Sci 1994; 107:2591–2597.

29. Romero-Graillet C, Aberdam E, Biagoli N, Massabni W, Ortonne J-P, Balloti R. Ultraviolet B radiation acts through the nitric oxide and cGMP signal transduction pathway to stimulate melanogenesis in human melanocytes. J Biol Chem 1996; 271:28,052–28,056.

30. Im S, Moro O, Peng F, et al. Activation of the cyclic AMP pathway by a-melanotropin mediates the response of human melanocytes to ultraviolet B radiation. Cancer Res 1998; 58:47–54.

31. Jimbow K, Uesugi T. New melanogenesis and photobiological processes in activation and proliferation of precursor melanocytes after UV-exposure: ultrastructural differentiation of precursor melanocytes from Langerhans cells. J Invest Dermatol 1982; 78:108–115.

32. Imokawa G, Kawai M, Mishima Y, Motegi I. Differential analysis of experimental hypermelanosis induced by UVB, UVA and contact dermatitis using a brownish guinea pig model. Arch Dermatol Res 1986; 278:352–362.

33. Pathak MA. Immediate and delayed pigmentary and other cutaneous response to solar UVA radiation (320–400 nm). In: Urbach F, Gange RW, eds. The Biological Effects of UVA Radiation. New York, New York: Praeger Pub, 1986:156–167.

34. Rosen CF, Seki Y, Farnelli W, et al. A comparison of the melanocyte response to narrow band UVA and UVB exposure in vivo. J Invest Dermatol 1987; 88:774–779.

35. Imokawa G, Yada Y, Kimura M, Morisaki N. Granulocyte/macrophage colony-stimulating factor is an intrinsic keratinocyte-derived growth factor for human melanocytes in UVA-induced melanosis. Biochem J 1996; 313:625–631.

36. Stary A, Robert C, Sarasin A. Deleterious effects of ultraviolet A radiation in human cells. Mutation Res 1997; 383:1–8.

37. Krutmann J. Ultraviolet A radiation-induced biological effects in human relevance for photoaging and photodermatosis. J Dermatol Sci 2000; 23:22–26.

38. Pathak MA, Fanselow DL. Photobiology of melanin pigmentation: dose/ response of skin to sunlight and its contents. J Am Acad Dermatol 1983; 9:724–733.
39. Schmidt R, Krien P, Régnier M. The use of diethylaminoethyl cellulose membrane filters in a bioassay to quantify melanin synthesis. Anal Biochem 1996; 235:113–118.
40. Duval C, Régnier M, Schmidt R. Distinct melanogenic response of melanocytes in mono-culture, co-cultured with keratinocytes, and in reconstructed human pigmented epidermis to UV-irradiation. Pigment Cell Res 2001; 14:348–355.
41. Bastiaens M, Hoefnagel J, Westendorp R, Vermeer BJ, Bouwes Bavinck JN. Solar lentigines are strongly related to sun exposure in contrast to ephelides. Pigment Cell Res 2004; 17:225–229.
42. Nouveau-Richard S, Yang Z, Mac-Mary S, et al. Skin ageing: a comparison between Chinese and European populations. A pilot study. J Dermatol Sci 2005; 40:187–193.
43. Ortonne JP. Pigmentary changes of the ageing skin. Br J Dermatol 1990; 122(S35):21–28.
44. Yang ZL, Qian BY, de Lacharrière O. Study on facial skin features in 304 Chinese women. Chinese J Dermatol 2001; 4:R75.
45. Li L, de Lacharrière O, Lian S, et al. Pigmented spots on face and hands: specific features in Chinese skin. A clinical study on 2000 Chinese women. World Congress of Dermatology, Paris, France, July 2002. Ann Dermatol Venereol 2002; 129:1S81–1S141.
46. Sanchez NP, Pathak MA, Sato S, Fitzpatrick TB, Sanchez L, Mihm MC Jr. Malasma: a clinical, light microscopic, ultrastructural and immunofluorescence study. J Am Acad Dermatol 1981; 4:698–710.
47. Nouveau S, Lam CY, Yang ZL, Qian BY, Wang BT, de Lacharrière O. Assessment of Asianphotoaging—UV versus polarized light photography. IV World Congress of the International Academy of Cosmetic Dermatology, Paris, France, July 2005.
48. Griffiths CE, Finkel LJ, Ditre CM, Hamilton TA, Ellis CN, Voorhees JJ. Topical tretinoin improves melasma. A vehicle-controlled clinical trial. Br J Dermatol 1993; 129(4):415–421.
49. Kauh YC, Zachian TF. Melasma. Adv Exp Med Biol 1999; 455:491–499.
50. Kimbrough-Green CK, Griffiths CE, Finkel LJ, et al. Topical retinoic acid for melasma in black patients. A vehicle-controlled clinical trial. Arch Dermatol 1994; 130(6):727–733.
51. Sivayathorn A. Melasma in orientals. Clin Drug Invest 1995; 10(S2):24–40.
52. De Lacharrière O, Li YH, Cheng L, et al. New trends on skin pigmentation in Chinese women. IX International Congress of Dermatology, Beijing, China, May 2004.

18

Sensitive Skin—An Ethnic Overview

Olivier de Lacharrière

Life Sciences, L'Oréal Recherche, Clichy, France

INTRODUCTION

In 1989, Maibach et al. (1) stated that, "the plausibility of the concept of the sensitive skin evokes discussion and often amusement because of the variance of the number of opinions compared with the amount of data, at least until recently." In fact, more than 30 years after the first publications (2) on sensitive skin, all the authors agree with the idea that the sensitive skin is a real syndrome.

In the last 15 years, several studies allow to better define the constitutional sensitive skin and to give key points about its clinical signs and its prevalence. In addition, some new data exist on the etiology and the mechanisms involved in sensitive skin.

CLINICAL FEATURES OF SENSITIVE SKIN

Clinical Signs

Sensitive skin is clinically characterized by sensorial signs perceived by the consumers. These self-perceived facial discomforts could be burning, stinging, or itching. They occur in specific situations provoked by climatic factors such as wind or sudden changes in temperature or by topical application usually well tolerated on skin. It clearly appears that sensitive skin is a term used by individuals who perceived their skin being more intolerant or

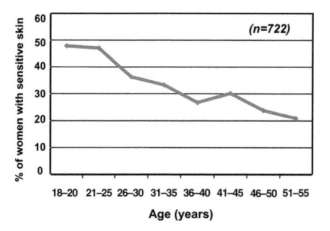

Figure 1 Evolution according to the age of prevalence of sensitive skin (study done in China).

reactive than the general population. Consequently, sensitive skin could be defined as a hyperreactive skin characterized by exaggerated sensorial reaction to environmental or topical factors, including hard water and cosmetics. This skin condition is highly more frequent in young women. With age, skin reactivity decreases. The same is the case with European or Chinese women (Fig. 1). For men, few studies have been performed; however, there is enough data to admit that sensitive skin is also a condition observed on men, but with a slighter prevalence (3).

Clinical Subgroups of Sensitive Skin

Several subgroups could be distinguish according to the severity of sensitive skin and the provocative factors: (i) severe sensitive skin (SSS), (ii) sensitive skin to environment (SSE), and (iii) sensitive skin to topical factors (Fig. 2) (4).

Severe Sensitive Skin

The SSS clinical form demonstrates very high facial skin reactivity to all kinds of factors: topical, environmental, including atmospheric pollution as also internal factors such as stress and tiredness. According to European cohort, SSS concerns 10% to 18% of women (3,5) and only 6% of men (3).

Skin Sensitive to Environment

A subject with SSE demonstrates high facial skin reactivity to heat or fast changes in temperature. These women complain frequently of sun intolerance. It is among this subgroup of sensitive skin that dry skin and blushing

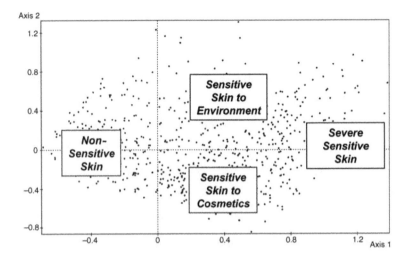

Figure 2 (*See color insert*) Projection of the subjects according to their severity and type of sensitive skin. Each point corresponds to one subject (study done in the United Kingdom, $n = 1023$). Abcisse axis gives the intensity of the skin reactivity of subgroups. Ordonate axis gives the reactivity factors with which the skin reacts.

skin are encountered. According to European cohort, around 15% to 20% of women are concerned.

Skin Sensitive to Cosmetics

In this subgroup of sensitive skin, the provocative factor is represented by the application of product on skin. It is important to underline that the observed intolerance appears immediately or in the minutes following the application. In some cases, the reaction occurs after the first application of the incriminated. According to European cohort, around 25% of women are concerned.

Diathesis Factors

In most cases of sensitive skin, skin hyperreactivity is constitutional. Thiers (6), who was the first to describe this syndrome, has suggested that diathesis features could exist. Sensitive skin appears preferentially in fair skin type. We also found that familial history of sensitive skin exists. In our studies we do not observe an exclusive link of sensitive skin to a specific skin type. Severe dry skin or severe oily skin could be equally concerned with skin hyperreactivity defining sensitive skin.

 Acquired skin hyperreactivity could mimic the signs observed during sensitive skin syndrome. This acquired "sensitive skin," characterized by a temporary decrease of the threshold of sensorial reactivity of the skin, could be linked to topical irritants improperly applied such as retinoids or hydroxy-acids. In those cases, it is possible that a skin, which is usually "nonreactive," becomes "reactive" for a period of time.

The presence of active facial dermatitis such as seborrheic dermatitis or rosacea could also reduce, during a period of time, the threshold of the skin reactivity. However, though a facial outbreak of atopic dermatitis increases the skin reactivity, it is not correct to consider all sensitive skins as atopic skin. In fact, in the sensitive skin population, we found 49% of atopic subjects and 51% of nonatopic in a European cohort of 2000 women (3). In addition, similar results of the absence of link between atopy and sensitive skin were found in a Chinese cohort of 2000 women.

The absence of link between a specific immuno-allergologic status and sensitive skin has been controversial. However, recent reports (5) give definite support to not sustain this hypothesis.

SENSITIVE SKIN IN THE WORLD POPULATION

Most of the studies on sensitive skin were performed in western countries on European subjects, but some recent works were devoted to Asian sensitive skin and comparison to African American, Hispanic, Asian, and European sensitive skins.

It is important to consider that population differences in the skin physiology exist. The published data compared mostly Euro-American and African American skins in the United States. There are very few publications on Asian skins.

Although the stratum corneum thickness is equal in African Americans and Euro-Americans, the number of cell layers is increased for African Americans (7). Irritation tests demonstrate that skin of Euro-Americans is more irritable than that of African Americans. Because it depends on the substances tested, the penetration differences between black and white skins are less clear (8,9).

Berardesca and Maibach explored the skin response to sodium-laurylsulphate (SLS) in three groups (Europeans, African Americans, and South Americans) by measuring transepidermal water loss (TEWL) and blood flow (Laser Doppler Velocimetry) (10,11). African Americans have a more intense TEWL response; on the other hand they show less intense reactivity of blood flow with low levels of erythema (12).

Aramaki et al. (13) compared skin response to SLS on Japanese and European healthy women living in Germany. They measured the TEWL and blood flow (Laser Doppler Velocimetry). No differences of the barrier function between the two groups were observed. Aramaki et al. also appreciated the complaints of these two groups during the test. They found significant subjective sensory differences between Japanese and German women: the Japanese women complained about stronger sensations. The authors suggested that it could be linked to cultural behavior. However, physiological differences must be also considered. Although there are some differences in the population regarding skin irritation, it must be kept in mind that irritation does not exactly reflect what sensitive skin is.

Sensitive Skin in Europe

According to several studies done in the United Kingdom (3) and France (14) on a certain number of subjects (more than 2000 and 1000, respectively), the prevalence of self-declared sensitive skin for women is estimated between 51% and 56% in Europe (3,14,15). Self-perceived SSS, which reflects the real importance of this disorder, concerned around 10% of the women. For men, only one study gave data (3) collected on 300 men; the reported prevalence was 38%.

Sensitive Skin in Subgroups of Population in the United States

The prevalence and the clinical forms of sensitive skin in four ethnic subgroups (African Americans, Asian-American, Euro-Americans, and Hispanics) of the San Francisco population have been studied on 811 women (16). Each group had at least 200 subjects.

The prevalence was 52%. The prevalence in each group was equivalent: 52% for African American, 51% for Asians, 50% for Euro-Americans, and 54% for Hispanics.

Although the prevalence of sensitive skin was the same in the different subgroups of population, there were some population variations in the clinical presentation and the factors of skin reactivity.

According to the clinical signs, the variations observed are

- The prevalence of itching was significantly higher in Asians (42% compared to 34% mean of all populations).
- Facial redness was less frequent in African American (29% compared to 41% mean of all populations).
- The prevalence of stinging and burning was equivalent in the different subgroups.

The factors for skin reactivity are also varied

- African Americans were the subgroup who had less skin reactivity to environmental factors such as wind, cold weather, sudden changes of temperature, and air pollution.
- Euro-Americans and Asian-Americans were the subgroup with the highest skin reactivity to climatic factors such as wind and sudden changes of temperature.
- The frequency of skin reactivity to alcoholic beverages was significantly lower in the African American and Hispanic sensitive-skin subgroup and higher in the Asian sensitive-skin subgroup.

- In addition, higher skin reactivity to spicy food was reported for Asian sensitive-skin subgroup.

It is not possible to extrapolate the prevalence of sensitive skin in this studied population to those of other countries, especially Asia or Africa, because all the interviewed subjects lived in the same American city.

Sensitive Skin in Japan

The reported prevalence of sensitive skin in Japan is around 50% (17,18). As found in Europe, there is a decrease of the prevalence of sensitive skin with age. In addition, sensitive skin is less frequent with phototype IV (19). For Japanese women, the vascular reactivity of the facial skin (i.e., erythema provoked by external factors) was not considered as a sign of sensitive skin.

In Japan, several authors have reported investigations focused on the causes of sensitive skin (17,18,20). Interestingly, some of them underline the main role of epidermal sensitive nerves in the skin reactivity observed on sensitive skin (18).

Sensitive Skin in China

In China, sensitive skin prevalence has been estimated on a population sample of 2000 women (living in Beijing, Harbin, Chengdu, and Suzhou) (21). The prevalence was 36%. The prevalence decreased with age (47% at 21–25 years; 20.8% at 51–55 years).

A significantly higher prevalence (55.8%) of sensitive skin was found in Chengdu (Sichuan) where the food is very spicy. On the whole Chinese population sample, the link between spicy-food consumption and sensitive skin prevalence was confirmed.

It must be considered that chili contains capsaicin. Therefore, first demonstration of the link between sensitive skin and epidermal nerves was based on the higher skin reactivity to capsaicin of sensitive-skin subjects compared to the nonsensitive ones. In fact, the impact of chili consumption on skin reactivity could be explained by the neurological basis of sensitive skin.

Sensitive Skin and Socioeconomic Factors

It is often a common opinion to think that socioeconomic factors could have an impact on the self-perception of sensitive skin. This question has been recently studied (5) and it was shown that the prevalence was similar according to the level of education or annual income.

PHYSIOLOGICAL MECHANISMS INVOLVED IN SENSITIVE SKIN

The literature is still a little confused about the origin of sensitive skin. Classical opinions admit that sensitive skin could be linked to a barrier function weakness, an atopic pattern, or a subexpression of skin allergy. There is a real mix-up between the terms "sensitive" and "allergic". It is probably due to the common etymology of "sensitization" and "sensitive." For some authors (22), sensitive skin is only a subclinical form of allergy, but for others (23), there is no relation between "sensitive skin" and allergic phenomena. Recently, we report on the results obtained with patch tests and prick tests on self-perceived sensitive skin subjects versus nonsensitive skin subjects (5). The statistical analysis of the data clearly demonstrates that sensitive skin is not linked to an immunoallergologic status. On the same sample of volunteers, we clearly observe a statistical difference in skin reactivity between both groups to capsaicin. Capsaicin (Trans-8-methyl-N-vanillyl-6-nonenamide) is an irritant compound extracted from red pepper. It acts on nociceptive C-fibers on specific receptor and provokes the relapse of neuropeptides (substance P and calcitonin gene-related peptide). The capsaicin test allows the discrimination between sensitive skin subjects and nonsensitive skin subjects (6). Furthermore, there is a real parallelism between the severity of sensitive skin and the importance of the response to the capsaicin test (5).

Actually, two main hypotheses must be considered to explain and understand sensitive skin (i) alteration of the barrier function of the skin and (ii) lower threshold of excitability of the epidermal sensitive nerves (fiber C).

An increase of the TEWL, which quantifies the barrier function, has been reported in sensitive skin subjects (24). However, this increase is inconstant. We consider now that the weakness of the skin barrier function explains only a small part of sensitive skin subjects.

The neurosensorial signs such as the pattern of capsaicin reactivity of sensitive skin suggest a neurogenic origin (25). The recent data, which emphasized the role of the C-fibers in the itching process, must also be considered (26). More recently, new data give additional support to the hypothesis of a neurogenic origin to sensitive skin. It was shown that the thresholds to electric stimulation of the skin at 5 Hz are different between sensitive skin subjects and nonsensitive ones (18).

Presently, we have to consider that the key target to explain sensitive skin is the epidermal sensitive nerves. In fact, barrier function is also likely involved, but inconstantly and as a secondary target.

CONCLUSION

Sensitive skin is a syndrome observed all over the world. The prevalence of 50% is usual, which is quite significant. The key target involved in sensitive skin appears to be epidermal sensitive nerves. The specificity of sensitive skin according to the populations is the factors of skin reactivity and, to a lesser extent, its clinical symptoms. Euro-Americans were characterized by higher skin reactivity to the wind and tended to be less reactive to cosmetics. African Americans presented less skin reactivity to most environmental factors. Asians appeared to have greater skin reactivity to sudden changes in temperature and to the wind, and tended to suffer from itching more frequently. In addition, the impact of chili intake on the skin reactivity must be taken into account.

In the reported differences of constitutional sensitive skin, several factors must be considered: genetic patterns, differences in the climatic conditions, differences in the cosmetic habit, and differences in the nutritional habits.

REFERENCES

1. Maibach HI, Lammintausta K, Berardesca E, Freeman S. Tendency to irritation: sensitive skin. J Am Acad Dermatol 1989; 21:833–835.
2. Wilson WW, Queor R, Masters RJ. The search for a practical sunscreen. South Med J 1966; 59:1425–1430.
3. Willis CM, Shaw S, De Lacharriere O, et al. Sensitive skin: an epidemiological study. Br J Dermatol 2001; 145:258–263.
4. De Lacharrière O. Peaux sensibles, Peaux réactives. Encycl Med Chir Cosmétologie et Dermatologie Esthétique 2002; A10:50–220.
5. De Lacharrière O, Nouveau S, Querleux B, et al. Sensitive Skin, A neurological perspective. IFSCC, Osaka, Japan, 2006.
6. Thiers H. Peau Sensible. In: Thiers H. Les Cosmétiques (2ème ed), Masson (Paris), 1986:266–268.
7. Weigand DA, Haygood C, Gaylor JR. Cell layers and density of Negro and European stratum corneum. J Invest Dermatol 1974; 62:563–568.
8. Stoughton RB. Bioassay methods for measuring percutaneous absorption. In: Montagna W, Stoughton RB, Van Scott EJ, eds. Pharmacology of the skin. New York, New York: Appleton-Century-Crofts, 1969:542.
9. Berardesca E, Maibach HI. Population differences in pharmacodynamic response to nicotinates in vivo in human skin: black and white. Acta Derm Venereol 1990; 70:63–66.
10. Berardesca E, Maibach HI. Population differences in sodium-lauryl-sulphate induced cutaneous irritation: black and white. Contact Dermatitis 1988; 18:65–70.
11. Berardesca E, Maibach HI. Sodium lauryl sulphate induced irritation: comparison of white and South Americans subjects. Contact Dermatitis 1998; 19: 136–140.
12. Berardesca E, Maibach HI. Sensitive and ethnic skin. A need for special skincare agents? Dermatol Clin 1991; 9:89–92.
13. Aramaki J, Kawana S, Effendy I, Happle R, Loffler H. Differences of skin irritation between Japanese and European women. Br J Dermatol 2002; 146:1052–1056.
14. Misery L, Myon E, Martin N, Verriere F, Nocera T, Taieb C. Sensitive skin in France: an epidemiological approach. Ann Dermatol Venereol 2005; 132(5): 425–429.
15. Morizot F, Le Fur I, Tschachler E. Sensitive skin. Definitions, prevalence and possible causes. Cosm Toil 1998; 113:59–66.
16. Jourdain R, Lacharriere O, Bastien P, Maibach HI. Ethnic variations in self-perceived sensitive skin: epidemiological survey. Contact Dermatitis 2002; 46: 162–169.

17. Ota N. Sensitive skin: an approach based on corneocytes morphology. J Jap Cosm Sc Soc 2005; 29(1):28–34.
18. Yokota T. Classification of sensitive skin based on the analysis of dermo-physiological parameters. J Jap Cosm Sc Soc 2005; 29(1):44–49.
19. Morizot F, Le Fur I, Numagami K, et al. Self-reported sensitive skin: a study on 120 healthy Japanese women. Edinburg, Scotland: 22nd IFSCC Congress. 23–26 September 2002.
20. Hariya T. A characterization of sensitive skin. J Jap Cosm Sc Soc 2005; 29(1): 35–43.
21. Yang FZ, De Lacharriere O, Lian S, et al. Sensitive skin: specific features in Chinese skin. A clinical study on 2,000 Chinese women. Ann Dermatol Venereol 2002; 129:1S11–1S77.
22. Francomano M, Bertoni L, Seidenari S. Sensitive skin as a subclinical expression of contact allergy to nickel sulfate. Contact Dermatitis 2000; 42:169–170.
23. De Lacharriere O, Jourdain R, Bastien P, Garrigue JL. Sensitive skin is not a subclinical expression of contact allergy. Contact Dermatitis 2001; 44:131–132.
24. Seidenari S, Francomano M, Mantovani L. Baseline biophysical parameters in subjects with sensitive skin. Contact Dermatitis 1998; 38:311–315.
25. De Lacharriere O, Reiche L, Montastier C, et al. Skin reaction to capsaicin: a new way for the understanding of sensitive skin. Proceedings of the 19th World Congress of Dermatology (Sydney, Australia). Aust J Dermatol 1997; 38(S2):288.
26. Schmelz M, Schmidt R, Bickel, Handwerker HO, Torebjörk HE. Specific C-receptors for itch in human skin. J Neurosci 1997; 17:8003–8008.

19

Diversity of Hair Growth Parameters

Geneviève Loussouarn
L'Oréal Recherche, Clichy, France

INTRODUCTION

The human head of hair naturally shows a great variety of shape, color, and thickness. Its diversity is also reflected in hair growth parameters, which obviously change with age, according to hormonal status and genetics. Even in a single head, hair distribution, as an image of growth characteristics, may vary to a large extent from one area to another. For example, in case of male pattern baldness, head hair is sparse in the frontline and the temples, scattered on the top, whereas dense in the nape. Furthermore, when dealing with data on human hair, its unique mosaic nature must be kept in mind, i.e., each hair has an autonomous life cycle leading to dramatic differences of size, growth duration, and possible onset of miniaturization process from one hair to another (1,2). Human hair has been conventionally classified into three subtypes—African, Asian, and Caucasian. Most studies have addressed the various morphological features, structure, and mechanical properties (3–9). A number of investigations have also been reported on physiological growth aspects such as hair cycle, growth period, frequency of renewal, anagen/telogen ratio, i.e., ratio of growing hair to resting hair, in men and women, with or without alopecia process. Nevertheless, most of these studies have been conducted on Caucasian hair. Very few are comparative studies concerning various hair subtypes.

The purpose of this review was to go through most of the published data pertaining to the growth of human hair on the scalp and to identify

Table 1 African Subtype Hair Growth Parameters

	Method	Volunteers	Scalp sites	Hair density (hairs/cm^2)	Growth rate (μm/day)	Telogen count (%)
Sperling 1999 (10) United States	B	22 African American (12 M+10 W)	–	170 ± 40		6 ± 6
		21–56 yrs; mean 32 yrs		79–254		0–21
Loussouarn 2001 (11) France	PTG	38 African (19 M+19 W)	V+T+O	187 ± 43	260 ± 43	19 ± 9
		18–59 yrs; mean 27 yrs		112–290	150–363	2–46
Loussouarn et al. 2005 (12) France	PTG	216 African (106M+110W)	V+T+O	161 ± 50	280 ± 50	14 ± 9
		18–35 yrs; mean 25 yrs		49–390	129–436	0–57

Abbreviations: PTG, phototrichogram; V, vertex; T, temporal; O, occipital; B, biopsy.

possible subtype-related differences in spite of the variety of methods by which data were obtained and the heterogeneous samples they came from.

The whole data considered is shown in Table 1 (10–12) for African subtype, Table 2 (12–20) for Asian subtype, and Table 3 (10–12,14,17,21–37) for Caucasian subtype. When the subtype was not specified, it was assumed to be the predominant subtype living where the study took place. The papers are given in a chronological order, except for the publications of a same author, which are put together for convenience. Three parameters were retained for comparison between subtypes: hair density, rate of growth, and telogen percentage. The methods used to assess hair growth parameters have changed over the last 50 years (38). Early studies were based on direct observation and visual counts in very small areas of the scalp, providing hair density and rate of growth, and on trichogram (TG) method providing percentages of growing hair and resting hair. From the 1990s, a noninvasive technique, the videotrichogram (VTG) or phototrichogram (PTG) method, has been developed whereby the three main hair growth parameters can be evaluated. Moreover, some authors have used 4 mm scalp biopsies (B), from which they measured hair density and anagen and telogen counts.

HAIR GROWTH EVALUATION METHODS

From direct observation of the scalp using a microscope with various magnifications and/or an ocular micrometer (DO), hair density and rate of growth can be measured. The latter is obtained after shaving a small area

(*Text continues on page 252*)

Table 2 Asian Subtype Hair Growth Parameters

	Method	Volunteers	Scalp sites	Hair density (hairs/cm^2)	Growth rate (μm/day)	Telogen count (%)
Saitoh et al. (13) 1970 Japan	DO	12 M, 11 W 9 M	V T		445 390	
Cottington et al. (14) 1977 United States	DO	3 Chinese women 47–59 yrs; mean 51 yrs	T	128±32 95–159		
Hayashi et al. (15) 1991 Japan	VTG	10 men without alopecia 27–48 yrs; mean 39 yrs 10 men with alopecia 35–48 yrs; mean 43 yrs	V V	181±19 153–219 157±37 85–229	313±60 250–466 109±29 75–151	
Tsuji et al. (16) 1994 Japan	PTG	56 Japanese men with alopecia 23–56 yrs; mean 41 yrs	V	270±56 183–387		32 20–63
Sivayathorn et al. (17) 1995 Thailand	PTG	16 Thai men with alopecia 18–55 yrs	FV O	212±14 189±10	288±8 392±9	41 18
Ueki et al. (18) 1998 Japan	PTG	159 Japanese women with or without diffuse alopecia 17–70 yrs; mean 35 yrs	P	166–normal cluster 115–alopecia cluster	400–normal cluster 342–alopecia cluster	
Yoo et al. (19) 2002 Korea	PTG	42 Korean (16 M + 26 W) 17–58 yrs	V+O+T	126±19 63 –173	309±20	8
Lee et al. (20) 2002 Korea	B	35 Korean (19M + 16W) 16–57; mean 33 yrs "normal scalp"	O	128±29 63–198		6±6 0–20
Loussouarn (12) 2005 France	PTG	188 Chinese (92M + 96W) 18–35 yrs; mean 26 yrs	V+O+T	175±54 78–333	411±53 244–611	12±7 1–48

Abbreviations: DO, ocular micrometer; PTG, phototrichogram; VTG, videotrichogram; V, vertex; T, temporal; O, occipital; FV, frontovertex; P, parietal; B, biopsy.

Table 3 Caucasian Subtype Hair Growth Parameters

	Method	Volunteers	Scalp sites	Hair density (hairs/cm²)	Growth rate (μm/day)	Telogen count (%)
Myers and Hamilton (21) 1951 United States	DO	54 subjects (26 M + 28 F) 9–84 yrs	V / T		350 / 330	
Barman et al. (22) 1965 Argentina	TG / DO	39 volunteers (17M + 22 W) 16–46 yrs	F + P + C + O	223 ± 25 / 175–300	344	17 ± 9 / 13–23
Barman et al. (23) 1969		36 volunteers (27 M + 9W) 50–83 yrs; mean 62 yrs	F + P + C + O	164 ± 13 / 87–330	308	20 ± 23 / 0–87
Pelfini et al. (24) 1969 Italy	DO	32 volunteers (16 M + 16W) 40–79 yrs	O		350	
Cottington et al. (14) 1977 United States	DO	17 Caucasian women 24–42 yrs; mean 33 yrs	T	226 ± 41 / 145–295		
Rushton et al. (25) 1983 United Kingdom	UA-TG	20 normal Caucasians (10M + 10 W) 17–32 yrs; mean 22 yrs	F + O	291 ± 26 / 233–93		8 ± 1 / 1–15
		25 Caucasian with AG-alopecia (10 M + 15 W) 17–39 yrs; mean 24 yrs	F + O	181 ± 27 / 69–352		22 ± 8 / 8–57
Rushton et al. (26) 1990	UA-TG	20 Caucasian W without alopecia 17–49 yrs; mean 29 yrs	F + O	280 ± 41 / 231–376		11 / 2–16
		100 Caucasian W with diffuse alopecia 14–54 yrs; mean 32 yrs	F + O	207 ± 55 / 69–360		21 / 4–46
Rushton et al. (27) 1991	UA-TG	13 Caucasian M without alopecia 20–30 yrs; mean 24 yrs	F	301 ± 30 / 253–358		11 / 5–17
		26 Caucasian M with AG-alopecia 20–30 yrs; mean 26 yrs	FV	232 ± 51 / 144–346		39 / 10–73

Runme and Martin (28) 1986 Germany	TG	26 men with AG-Alopecia 20–33 yrs; mean 26 yrs	F	166±28	355±24	22
	DO		O	193±24	389±21	11
Friedel et al. (29) 1989 France	PTG	5 Men without alopecia 17–29 yrs	V	204±10	350±30	18±3
		35 Men with alopecia 19–45 yrs; mean 28 yrs	V	182–240	280–420	9–25
			V	187±8	275±23	40±2
Whiting (30) 1993 United States	B	22 normal control (13M+9W) 18–70 yrs; mean 43 yrs	V	317±83		7±8
				151–468		0–32
		106 Men with AG-Alopecia 16–70 yrs; mean 37 yrs	V	278±97		16
Lee et al. (31) 1995 Australia	B	10 control 6M+4W 30–60 yrs; mean 44 yrs	—	228±73		
				119–340		
		10 volunteers with AG-Alopecia (3M+7W) 26–78 yrs; mean 43 yrs	—	173±104		
				53–368		
Courtois et al. (32) 1995 France	PTG	16 Caucasian women without alopecia 19–60 yrs; mean 34 yrs	F + FP + V	252±67		12±8
		25 Caucasian women with alopecia 18–63 yrs; mean 41 yrs	F + FP + V	192±58		22±12
		13 Caucasian men with alopecia	F + FP + V	201±51		31±11
Courtois et al. (33) 1996	PTG	9 Caucasians without alopecia (6W+3M) 25–49 yrs; mean 36 yrs	FV	313±49		10±6
				243–411		1–17
		5 Caucasians with alopecia (1W+4M) 25–47 yrs; mean 38 yrs	FV	211±57		29±11
				152–279		18–45
Sivayathorn (17) 1995 Thailand	PTG	16 European men with alopecia 18–more than 46 yrs	FV	203±16	267±9	21
			O	198±9	300±10	14

(Continued)

Table 3 Caucasian Subtype Hair Growth Parameters (*Continued*)

	Method	Volunteers	Scalp sites	Hair density (hairs/cm^2)	Growth rate (µm/day)	Telogen count (%)
Sperling (10) 1999 United States	B	12 white Americans (4M+8W) 17–61 yrs; mean 35 yrs	–	282±44 206–357		5±5 0–16
Birch et al. (34) 2001 United Kingdom	PTG	377 women 18–99 yrs	FV	293±61 (at age 35 yrs) 211±55 (at age 70 yrs) 75–450		
Loussouarn (11) 2001 France	PTG	45 Caucasians (23W+22M) mean age 28 yrs	V+O	227±55 98–334	396±55 281–537	14±11 0–50
Loussouarn et al. (12) 2005	PTG	107 Caucasians (56M+51W) 18–35 yrs; mean 28 yrs	V+T+O	226±73 80–488	367±56 165–506	12±8 1–54

d'Amico et al. (35) 2001 Italy	VTG	28 healthy adults (20W + 8M) 18–35 yrs; mean 23 yrs	V	260 ±30 (men) 300 ±20 (women)	350 ±30 380 ±30	17 ±2 11 ±1
Vecchio et al. (36) 2002 Italy	VTG	109 men grade I to VI according Hamilton 17–78; mean 36 yrs	O P	127 67–260 110		
Van Neste (37) 2006 Belgium	DO	13 Women with Diffuse hair loss (D) 50 Women with Ludwig pattern (L) 29 Women with No visible hair loss (N) 12–76 yrs	V + O		367 ±34 (D) 389 ±45 (L) 395 ±48 (N)	

Abbreviations: DO, ocular micrometer; TG, trichogram; UA-TG, unit area TG; PTG, phototrichogram; VTG, videotrichogram; V, vertex; T, temporal; O, occipital; F, frontal; P, parietal; C, coronal; FP, frontoparietal; FV, frontovertex; B, biopsy.

and by measuring the increase of the hair length seven or 10 days later, either in situ on the scalp or after having collected the shaved fragments of hair.

The TG is based on a rapid plucking of about 50 hairs, which are then mounted between a glass slide and a cover slip for microscope observation of the bulbs. Visual assessment of the proximal part enables the classification of each hair with regard to the stage or phase of hair cycle, i.e., anagen or telogen. A variant of this technique, the unit area TG (UA-TG), consists in clipping all the hairs present within a standardized area in order to calculate the hair density not accessible with the classical TG.

PTG or videotrichogram consists in shaving hairs from a scalp area of around 1 cm^2, taking a picture of this area using a camera or video camera. Two days later, a picture of the same area is taken again. Comparing this set of pictures allows the differentiation between anagen hairs that have grown for these two days and telogen hairs that have not grown, and the measurement of the increase in the length of anagen hair. Using this method, the hair density can also be recorded.

Biopsies, particularly of horizontal section, have also been used to assess hair follicles according to their respective hair-cycle phase. Because they are performed with a specified punch size, this method enables the calculation of the hair density.

The size of the sample population in the papers included in this review varies from 3 to 216 volunteers of both genders. Factors that influence the hair growth such as age or scalp area are often mentioned. Seven various areas according to the designation of Moretti et al. (39) or Peccoraro and Astore (40) have been assessed: they include three on the top of the head, named vertex (V), coronal (C), and parietal (P) areas, one on the upper forehead, i.e., the frontal (F) area, one in-between area designated as frontovertex (FV) or frontoparietal (FP), one on the sides of the head called the temporal (T) area, and lastly one on the back of the head, i.e., the occipital (O) area, often used as a control area as regards the alopecia process.

HAIR DENSITY

African Subtype

The few studies on African hair summarized in Table 1 are quite in agreement, even if they have not been performed with the same methods. Sperling (10) found quite low values of hair density, with an average of 170 ± 40 hairs/cm^2 on scalp biopsies from 22 African Americans aged 21 to 56 years (area not specified). Low hair densities ca. 165 hairs/cm^2 have also been recorded by Loussouarn et al. (11,12) in 346 Africans from central or western Africa and South Africa, using the PTG technique on vertex, occipital, and temporal areas.

In the two latter studies, no difference was noticed between men and women. Hair density decreased significantly when moving from the vertex to the occipital area and then to the temporal area in both men and women. Ageing (11), like male alopecia in young adults (11,12), seemed to have little impact on hair density in the African subtype.

Asian Subtype

Average hair density from data published on the Asian subtype (Table 2) ranges from 126 to 181 hairs/cm^2 in normal scalp. The lowest mean values were found first in three Chinese women, 47 to 59 years of age, by Cottington et al. (14) (128 ± 32 hairs/cm^2) through DO in temporal areas, and then in Korean volunteers of both genders by Yoo et al. (19) (126 ± 19 hairs/cm^2) using PTG on three scalp areas—vertex, occipital, and temporal—of 42 volunteers and by Lee et al. (20) (128 ± 29 hairs/cm^2) from biopsy observations of the occipital area of 35 volunteers. Lee et al. (20) demonstrated a gender-related difference with a higher hair count in Korean women than in men whereas Yoo et al. (19) showed differences in hair density according to the area of the scalp, with lower densities at the temples in both genders and a weak decrease in hair counts with aging in women.

Using PTG, Loussouarn et al. (12) found an average density of 175 ± 54 hairs/cm^2 for the whole scalp in a cohort of 188 young Chinese adults, men and women, aged 18 to 35 years. However, the density was lower in the temporal area (119 ± 24 hairs/cm^2) and higher in the occipital and vertex areas (182 ± 34 and 224 ± 38 hairs/cm^2, respectively). No gender-related difference was noticed in this study. Hayashi et al. (15) compared vertex areas in 10 men with alopecia (mean age 43 years) versus 10 men without alopecia (mean age 39 years) in Tokyo. Using VTG, the authors demonstrated a clear decrease in hair density in the vertex of volunteers with alopecia (157 ± 37 vs. 181 ± 19 hairs/cm^2). Ueki et al. (18) drew a similar conclusion from a study in a large sample of Japanese women with diffuse alopecia on parietal areas of the scalp. About 159 volunteers, aged 17 to 70 years, were included in this study and a cluster analysis of PTG data showed a decrease in hair density in subjects with alopecia pattern compared to those with "normal" pattern (115 vs. 166 hairs/cm^2).

The highest hair density in the Asian subtype was paradoxically reported in two studies involving men with male pattern baldness, both of them using PTG. Tsuji et al. (16) enrolled 56 Japanese men, aged 23 to 56 years who were, for the most part, either at an early or midstage of male-pattern alopecia and they recorded a mean value of hair density as high as 270 ± 40 hairs/cm^2 at the vertex of these volunteers. Sivayathorn et al. (17) showed no difference in hair density according to scalp area in 16 Thai men with male pattern baldness, although the FV area tended to show higher counts of hair in comparison with occipital area (212 ± 14 vs. 189 ± 10 hairs/cm^2).

Caucasian Subtype

As far as Caucasian hair is concerned, a large amount of papers and data are available (Table 3). The earlier studies mostly focused on physiological aspects of hair growth, whereas in the 1980s to 1990s they pertained to the changes associated with male and female alopecia. The average reported hair density ranges from 164 to 317 hairs/cm^2. Barman et al. (22,23) found a decrease in hair density with aging, from 223 ± 25 to 164 ± 13 hairs/cm^2, by comparing two groups of volunteers of both genders, aged 16 to 46 years and 50 to 83 years, respectively. The data was recorded through DO of four scalp areas namely, frontal, parietal, coronal, and occipital. The study conducted by Cottington et al. (14) in 17 Caucasian women using the same method found an average hair density of 226 ± 41 hairs/cm^2 at the temporal area. In a similar way, Runne and Martin (28) showed a decrease in hair density according to the stage of androgenogenetic alopecia (AGA) in 26 men (aged 20 to 33 years) at the frontal area compared with occipital (166 ± 28 vs. 193 ± 24 hairs/cm^2).

Using the UA-TG, Rushton et al. (25–27) turned the attention to changes in hair growth parameters associated with alopecia in Caucasian adults. They compared a group of 10 men and 15 women (mean age 24 years) with AGA to a control group of 10 normal men and 10 normal women matched for age. They found an overall decrease in hair density at the frontal and occipital areas (181 ± 27 vs. 291 ± 26 hairs/cm^2) (25). They mainly explained the fact that they found higher density in normal volunteers than reported by Barman et al. (22,23) and Cottington et al. (14) by the different methods used for evaluation. In two further studies (26,27) they confirmed the decrease in hair density, both at the frontal and occipital areas in 100 women aged 14 to 54 years with diffuse alopecia, compared to 20 control women aged 17 to 49 years (average 207 ± 55 vs. 280 ± 41 hairs/cm^2) and in frontal-vertex area in 26 men aged 20 to 30 years showing male pattern baldness compared with 13 age-matched controls (average 232 ± 51 vs. 301 ± 30 hairs/cm^2).

The mean hair density data obtained from counts on biopsies from normal scalp varies from 228 to 317 hairs/cm^2. As regards diagnosis of male pattern AGA on the posterior vertex, Whiting (30) mentioned a mean hair density of 317 ± 83 hairs/cm^2 in 22 control subjects (13 men and 9 women; mean age 43 years) vs. 278 ± 97 hairs/cm^2 in 106 men with AGA (mean 37 years). In a similar comparison study, Lee et al. (31) recorded a mean density of 228 ± 73 hairs/cm^2 in control subjects (six men and four women aged 30 to 60 years) vs. 173 ± 104 hairs/cm^2 in subjects with AGA (three men and seven women aged 26 to 78 years). The area of the scalp was not specified by Sperling (10), who reported a hair density of 282 ± 44 hairs/cm^2 in 12 unaffected Caucasian American (four men and eight women aged 17 to 61 years).

Hair density assessed in normal scalp using VTG or PTG method ranges from 226 to 313 hairs/cm^2. Courtois et al. (32) demonstrated a decrease in hair counts at four scalp areas (FP, frontal, anterior-vertex, and posterior-vertex) in 25 women with alopecia, aged 18 to 63 years compared to 16 women without alopecia, aged 19 to 60 years (average hair density 252 ± 67 vs. 192 ± 58 hairs/cm^2). In a second study about seasonality of hair shedding, Courtois et al. (33) reported data in 14 volunteers, gender-matched, at the FV area showing variation according to the stage of alopecia from an average density of 313 ± 49 hairs/cm^2 in normal scalp down to 211 ± 57 hairs/cm^2. Birch et al. (34) described a decrease in hair density at the FV area with aging in 377 women (from 293 ± 61 hairs/cm^2 at 35 years of age to 211 ± 55 hairs/cm^2 at 70 years of age). Loussouarn et al. (11,12) studied hair growth parameters first at the vertex and occipital areas of 45 young Caucasian adults (mean age 28 years) then at the vertex, occipital, and temporal areas of 107 young Caucasian adults of both gender (mean age 28 years). The average hair densities in the whole scalp were 227 ± 55 and 226 ± 73 hairs/cm^2. Like in African and Chinese volunteers, the authors demonstrated that hair density was higher at the vertex than at the occipital area, which in its turn was higher than at the temporal area. Significantly lower density was found in men than in women, which is partially explained by the higher prevalence of alopecia in Caucasian men. D'Amico et al. (35) also found a difference in average hair density of the vertex between men (260 ± 30 hairs/cm^2) and women (300 ± 20 hairs/cm^2), in a group of 28 healthy young adults. In male AGA, a decrease in hair density (187 ± 8 vs. 204 ± 10 hair/cm^2) was shown by Friedel et al. (29), by comparing data of vertex area in two groups of men, with and without alopecia. In 109 men with or without alopecia (mean age 36 years), Vecchio et al. (36) observed an average occipital density of 127 hairs/cm^2 whereas parietal density was 110 hairs/cm^2. Lastly Sivayathorn et al. (17) measured hair density in 16 European men with male pattern baldness and found very close average density at the FV and occipital areas (203 ± 16 and 198 ± 9 hairs/cm^2, respectively).

RATE OF HAIR GROWTH

African Subtype

In African volunteers, Loussouarn (11) found quite a low average growth rate of 260 ± 43 μm/day, which was confirmed in a larger sample (12) with a mean value of 280 ± 50 μm/day. No difference was observed between men and women (11,12). Lower rates were noticed at the occipital area and growth rate seemed to decrease in case of alopecia (12).

Asian Subtype

In Asian volunteers, reported rate of growth ranges from 309 to 445 μm/day in normal scalp (Table 2). From DO using capillary tubes in a group of 23 Japanese volunteers, Saitoh et al. (13) found an average rate of 445 μm/day at the vertex area in both men and women. At the temporal area, the rate of growth was only measured in nine men and the average rate was 390 μm/day. Hayashi et al. (15) found a much lower rate of growth (313 ± 60 μm/day) using VTG at the vertex area of men without alopecia, and a strong decrease in men with alopecia (mean value 109 ± 29 μm/day). Ueki et al. (18) also separated normal state versus alopecia state in Japanese women as regards rate of growth (400 vs. 342 μm/day). In Korean volunteers, Yoo et al. (19) found a rate of growth of 309 ± 20 μm/day, with a lower rate at the temporal area compared with vertex and occipital areas. In Chinese volunteers, Loussouarn et al. (12) recorded a rate of growth of 411 ± 53 μm/day, with slightly lower values at the temporal area (400 ± 51 μm/day) compared with vertex and occipital areas (421 ± 53 μm/day and 414 ± 52 μm/day, respectively). No difference between men and women was reported. Otherwise, Sivayathorn et al. (17) showed a decrease in rate of growth at the vertex versus occipital area in 16 Thai men with alopecia (288 ± 8 vs. 392 ± 9 μm/day).

Caucasian Subtype

The rate of growth reported in Caucasians with normal scalp condition ranges from 308 to 396 μm/day (Table 3). From DO in 54 subjects, Meyers and Hamilton (21) found 350 μm/day at the crown and 330 μm/day at the temporal area. They reported higher rates in women than in men. Barman et al. (22,23) showed a decrease with aging, i.e., 344 μm/day in young adults versus 308 μm/day in subjects over 50. Pelfini et al. (24) measured an average growth rate of 350 μm/day at the occipital area of 32 healthy subjects of both genders. Friedel et al. (29) observed a decrease in rate of growth at the vertex of men with AGA compared with unaffected men (275 ± 23 vs. 350 ± 30 μm/day). Loussouarn et al. (11,12) found mean values of 396 ± 55 and 367 ± 56 μm/day in two studies involving both men and women. They did not notice any difference according to gender, whereas d'Amico et al. (35), in a smaller group, observed a gender-related difference with a faster rate of growth in women (380 ± 30 μm/day) than in men (350 ± 30 μm/day). In 29 women with no visible hair loss, Van Neste (37) recorded an average 395 ± 48 μm/day at the occipital and vertex areas. He particularly showed a decrease in women with diffuse hair loss (367 ± 34 μm/day). Lastly, in men with ongoing alopecia, Syvayarthorn et al. (17) like Runne and Martin (28) demonstrated a difference of rate of growth between frontal area and occipital area, which is not affected by baldness [267 ± 9 vs. 300 ± 10 μm/day (17) and 355 ± 24 vs. 389 ± 21 μm/day (28)].

TELOGEN PERCENTAGE

Irrespective of hair subtypes, reported telogen counts range between 5% and 20% in the normal scalp (10–12,19,20,22,23,25,27,29,30,32,33,35).

They tend to be higher in men than in women in the three subtypes (10–12,22,23,35).

When volunteers with and without hair pattern alopecia (11,12,25–27,29,32,33) are compared, or when affected and unaffected areas are compared on the same head (17,28), an increase over 20% telogen hairs has been found, associated with ongoing alopecia process in the three hair subtypes. An increase in telogen counts with aging was reported in both Asians (16) and Caucasians (23).

COMPARISON OF THE THREE HAIR SUBTYPES

Data reported on the main hair growth parameters in normal human scalp, i.e., unaffected by hair loss, in the tree hair subtypes is summarized in Figure 1 (hair density), Figure 2 (rate of growth), and Figure 3 (telogen percentage). Even if the size and nature of sample population varied to a large extent and different methods were used to get the data, it appears from the graphs that despite some subtype-related differences as regards hair density and rate of growth, data on telogen percentage are fairly similar in the three subtypes.

It seems that higher hair densities are found in Caucasians whereas Asians and Africans look closely similar with lower hair densities. Moreover, on the whole, higher rates of growth are reported in Asians and lower rates in Africans, whereas Caucasians show intermediate values. Among all papers included in this review, only four intended to compare hair growth

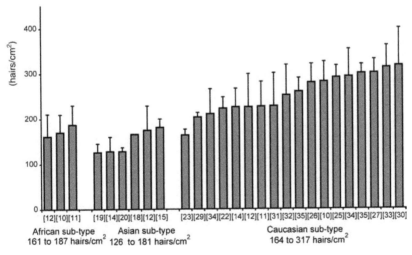

Figure 1 Average hair densities of normal scalp (+SD, if available) reported in the three hair subtypes.

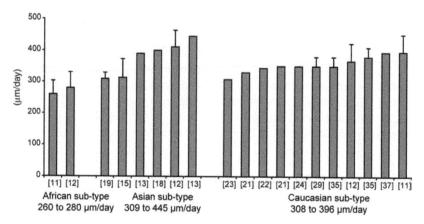

Figure 2 Average rates of growth of normal scalp (+SD, if available) reported in the three hair subtypes.

parameters according to ethnic origin, and one reported an accidental observation. These studies are summarized together in Table 4, and give consistent data overall.

Cottington et al. (14), within the context of a paper focused on observations on female hair scalp, noticed that the three Chinese women included in the study showed a lower hair density than the Caucasian ones. However, the authors could not identify whether the differences were related to ethnic subtype or to aging because Chinese volunteers were older than Caucasian. Lee et al. (20) and Loussouarn et al. (12) investigated volunteers better matched for age and confirmed significant lower density in Koreans or

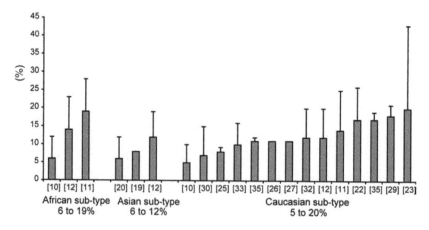

Figure 3 Average telogen percentages of normal scalp (+SD, if available) reported in the three hair subtypes.

Table 4 Hair Subtypes Comparative Studies

References	Cottington et al. (14) 1977		Sivayathorn et al. (17) 1995				Sperling (10) and Lee et al. (20) 1999 and 2002				Loussouarn et al. (12) 2005		
Method	DO		PTG				B				PTG		
Volunteers	17 Caucasians	3 Chinese	16 Thais with alopecia		16 Europeans with alopecia		22 African Americans	12 white Americans	22 normal controls	35 Koreans	216 Africans	188 Chinese	107 Caucasians
Age (yrs)	Mean 33	Mean 51	18–55		18±46		Mean 32	Mean 35	Mean 43	Mean 33	Mean 25	Mean 26	Mean 28
Scalp area	T	T	FV	O	FV	O	—	—	V	O	V+O+T	V+O+T	V+O+T
Hair density (hairs/cm²)	226±41 145–295	128±32 95–159	212±14	189±10	203±16	198±9	170±40 79–254	282±44 206–357	317±83 151–468	128±29 63–198	161±50 49–390	175±54 78–333	226±73 80–488
Telogen count (%)			41	18	21	11	6±6 0–21	5±5 0–16	7±8 0–32	6±6 0–20	14±9 0–57	12±7 1–48	12±8 1–54
Growth rate (µm/day)			288±8	392±9	267±9	300±10					280±50 129–436	411±53 244–611	367±56 165–506

Abbreviations: DO, ocular micrometer; PTG, phototrichogram; V, vertex; T, temporal; O, occipital; FV, frontovertex.

Chinese compared to Caucasians. Sivayathorn et al. (17) did not notice such a difference between Thai and European volunteers with alopecia, but they reported that Thai hair grew more rapidly compared to European hair; they suggested it may be related to genetics or to climate. Loussouarn et al. (12) confirmed a faster growth rate in Asian hair compared to Caucasian hair. Concerning African hair, Sperling (10) like Loussouarn et al. (12) found significant lower hair density than in Caucasian hair. Rate of growth of African hair was significantly lower than that of Caucasian hair (12).

As far as telogen percentage is concerned, it seems that Thai (17) and African (12) subjects tended to have higher values, which could indicate shorter hair cycle.

CONCLUSION

In spite of the variety of sources of data, methods, and samples, some characteristic features emerge in conventional hair subtypes: African hair seems to be characterized by low density and low rate of growth, Asian hair by low density and fast rate of growth, and Caucasian hair by high density.

The actual picture is likely to be contrasting and the subtype concept probably obscures wide interindividual variations. Increased migration and mixing of populations lead to a still higher degree of diversity. It has been shown that all intermediate hair types can be found all around the world and that the subtype classification is an oversimplification of the reality, which rather displays a continuum of mixed types of hair (41). Thus subtype likely represents only a dominant trend, even here where the diversity of hair growth parameters reflects as many levels as individual or family histories.

ACKNOWLEDGMENT

The advice and the critical review of C. Bouillon are gratefully acknowledged.

REFERENCES

1. Courtois M, Loussouarn G, Hourseau C, Grollier JF. Ageing and hair cycles. Br J Dermatol 1995; 132:86–93.
2. Courtois M, Loussouarn G, Hourseau C, Grollier JF. Hair cycle in alopecia. Skin Pharmacol 1994; 7:84–89.
3. Menkart J, Wolfram L, Mao I. Caucasian hair. Negro hair and wool: similarities and differences. J Soc Cosmet Chem 1966; 17:769–787.
4. Lindelöf B, Forslind B, Hedblad MA, Kaveus U. Human hair form revealed by light and scanning electron microscopy and computer aided three-dimensional reconstitution. Arch Dermatol 1988; 124:1359–1363.
5. Dekio S, Jidoi J. Amounts of fibrous proteins and matrix substances in hairs of different races. J Dermatol 1990; 17:62–64.

6. Franbourg A, Hallegot P, Baltenneck F, Toutain C, Leroy F. Current research on ethnic hair. J Am Acad Dermatol 2003; 48:S115–S119.
7. Bernard BA. Hair shape of curly hair. J Am Acad Dermatol 2003; 48:S120–S126.
8. Thibaut S, Bernard BA. The biology of hair shape. Int J Dermatol 2005; 44(suppl 1):2–3.
9. Franbourg A, Leroy F. Hair structure, function and physicochemical properties. In: Bouillon C, Wilkinson J, eds. The Science of Hair Care. Boca Raton, Florida: Taylor & Francis, 2005:1.
10. Sperling L. Hair density in African Americans. Arch Dermatol 1999; 135: 656–658.
11. Loussouarn G. African hair growth parameters. Br J Dermatol 2001; 145: 294–297.
12. Loussouarn G, El Rawadi C, Genain G. Diversity of hair growth profiles. Int J Dermatol 2005; 44(suppl 1):6–9.
13. Saitoh M, Uzuka M, Sakamoto M, Kobori T. Rate of hair growth. In: Montagna W, Dobson RL, eds. Hair Growth. Oxford, Pergamon, England: 1969:183–201.
14. Cottington E, Kissinger R, Tolgyesi W. Observations on female scalp hair population, distribution and diameter. J Soc Cosmet Chem 1977; 28:219–229.
15. Hayashi S, Miyamoto I, Takeda K. Measurement of human hair growth by optical microscopy and image analysis. Br J Dermatol 1991; 125:123–129.
16. Tsuji Y, Ishino A, Hanzawa N, et al. Quantitative evaluations of male pattern baldness. J Dermatol Sci 1994; 7(suppl):S136–S141.
17. Sivayathorn A, Perkins T, Pisuttinusart P, et al. A comparison of the hair growth characteristics of Thai and Caucasian men with male pattern baldness. In: Van Neste DJJ, Randall VA, eds. Hair Research for the Next Millennium. Amsterdam: Elsevier Science BV, 1996:341–344.
18. Ueki R, Tsuboi R, Inaba Y, Ogawa H. Phototrichogram analysis of Japanese female subjects with chronic diffuse hair loss. J Invest Dermatol 2003; 8(1):116–120.
19. Yoo JH, Park HY, Park TH, Kim KJ. Quantitative analysis on the scalp hair characteristics in Koreans using phototrichogram. Korean J Dermatol 2002; 40(9):1035–1043.
20. Lee HJ, Ha SJ, Lee JH, Kim JW, Kim HO, Whiting D. Hair counts from scalp biopsy specimens in Asians. J Am Acad Dermatol 2002; 46:218–221.
21. Myers R, Hamilton J. Regeneration and rate of growth of hairs in man. Ann NY Acad Sci 1951; 53:562–568.
22. Barman J, Astore I, Pecoraro V. The normal trichogram of the adult. J Invest Dermatol 1965; 44:233–236.
23. Barman J, Astore I, Pecoraro V. The normal trichogram of people over 50 years apparently not bald. In: Montagna W, Dobson RL, eds. Hair Growth. Oxford, Pergamon, England: 1969:211–220.
24. Pelfini C, Cerimele D, Pisanu G. Aging of the skin and hair growth in man. In: Montagna W, Dobson RL, eds. Hair Growth. Oxford, Pergamon, England: 1969:153–160.
25. Rushton D, James K, Mortimer C. The unit area trichogram in the assessment of androgen-dependent alopecia. Br J Dermatol 1983; 109:429–437.

26. Rushton D, Ramsay I, James K, Norris M, Gilkes J. Biochemical and trichological characterization of diffuse alopecia in women. Br J Dermatol 1990; 123: 187–197.
27. Rushton D, Ramsay I, Norris M, Gilkes J. Natural progression of male pattern baldness in youg men. Clin Exp Dermatol 1991; 16:188–192.
28. Runne U, Martin H. Veränderungen von den Telogenrate, Haardichte, Haarduchmensser, und Wachstumsgeschwindigkeit bei der androgenetischen Alopezie des Mannes. Hautarzt 1986; 37:198–204.
29. Friedel J, Will F, Grosshans E. Le phototrichogramme adaptation, standardisation et applications. Ann Dermatol Venereol 1989; 116:629–636.
30. Whiting D. Diagnostic and predictive value of horizontal sections of scalp biopsy specimens in male pattern androgenetic alopecia. J Am Acad Dermatol 1993; 28:755–763.
31. Lee MS, Kossard S, Wilkinson B, Doyle J. Quantification of hair follicle parameters using computer image analysis: a comparison of androgenetic alopecia with normal scalp biopsies. Aus J Dermatol 1995; 36:143–147.
32. Courtois M, Courbière C, Loussouarn G, Hourseau C. La formule pilaire dans l'alopécie féminine. B. e. d. c. 1995; 3(1):37–43.
33. Courtois M, Loussouarn G, Hourseau C, Grollier JF. Periodicity in the growth and shedding of hair. Br J Dermatol 1996; 134:47–54.
34. Birch MP, Messenger JF, Messenger AG. Hair density, hair diameter and the prevalence of female pattern hair loss. Br J Dermatol 2001; 144:297–304.
35. D'Amico D, Vaccaro M, Guarneri F, Borgia F, Cannavo S, Guarneri B. Phototrichogram using videomicroscopy: a useful technique in evaluation of scalp hair. Eur J Dermatol 2001; 11:17–20.
36. Vecchio F, Guarrera M, Rebora A. Perception of baldness and hair density. Dermatology 2002; 204:33–36.
37. Van Neste D. Female patients complaining about hair loss: documentation of defective scalp hair dynamics with contrast-enhanced phototrichogram. Skin Res Technol 2006; 12:83–89.
38. Piérard GE, Piérard-Franchimont C, Marks R. Elsner and the EEMCO group, EEMCO guidance for the assessment of hair shedding and alopecia. Skin Pharmacol Physiol 2004; 17:98–110.
39. Moretti G, Baccaredda-Boy A, Rebora A. Biochemical aspects of hair growth. In: Montagna W, Dobson RL, eds. Hair Growth. Oxford, Pergamon, England: 1969:535–553.
40. Pecoraro V, Astore IPL. Measurements of hair growth under physiological conditions. In: Orfanos CE, Happle R, eds. Hair and Hair Diseases. Berlin Heidelberg: Springer-Verlag, 1990:10.
41. de la Mettrie R, Saint-Léger D, Loussouarn G, Garcel AL, Porter C, Langaney A. Shape variability and classification of human hair: a worldwide approach. (In press).

Index

Acne
  clinical features, 199
  inflammatory, 200
  light-based therapies for, 203
  nodulocystic, 199, 200
  products for, 216
  scarring, 200
  in skin, of color patients, 201
  treatment, 201
Acne hyperpigmented macules
    (AHMs), 199
Acne-induced postinflammatory
    hyperpigmentation
  in dark skin, 201
  treatment of, 201, 203
    chemical peels in, 202
Acne keloid, 182
Acne vulgaris, 197
  in black skin, 199
  epidemiology of, 198
  lesions of, 199
  pathogenesis of, 198
  treatment of, 200
Acral lentiginous melanomas, mortality
    of, 190
Actinic lentigos, 227–229
Actinic lichen planus (ALP), 137–138
Adsorbosilplus-1, 171
Aging, chronological, 150

Aging-associated skin changes
  severities of, 142
  type of, 142
Allergic contact dermatitis
  case of, 130
  racial differences in susceptibility
    to, 128–129
Alopecia, 72, 183
  central centrifugal cicatricial, 72
  classification of, 72
Amyloidosis
  cutaneous, 136
  lichen, 136
Anagen hair, 252
Androgenogenetic alopecia
    (AGA), 254
Anisotropy index, 148
  evolution of, with age, 149
  variation, 148
Antiacne treatments, 214
Ashy skin, 42
Asian skin reactivity, 170
Atopic dermatitis (AD), 130, 135–136
  racial differences in, 129–130

Beauty imaging system
    (BIS), 109
Biopolymers, heterogeneous, 223

Body hair, 69
Bullous disease, 185

C-fibers, role of, 241
Caucasian skin, 20
Cellulitis, dissecting, 74
Central scarring alopecia,
    centrifugal, 183
Chinese herbal balls, 188
Chloasma, 229
Cholesterol sulphate, 174
Collagen
    bundles, visualization of, 39
    distribution of, 37
Contact dermatitis, 211
    allergic
        case of, 130
        racial differences in susceptibility
            to, 128–129
Corneocytes, 170
Corneometer CM 825PC, 113
Cutaneous disease, 180
    clinical appearances of, 180
    culture, 185
    depositional, 184
    epidemiology of, 190
    facial lentigo, 187
    race impact of, 180–181
Cutaneous inflammatory
        diseases, 184–185
Cytoplasmic pigment granules, 106

Deoxyhemoglobin, 34
Dermatitis
    atopic, 130
    facial, 238
    herpetiformis, 185
Desmoglein mutations, 182
Dihydroxyphenylalanine (DOPA), 21
Dihydroxyphenylalanine (DOPA)-
        positive melanocytes, 10
Doppler flowmetry, laser, 106
Dyschromias, in Mongoloid race, 181

Eczema, 182
Elastin matrix, 39

Emollients, greasy, 186
Endothelin receptor inhibitors, 214
Epidermal lipid synthesis, 176
Epidermal melanin,
        dispersion of, 201
Epidermal melanin pigmentation
        (EMP), 20
    absorption spectrum of, 23
    concentration of, 20
    constituents, 21
    estimation of, 20
    intensity of, 20
    melanin absorption, 24
Erythema nodosum, 184
Evaporimetry measurements, 172

Facial dermatitis, 238
Facial hair, 69
Facial lentigo, 187
Facial wrinkling, differences
        in, 109–113
Facultative pigmentation, 28
    spectral signatures of, 33
Folliculitis barbae, 73
Folliculitis keloidalis, 74
Folliculitis papillaris capillitii, 182
Fraternity keloid, 187

Hair
    amino acid analyses of, 60–61
    anagen, 252
    beard, 212
    body and facial, 69
    care, products for, 215
    cell fusion, 59
    chemical composition, 60
    color, 64
    component of, 59
    cortex, 59
    cross-sectional parameters
        of, 64
    curliness
        cause for, 63
        origins of, 89–90
    cuticle of, 57, 59
    cuticular bands, 59
    density, 68–69

[Hair]
dry brittle, treatment, 213
enthalpies, 62
epicuticle of, 59
ethnic, 70
geometry, 63
growth, 69
evaluation methods, 246, 252
structures of, 56
hair diameter, definitions of, 81
keratin fibers, structure of, 60
laser removal of, 73
mechanical properties, 65
microfibrils, 59
transmission electron micrograph
of, 60
pathologies of, 70
physical properties, 62
racial differences in, 206
scalp, 56
scanning electron micrograph
of, 57–58
solubilized, keratose fractions of, 62
straightening
agents, 212
chemical, 70
thermal, 70
structure of, 209
subtypes, comparison of, 257–260
telogen percentage, 256–257
temperatures, 62
transmission electron
micrograph of, 58
treatment products, 218
types, 56
Hair, black
problems of
African Americans, 211
brittle hair, 212
hair breakage, 212
hair loss, 212
Hair bulb, pigmentary activity of, 64
Hair density
subtype
African, 252–253
Asian, 253
Caucasian, 254

Hair growth, rate of, 255
subtype
African, 255
Asian, 255–256
Caucasian, 256
Hair-growth parameters
diversity of, 245
subtype, 246
African, 246
Asian, 247
Caucasian, 248
Hair on water-keratin interaction,
influence of ethnic origin of, 93
equilibrium in water, 101–102
equilibrium kinetics, 102
measurement of enthalpy, 97–98
sorption isotherms, 97
sorption kinetics, 98
swelling in water, 98–100
water swelling of hair, 95
water vapor sorption analysis, 94–95
Hair-shaft damage, forms of, 70
Hair's transverse dimensions
effect of, 81–82
evaluation of, 84
methods for measuring, 82
race and ethnicity, 80–81
Head hair, 79
types
Caucasoid—finer, 80
Mongoloid—coarse, 80
Negroid—coarse, 80
Hydroquinone, applications of, 185
Hyperpigmentation
differences in, 113
perifollicular, 27
cause for, 28
structure of, 28
Hypersensitivity
delayed-type, 130
immediate-type, 129

Itch
ehnic, 135
in ethnic populations, 135–138
studies in, 138

Itchy dermatosis, in Japanese
   skin, 136–137

Kagoshima, 111
Kawasaki's disease, 184
Keloidal scars, risk of, 200
Keratinocytes, 21, 24, 224
   dermal–epidermal junction, 24, 25
   in epidermis, 21
   role of, 225
   suprabasal, 25

Laser-scan micrometer (LSM), 84
   application of, 82
Laser Doppler flowmetry, 106
Laser Doppler velocimetry (LDV), 16
Lentigos, actinic, 227–229
Lesions
   pigmented, 227–229
   skin pigmented, 226–227
Lichen amyloidosis, 136
Linnaeus's classification, 5–6
Lipids extraction, 171
Liposomal stratum corneum lipids, 176

Malassezia furfur, 181
Mast cells, in black skin, 211
Melanin, 223–224
   absorption spectra of, 22
   composition modulators, 213
   and dermatoses, in ethnic skin, 188
   distribution, 24
      in basal keratinocytes, 25
      in dark skin, 24
   dust, 24
   effects of, 50
   enzymatic, 23
   epidermal glyphics on, 27
   ethnic differences in biology of, 48–49
   function of, 50
   granules, 37
   photoprotective role of, 164
   pigment, 39
   production, 21
      inducer of, 226
   role of, 15, 106

[Melanin]
   in skin, 21
   and skin types, 19
   solid, 20
   synthesis, rate of, 227
Melanin-bearing keratinocytes, 25
Melanin-laden keratinocytes, 26
Melanization, 23
Melanocytes, 208, 224
   assessment of, 48
   cytotoxic agents, 214
   DOPA-positive, 10
   eumelanin, 208
   morphology of, 225
   pheomelanin, 208
   secretory products, 64
   tyrosinase induction in, 201
Melanoma, development of, 50
Melanosome transfer inhibitors, 214
Melanosomes, 22, 49, 106, 224
   distribution of, 24, 48, 50
   ellipsoidal, 208
   function of, 50
   spherical, 208
Melasma, 229–230
Methylene blue staining technique, 59
Microdermabrasion, in skin
      complexions, 202
Micro relief lines, 156
Micro-sensors, 156
Microtopography, skin, 142
Minimal erythema dose
      (MED), 29, 47, 106

Nagashima's disease, 136–137
Nail, black
   hyperpigmentation of, 212
   problems, 211
Neapolitan disease, 4
Nodosum, erythema, 184

Oxyhemoglobin, 34

Para-phenylenediamine, 187
Petrolatum, 186
Pheomelanin (red-melanin), 21

Photoaging, racial differences, 51
Photo-aging effect, 164
Photobleaching process, 64
Photodynamic therapy (PDT), 24
Photosensitization
  chronic exposure, 28
  risk of, 28
Phototrichogram (PTG)
    method, 246, 252
Pigment production, induction of, 30
Pigmentary disorders, 210
Pigmentation, cutaneous, evolution
    of, 9
Pigmented lesions, 227–229
Pityriasis rosea, lesions of, 189
Plastic occlusion stress test (POST), 170
  and delipidization, 176
  measurements, 171
Polar lipids, 176
Pomade acne, 186
  diagnosis of, 200
Postinflammatory hyperpigmentation
    (PIH), 197, 199
Principal component analysis (PCA),
    146–147
Propionibacterium acnes, 198, 214
Prurigo mitis, 136
Prurigo pigmentosa, 136–137
Pseudofolliculitis barbae, 73, 210
Psoralen plus UVA (PUVA), 35

Races, modern, classification of, 56
Razor bumps, products for, 217
Rosacea, 238

Sarcoidosis, 183
SAS® software, 146
Scalp hair, 56
Scarring follicular diseases, 182
Sebaceous glands, 208
Seborrheic dermatitis, 72, 238
Sensitive skin
  clinical features of, 235–238
    diathesis factors, 237–238
  clinical signs, 235–236

[Sensitive skin]
  clinical subgroups of, 236–237
  physiological mechanisms involved
    in, 240–241
  prevalenc of, 240
  sensorial reactivity of, 237
  and socioeconomic factors, 240
  in world population, 238–240
Sensitive skin to environment (SSE), 236
Sensory irritation, racial differences
    in, 130
Severe sensitive skin (SSS), 236
Silfo®, 143
Sin-Luk pill, 188
Skin
  age-associated changes, 150
  aging, 141, 227–229
    occurrence, 150
    severity of, 150
    signs of, 150
  allergy, manifestation of, 129
  ashy
    products for, 217
    treatment of, 213
  black, 210
    ashy skin, 210
    contact dermatitis, 211
    cosmetic ingredients, 213
    irritation, 211
    keloids, 210
    pigmentary disorders in, 210
    problems of, African
        Americans, 211
    scarring, 210
    vitiligo, 211
  cancer
    incidence of, 50
    racial differences in, 50–51
  care, products for, 215
  conductance, racial differences in, 15
  dermal structure, 207
  disease, in ethnic skin, 180
  epidermal structure
    stratum granulosum, 207
    stratum lucidum, 207
  fibroblasts in, 207
  hydration, differences in, 113–115

[Skin]
  hyperreactivity, 237
  irritation
    chemical-induced, 125
    cumulative, 170
    racial differences in susceptibility
      to, 125–128
  light distribution in, 36
  lines, changes in, 148
  lipids
    role of, 15
    content of, 207
  lymphatic vessels in, 207
  micro relief, 154
    analysis of, 148
    characteristics, 162
    changes, 142
    corner density (CD) of, 157
    directions angle difference of, 157
    hair follicles effect in, 159
    inter- and intraethnic
      differences, 153
    investigation, 154, 164
    line density of, 157, 159
    measurements, 162
    parameters, 143, 148, 157, 159
    statistical analysis, 157–158
  microtopography, 142, 150
    comparison, 150
  occlusion, 175
  oily, 211
    products for, 216
  parameters, differences in, 116–120
  permeability, by TEWL, 106
  pH meter, 116
  pigmentation, 48, 223–224
    constitutive, 50
  pigmentation disorders, for black
    skin, 219
  pigmented lesions, 226–227
  racial differences in, 206
  reactivity, factors for, 239
  replicas, 143
    analysis of, 143
    images of, 149
  responsiveness, 170
  sensitivity, 128–129

[Skin]
  comparison, 31
    to cosmetics, 237
    self-assessed, 130
  shades, 20
  sites, images of, 38
  surface
    analysis of, 145
    lipids, 171
  topography, 109
  types, 19
Skin, ethnic
  characterization, 19
  biophysical properties of
    barrier function, 13–14
    biophysical parameters, 15–16
    irritation, 16
  definition, 43
  etymology, 179
  light penetration, 21
  melanin and dermatoses in, 188
  melanin content, 21
  pain studies in, 138
  sensitivity, 19
Skin color, 9–10, 19, 106, 179–180
  anthropology of, 1, 9
    Blumenbach and Caucasians, 6–8
    NOAH'S children, 8
    racism and medicine, 3–4
  constitutive, definition of48
  documentation of, 40–43
  and ethnical melanocyte specificities,
    224–226
  facultative, 48
  hyperpigmentation, treatment of, 213
  racial and ethnic differences in, 48
Skin photo type (SPT), 47
SkinVisiometer®, 161
Sodium dodecyl sulfate (SDS), 126, 128
Sodium lauryl sulphate (SLS), 16, 238
Solar erythema reaction, 30
Soret bands, 39
Spearman correlation coeficient, 147
Staphylococcus aureus, 75, 182
Stratum corneum, 13, 170
  hydration, 113
  lipid composition, 174

[Stratum corneum]
lipids and water holding capacity, 169
lipids removal from, 171
properties of, 175
removal, in blacks, 206
structural variations, 170
structure of, 207
TEWL measurements in, 171
Sulfanilamide, effects of, 4
Sun-damaged skin, 150
Sweat glands
apocrine, 208
eccrine, 208

Telogen hairs, 252, 257
Tewameter, 171
Thin layer chromatography, 171–172
Tinea capitis, 184
Traction alopecia, 71
Traction folliculitis, in children, 71
Transepidermal water loss (TEWL),
14–16, 170, 238
on control site, 174
on delipidized site, 173
measurements, 171
values for different races, 175

Transient congenital mongolian
spots, 181
Trichogram (TG) method, 246, 252
Trichophyton tonsurans infections, 184
Trichorrhexis nodosa, acquired, 70
Tyrosinase, activity of, 49

Ultraviolet (UV)-induced pigment, 32
Ultraviolet light, penetration of, 10
Ultraviolet (UV) radiation, 111, 106, 226

Vasoactive compound, application
of, 14
Vertical scanning interferometry
(VSI), 143
Videotrichogram (VTG)
method, 246, 252

Water holding capacity (WHC), 170
White-light interferometry. *See* Vertical
scanning interferometry (VSI)
Wrinkle area fraction, 110

Xerotic skin, 186